T0324668

Perinatal HIV Infection

Guest Editors

ATHENA P. KOURTIS, MD, PhD, MPH
MARC BULTERYS, MD, PhD

CLINICS IN PERINATOLOGY

www.perinatology.theclinics.com

Consulting Editor

LUCKY JAIN, MD, MBA

December 2010 • Volume 37 • Number 4

SAUNDERS an imprint of ELSEVIER, Inc.

W.B. SAUNDERS COMPANY
A Division of Elsevier Inc.

Elsevier, Inc. • 1600 John F. Kennedy Blvd. • Suite 1800 • Philadelphia, PA 19103-2899

http://www.theclinics.com

CLINICS IN PERINATOLOGY Volume 37, Number 4
December 2010 ISSN 0095-5108, ISBN-13: 978-1-4377-2480-6

Editor: Carla Holloway
Developmental Editor: Jessica Demetriou

Clinics in Perinatology (ISSN 0095-5108) is published quarterly by Elsevier Inc., 360 Park Avenue South, New York, NY 10010-1710. Months of issue are March, June, September, and December. Business and Editorial Offices: 1600 John F. Kennedy Blvd., Ste. 1800, Philadelphia, PA 19103-2899. Customer Service Office: 3251 Riverport Lane, Maryland Heights, MO 63043. Periodicals postage paid at New York, NY and additional mailing offices. Subscription prices are $256.00 per year (US individuals), $382.00 per year (US institutions), $306.00 per year (Canadian individuals), $485.00 per year (Canadian institutions), $376.00 per year (foreign individuals), $485.00 per year (foreign institutions) $122.00 per year (US students), and $176.00 per year (Canadian and foreign students). Foreign air speed delivery is included in all Clinics subscription prices. All prices are subject to change without notice. **POSTMASTER:** Send address changes to *Clinics in Perinatology*, Elsevier Health Sciences Division, Subscription Customer Service, 3251 Riverport Lane, Maryland Heights, MO 63043. **Customer Service: Telephone: 1-800-654-2452** (U.S. and Canada); **1-314-447-8871** (outside U.S. and Canada). **Fax: 1-314-447-8029. E-mail: journalscustomerservice-usa@elsevier.com** (for print support); **journalsonlinesupport-usa@elsevier.com** (for online support).

Reprints. For copies of 100 or more, of articles in this publication, please contact the Commercial Reprints Department, Elsevier Inc., 360 Park Avenue South, New York, NY 10010-1710. Tel. (212) 633-3812; Fax: (212) 482-1935; email: reprints@elsevier.com.

Clinics in Perinatology is also published in Spanish by McGraw-Hill Interamericana Editores S.A., P.O. Box 5-237, 06500 Mexico D.F., Mexico.

Clinics in Perinatology is covered in *MEDLINE/PubMed (Index Medicus) Current Contents, Excepta Medica, BIOSIS* and *ISI/BIOMED.*

Printed and bound in the United States of America
Transferred to Digital Print 2011

Contributors

CONSULTING EDITOR

LUCKY JAIN, MD, MBA
Richard Blumberg Professor and Executive Vice Chairman, Department of Pediatrics,
Emory University School of Medicine, Atlanta, Georgia

GUEST EDITORS

ATHENA P. KOURTIS, MD, PhD, MPH
Senior Service Fellow, Division of Reproductive Health, National Center for Chronic
Disease Prevention and Health Promotion, Centers for Disease Control and Prevention,
Atlanta; Associate Professor of Pediatrics, Department of Pediatrics, Emory University
School of Medicine, Atlanta, Georgia; Associate Professor of Obstetrics/Gynecology,
Department of Obstetrics and Gynecology, Eastern Virginia Medical School,
Norfolk, Virginia

MARC BULTERYS, MD, PhD
Division of HIV/AIDS, Center for Global Health, Centers for Disease Control and
Prevention (CDC), Atlanta, Georgia; Director, Centers of Disease Control and Prevention
Global AIDS Program, China, Beijing, China

AUTHORS

GRACE ALDROVANDI, MD
Associate Professor of Pediatrics, Department of Pediatrics, Children's Hospital
Los Angeles, University of Southern California, Los Angeles, California

BROOKIE M. BEST, PharmD, MAS
Department of Pediatrics, Rady Children's Hospital San Diego, Skaggs School
of Pharmacy and Pharmaceutical Sciences, University of California, La Jolla,
San Diego, California

MARC BULTERYS, MD, PhD
Division of HIV/AIDS, Center for Global Health, Centers for Disease Control and
Prevention (CDC), Atlanta, Georgia; Director, Centers of Disease Control and Prevention
Global AIDS Program, China, Beijing, China

PHILIP L. BULTERYS, BSc
Department of Biology, Stanford University, Stanford; David Geffen School of Medicine,
University of California Los Angeles, Los Angeles, California

ANDRES F. CAMACHO-GONZALEZ, MD
Pediatric Infectious Disease Fellow, Division of Pediatric Infectious Diseases,
Department of Pediatrics, Children's Healthcare of Atlanta, Emory University,
Atlanta, Georgia

RANA CHAKRABORTY, MD, PhD
Associate Professor of Pediatrics, Director of the Ponce HIV Family and Youth Clinic,
Division of Pediatric Infectious Diseases, Department of Pediatrics, Children's
Healthcare of Atlanta, Emory University, Atlanta, Georgia

DIANA F. CLARKE, PharmD
Section of Pediatric Infectious Diseases, Department of Pediatrics, Boston Medical
Center, Boston, Massachusetts

SUDEB C. DALAI, MSc
Division of Infectious Disease, Stanford University Medical Center, Stanford University
School of Medicine, Stanford; Division of Epidemiology, University of California-Berkeley,
School of Public Health, Berkeley, California

MARGERY DONOVAN, ND, APRN, PNP-BC
Family HIV Program, Dartmouth-Hitchcock-Medical Center, Lebanon, New Hampshire

SASCHA ELLINGTON, MSPH
Division of Reproductive Health, National Center for Chronic Disease Prevention and
Health Promotion, Centers for Disease Control and Prevention, Atlanta, Georgia

MONICA ETIMA, MBChB, MMed
Senior Pediatrician and Investigator, Makerere University-Johns Hopkins University
Research Collaboration, Upper Mulago Hill Road, Kampala, Uganda

ARACELIS D. FERNANDEZ, MD
Assistant Professor of Clinical Pediatrics, Department of Pediatrics, Columbia University,
The Affiliation at Harlem Hospital, New York, New York

ALICIA R. GABLE, MPH
Research Associate, Department of Pathology, The Johns Hopkins University School
of Medicine, Baltimore, Maryland

MARY GLENN FOWLER, MD, MPH
Professor, Department of Pathology, The Johns Hopkins University School of Medicine,
Baltimore, Maryland; On-site Investigator, Makerere University-Johns Hopkins University
Research Collaboration, Kampala, Uganda

LUCKY JAIN, MD, MBA
Richard Blumberg Professor and Executive Vice Chairman, Department of Pediatrics,
Emory University School of Medicine, Atlanta, Georgia

DENISE J. JAMIESON, MD, MPH
Division of Reproductive Health, National Center for Chronic Disease Prevention and
Health Promotion, Centers for Disease Control and Prevention, Atlanta, Georgia

DAVID A. KATZENSTEIN, MD
Division of Infectious Disease, Stanford University Medical Center, Stanford University
School of Medicine, Stanford, California

ATHENA P. KOURTIS, MD, PhD, MPH
Senior Service Fellow, Division of Reproductive Health, National Center for Chronic
Disease Prevention and Health Promotion, Centers for Disease Control and Prevention,
Atlanta; Associate Professor of Pediatrics, Department of Pediatrics, Emory University
School of Medicine, Atlanta, Georgia; Associate Professor of Obstetrics/Gynecology, De-
partment of Obstetrics and Gynecology, Eastern Virginia Medical School, Norfolk, Virginia

LOUISE KUHN, PhD
Professor of Epidemiology, Gertrude H. Sergievsky Center, College of Physicians and Surgeons; Department of Epidemiology, Mailman School of Public Health, Columbia University, New York, New York

MARGARET A. LAMPE, RN, MPH
Health Education Specialist, Division of HIV/AIDS Prevention, Epidemiology Branch, National Center for HIV/AIDS, Viral Hepatitis, STD and TB Prevention, Centers for Disease Control and Prevention, Atlanta, Georgia

JENNIFER K. LEGARDY-WILLIAMS, MPH
Division of Reproductive Health, National Center for Chronic Disease Prevention and Health Promotion, Centers for Disease Control and Prevention, Atlanta, Georgia

BARB LOHMAN-PAYNE, PhD
Department of Paediatrics and Child Health, University of Nairobi, Nairobi, Kenya; Research Assistant Professor, Department of Medicine; Adjunct Research Assistant Professor, Department of Global Health, University of Washington, Seattle, Washington

MARK MIROCHNICK, MD
Division of Neonatology, Department of Pediatrics, Boston University School of Medicine, Boston, Massachusetts

JULIE MIRPURI, MD
Division of Neonatal-Perinatal Medicine, Department of Pediatrics, Emory University School of Medicine, Atlanta, Georgia

STEVEN NESHEIM, MD
Epidemiology Branch, Division of HIV/AIDS Prevention, National Center for HIV, Viral Hepatitis, STD, and TB Prevention, Centers for Disease Control and Prevention, Atlanta, Georgia

MAXENSIA OWOR, MBChB, MMed
Clinic Director and Investigator, Makerere University-Johns Hopkins University Research Collaboration, Kampala, Uganda

PAUL PALUMBO, MD
Professor of Medicine and Pediatrics, Dartmouth-Hitchcock-Medical Center, Dartmouth Medical School, Lebanon, New Hampshire

JENNIFER S. READ, MD, MS, MPH, DTM&H
Medical Officer, Pediatric, Adolescent, and Maternal AIDS Branch, Center for Research for Mothers and Children, Eunice Kennedy Shriver National Institute of Child Health and Human Development, National Institutes of Health, Bethesda, Maryland

LISA-GAYE E. ROBINSON, MD
Assistant Professor of Clinical Pediatrics, Department of Pediatrics, Columbia University, The Affiliation at Harlem Hospital, New York, New York

ALLISON C. ROSS, MD
Assistant Professor of Pediatrics, Division of Pediatric Infectious Diseases, Department of Pediatrics, Children's Healthcare of Atlanta, Emory University, Atlanta, Georgia

SARAH L. ROWLAND-JONES, MA (Cantab), BM, BCh, DM (Oxon)
Professor of Immunology and Honorary Consultant in Infectious Diseases, Nuffield Department of Medicine, John Radcliffe Hospital, Oxford University, Oxford, United Kingdom

JENNIFER SLYKER, PhD
Acting Instructor, Department of Global Health; Department of Medicine, University of Washington, Seattle, Washington; Nuffield Department of Medicine, John Radcliffe Hospital, Oxford, United Kingdom

PAUL J. WEIDLE, PharmD, MPH
Epidemiology Branch, Division of HIV/AIDS Prevention, National Center for HIV, Viral Hepatitis, STD, and TB Prevention, Centers for Disease Control and Prevention, Atlanta, Georgia

Contents

This article reviews the epidemiology of perinatal (HIV)-1 in the United
States in the past 2 decades and the international HIV epidemic among
pregnant women and their infants. Since the peak of 1700 reported cases
of pediatric AIDS in 1992, there has been dramatic progress in decreasing
perinatal HIV transmission in the United States with fewer than 50 new
cases of AIDS annually (>96% reduction) and fewer than 300 annual perinatal HIV transmissions in 2005. This success has been due to use of combination antiretrovirals given to mothers during pregnancy and labor/
delivery, obstetric interventions that reduce the risk of transmission, provision of zidovudine (ZDV) prophylaxis for 6 weeks to HIV-exposed newborns and use of formula. Internationally, the burden of mother-to-child
HIV transmission remains heavy with 2.1 million children less than 15 years
of age estimated to be living with HIV and 430,000 new HIV infections in
infants occurring each year, with most cases occurring in Africa. Current
international efforts are directed at scaling up successful prevention of
mother-to-child transmission interventions and new research directed at
making breastfeeding safer using antiretroviral prophylaxis to either
mothers or their infants.

More than 400,000 children were infected with (HIV-1) worldwide in 2008,
or more than 1000 children per day. Mother-to-child transmission (MTCT)
of HIV-1 is the most important mode of HIV acquisition in infants and children. MTCT of HIV-1 can occur in utero, intrapartum, and postnatally
through breastfeeding. Great progress has been made in preventing
such transmission, through the use of antiretroviral prophylactic regimens
to the mother during gestation and labor and delivery and to either mother
or infant during breast feeding. The timing and mechanisms of transmission, however, are multifactorial and remain incompletely understood.
This article summarizes what is known about the pathogenetic mechanisms and routes of MTCT of HIV-1, and includes virologic, immunologic,
genetic, and mucosal aspects of transmission.

Great progress has been made in understanding the pathogenesis, treatment, and transmission of HIV and the factors influencing the risk of mother-to-child transmission (MTCT). Many questions regarding the molecular evolution and genetic diversity of HIV in the context of MTCT remain unanswered. Further research to identify the selective factors governing which variants are transmitted, how the compartmentalization of HIV in different cells and tissues contributes to transmission, and the influence of host immunity, viral diversity, and recombination on MTCT may provide insight into new prevention strategies and the development of an effective HIV vaccine.

Diagnosis and management of perinatally acquired human immunodeficiency virus infection poses many challenges in the areas of diagnosis, clinical and psychosocial intervention, and public health policy. Diagnostic tests have evolved over the years and many are currently used in the perinatal setting. Considerable progress has been realized in each of these areas through cooperative efforts of laboratory scientists, clinical teams, and stakeholders. However, there remain multiple challenges to address in the future.

The World Health Organization's Strategic Approaches to the Prevention of HIV Infection in Infants includes 4 components: primary prevention of HIV-1 infection; prevention of unintended pregnancies among HIV-1–infected women; prevention of transmission of HIV-1 infection from mothers to children; and provision of ongoing support, care, and treatment to HIV-1–infected women and their families. This review focuses on antiretrovirals for secondary prevention of HIV-1 infection–prevention of HIV-1 transmission from an HIV-1–infected woman to her child. Antiretroviral strategies to prevent the mother-to-child transmission of HIV-1 in nonbreastfeeding populations comprise antiretroviral treatment of HIV-1–infected pregnant women needing antiretrovirals for their own health, antiretroviral prophylaxis for HIV-1–infected pregnant women not yet meeting criteria for treatment, and antiretroviral prophylaxis for infants of HIV-1–infected mothers. The review primarily addresses antiretroviral strategies for nonbreastfeeding, HIV-1–infected women and their infants in resource-rich settings, such as the United States. Antiretroviral strategies to prevent antepartum, intrapartum, and early postnatal transmission in resource-poor settings are also addressed, albeit more briefly.

The risk of mother-to-child transmission (MTCT) of HIV can be reduced through cesarean delivery prior to the onset of labor and prior to rupture of the membranes (elective cesarean delivery [ECD]). As a result of this evidence, the American College of Obstetricians and Gynecologists and the Department of Health and Human Services Panel on Treatment of HIV-Infected Pregnant Women and Prevention of Perinatal Transmission developed guidelines recommending ECD for HIV-infected women with plasma viral loads of more than 1000 copies/mL. Since the release of the recommendations, an increase in ECD has been seen among HIV-infected women in the United States. This article discusses the evidence on efficacy of ECD, current recommendations in the United States, and risks and morbidity related to ECD. Although the benefit of ECD in preventing MTCT of HIV is substantial, some questions remain. Specifically, the benefit of ECD for women with very low viral loads or for women using combination antiretroviral regimens is unclear, as is the timeframe after onset of labor or rupture of membranes within which ECD will still confer preventive benefits.

Despite more than 2 decades of research, an effective vaccine that can prevent HIV-1 infection in populations exposed to the virus remains elusive. In the pursuit of an HIV-1 vaccine, does prevention of exposure to maternal HIV-1 in utero, at birth or in early life through breast milk require special consideration? This article reviews what is known about the immune mechanisms of susceptibility and resistance to mother-to-child transmission (MTCT) of HIV-1 and summarizes studies that have used passive or active immunization strategies to interrupt MTCT of HIV-1. Potentially modifiable infectious cofactors that may enhance transmission and/or disease progression (especially in the developing world) are described. An effective prophylactic vaccine against HIV-1 infection needs to be deployed as part of the Extended Program of Immunization recommended by the World Health Organization for use in developing countries, so it is important to understand how the infant immune system responds to HIV-1 antigens, both in natural infection and presented by candidate vaccines.

Breastfeeding accounts for about 40% of mother-to-child transmission of HIV-1 worldwide and carries an estimated risk of transmission of 0.9% per month after the first month of breastfeeding. It is recommended that HIV-1–infected women completely avoid breastfeeding in settings where safe feeding alternatives exist. However, as replacement feeding is not safely available in many parts of the world, and because breastfeeding provides optimal nutrition and protection against other infant infections, there is intense ongoing research to make breastfeeding safe for HIV-1–infected

pertinent management considerations needed for clinicians to provide optimal care to the HIV-exposed infant.

Despite well-established strategies to decrease the mother-to-child transmission of HIV-1, new perinatal infections continue to occur globally, reflecting marked disparities in access to health care. Once HIV-1 infection has been established in an infant, the combination of early initiation of antiretroviral therapy and prophylaxis against *Pneumocystis jiroveci* pneumonia is paramount to reducing disease progression. This article reviews the recommendations and evidence for the treatment of HIV-1–infected infants.

Prematurity and HIV present a complex challenge, with biologic underpinnings that are often confounded by a myriad of other factors that coexist in this high-risk population. Furthermore, many of the current management options designed to reduce mother-to-infant transmission, including antiretroviral therapy and cesarean birth, may each have an independent effect on prematurity. These issues notwithstanding, knowledge gained from randomized controlled trials and epidemiologic studies has made a significant impact on the approach to this challenging public health problem worldwide. This article discusses the significance, contribution, and management of perinatal transmission of HIV in prematurity.

Antiretrovirals may be used in pregnant women infected with the HIV and their newborns both for treatment of maternal HIV disease and for prevention of mother-to-child transmission of HIV. More than 25 antiretroviral agents in 5 classes have been approved, with new drugs and classes in development. This article reviews current knowledge of the pharmacology of these drugs during pregnancy and in the newborn period, highlighting those pharmacologic issues critical to the safe and effective use of antiretrovirals in these populations.

GOAL STATEMENT

The goal of *Clinics in Perinatology* is to keep practicing neonatologists and maternal-fetal medicine specialists up to date with current clinical practice in perinatology by providing timely articles reviewing the state of the art in patient care.

ACCREDITATION

The *Clinics in Perinatology* is planned and implemented in accordance with the Essential Areas and Policies of the Accreditation Council for Continuing Medical Education (ACCME) through the joint sponsorship of the University of Virginia School of Medicine and Elsevier. The University of Virginia School of Medicine is accredited by the ACCME to provide continuing medical education for physicians.

The University of Virginia School of Medicine designates this educational activity for a maximum of 15 *AMA PRA Category 1 Credits*™ for each issue, 60 credits per year. Physicians should only claim credit commensurate with the extent of their participation in the activity.

The American Medical Association has determined that physicians not licensed in the US who participate in this CME activity are eligible for a maximum of 15 *AMA PRA Category 1 Credits*™ for each issue, 60 credits per year.

Credit can be earned by reading the text material, taking the CME examination online at http://www.theclinics.com/home/cme, and completing the evaluation. After taking the test, you will be required to review any and all incorrect answers. Following completion of the test and evaluation, your credit will be awarded and you may print your certificate.

FACULTY DISCLOSURE/CONFLICT OF INTEREST

The University of Virginia School of Medicine, as an ACCME accredited provider, endorses and strives to comply with the Accreditation Council for Continuing Medical Education (ACCME) Standards of Commercial Support, Commonwealth of Virginia statutes, University of Virginia policies and procedures, and associated federal and private regulations and guidelines on the need for disclosure and monitoring of proprietary and financial interests that may affect the scientific integrity and balance of content delivered in continuing medical education activities under our auspices.

The University of Virginia School of Medicine requires that all CME activities accredited through this institution be developed independently and be scientifically rigorous, balanced and objective in the presentation/discussion of its content, theories and practices.

All authors/editors participating in an accredited CME activity are expected to disclose to the readers relevant financial relationships with commercial entities occurring within the past 12 months (such as grants or research support, employee, consultant, stock holder, member of speakers bureau, etc.). The University of Virginia School of Medicine will employ appropriate mechanisms to resolve potential conflicts of interest to maintain the standards of fair and balanced education to the reader. Questions about specific strategies can be directed to the Office of Continuing Medical Education, University of Virginia School of Medicine, Charlottesville, Virginia.

The faculty and staff of the University of Virginia Office of Continuing Medical Education have no financial affiliations to disclose.

The authors/editors listed below have identified no professional or financial affiliations for themselves or their spouse/partner:

Grace Aldrovandi, MD; Robert Boyle, MD (Test Author); Marc Bulterys, MD, PhD (Guest Editor); Philip L. Bulterys, BSc; Rana Chakraborty, MD, PhD; Diana F. Clarke, PharmD; Sudeb C. Dalai, MSc; Margery Donovan, ND, APRN, PNP-BC; Sascha Ellington, MSPH; Monica Etima, MBChB, MMed; Aracelis D. Fernandez, MD; Mary Glenn Fowler, MD, MPH; Alicia R. Gable, MPH; Carla Holloway (Acquisitions Editor); Lucky Jain, MD, MBA (Consulting Editor); Denise J. Jamieson, MD, MPH; David A. Katzenstein, MD; Athena P. Kourtis, MD, PhD, MPH (Guest Editor); Louise Kuhn, PhD; Margaret A. Lampe, RN, MPH; Jennifer K. Legardy-Williams, MPH; Barb Lohman-Payne, PhD; Mark Mirochnick, MD; Julie Mirpuri, MD; Steven Nesheim, MD; Maxensia Owor, MBChB, MMed; Paul Palumbo, MD; Jennifer S. Read, MD, MS, MPH, DTM&H; Lisa-Gaye E. Robinson, MD; Jennifer Slyker, PhD; and Paul J. Weidle, PharmD, MPH.

The authors/editors listed below identified the following professional or financial affiliations for themselves or their spouse/partner:

Brookie M. Best, PharmD, MAS is the Principal Investigator of a grant from Millenium Laboratories.
Andres F. Camacho-Gonzalez, MD is an industry funded research/investigator for Bristol Myers Squibb.
Allison C. Ross, MD is an industry funded research/investigator for GlaxoSmithKline and Cubist Pharmaceuticals.
Sarah L. Rowland-Jones, MA (Cantab), BM BCh, DM (Oxon) 's spouse owns stock in G-Nostics.

Disclosure of Discussion of Non-FDA Approved Uses for Pharmaceutical Products and/or Medical Devices.
The University of Virginia School of Medicine, as an ACCME provider, requires that all faculty presenters identify and disclose any off-label uses for pharmaceutical and medical device products. The University of Virginia School of Medicine recommends that each physician fully review all the available data on new products or procedures prior to clinical use.

TO ENROLL

To enroll in the Clinics in Perinatology Continuing Medical Education program, call customer service at 1-800-654-2452 or visit us online at www.theclinics.com/home/cme. The CME program is available to subscribers for an additional fee of $196.00

THE CLINICS ARE NOW AVAILABLE ONLINE!

Access your subscription at:
www.theclinics.com

Foreword

Perinatal HIV Infection: Time to Rejoice or Call to Action?

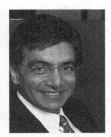

Lucky Jain, MD, MBA
Consulting Editor

One of the greatest challenges in clinical medicine is the excruciatingly long gap between the timing of medical innovations and their implementation into day-to-day practice. Estimates vary, but most experts agree that it takes as many as 15–20 years for recommendations emerging from sound science (such as randomized controlled trials) to become standard of care.[1] Efforts to reduce perinatal HIV transmission are, however, a shining example of how this paradigm can be changed. Recommendations emerging from the *Pediatric AIDS Clinical Trials Group 076 (PACTG076) protocol*, which was published in 1994, and subsequent studies to reduce mother-to-child transmission of HIV have been widely embraced and incorporated into practice where resources are available.[2] Using a combination of interventions including antiretroviral treatment and avoidance of breastfeeding, transmission rates in resource-rich countries are down to 1–2%.[3] The resulting global public health impact has been enormous. While gaps remain, the many articles in this issue of the *Clinics of Perinatology* highlight the significant progress that has been made in this field.

The gaps are restricted, for the most part, to resource-poor nations, and to the impoverished segments within more industrialized nations.[4] The same factors which have allowed well-resourced nations to achieve a remarkable public health success are standing in the way of duplication of this success in poorer areas. These regions not only have high prevalence of HIV, infections are often not picked up until late in gestation, limiting the opportunities for intervention. Restriction of breastfeeding has its own limitations and consequences, given the expense associated with formula feeds and risk of diarrhea and malnutrition. **Fig. 1** reminds us of the striking differences in the percentage of adult females (15 years plus) living with HIV in various parts of the world.[4] It also reminds us of the association between a nation's per capita gross domestic product (GDP) and infant mortality. Globally, the availability of basic health services and infrastructure tends to decline precipitously when the per capita GDP falls

Clin Perinatol 37 (2010) xv–xvii
doi:10.1016/j.clp.2010.09.003
0095-5108/10/$ – see front matter © 2010 Elsevier Inc. All rights reserved.

perinatology.theclinics.com

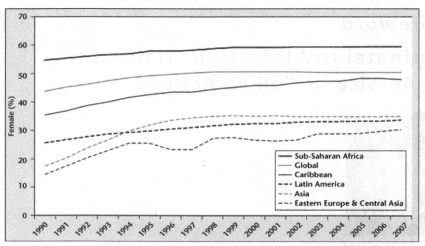

Fig. 1. Percentage of female adults (age 15 years +) living with human immunodeficiency virus (1990–2007). (*From* UNAIDS/WHO. AIDS epidemic update, November 2009. Geneva; UNAIDS: 2009. Available at: http://www.who.int/hiv/pub/epidemiology/epidemic/en/index.html; with permission.)

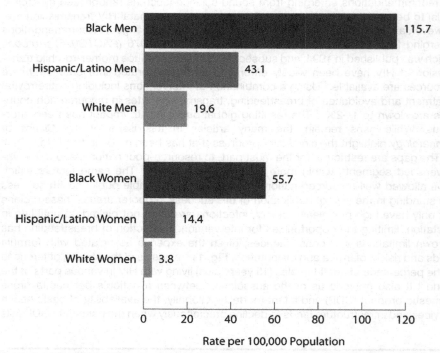

Fig. 2. Racial/ethnic differences in HIV incidence in the US. (*From* the CDC. Subpopulation Estimates from the HIV Incidence Surveillance System—United States, 2006. MMWR 2008;57(36):985–9.)

below $3,000; the associated rise in infant mortality is astronomical. A nation's lack of prosperity is also a marker of a multitude of other problems such as lack of food, sanitation, illiteracy, and overall poor access to healthcare services. HIV continues to have a serious impact on infant mortality in many poor nations, particularly those in the sub-Saharan Africa. The loss of life and productivity in these nations (as a direct result of HIV) is unprecedented; it is particularly distressing, given how it could have been prevented with relatively simple interventions.

A similar divide exists, albeit to a lesser degree, in our own backyard. **Fig. 2** shows the ethnic divide in HIV prevalence in the United States.[5] Black men and women, many in the child-bearing ages, carry a disproportionate share of this burden. Health disparities extend to other areas as well, but are particularly striking when it comes to women's health and childbirth. Prematurity rates continue to be high among black women, as do rates of maternal and infant mortality.[6] The racial gap has narrowed when it comes to perinatal HIV transmission; however, late and/or inadequate prenatal care and lack of universal screening for HIV are public health issues that need to be addressed. These, and many other issues, have been covered in great detail in this issue of the *Clinics* and Drs Kourtis and Bulterys are to be congratulated for putting together a superb state-of-the-art offering on this important subject.

Lucky Jain, MD, MBA
Department of Pediatrics
Emory University School of Medicine
2015 Uppergate Drive
Atlanta, GA 30322, USA

E-mail address:
ljain@emory.edu

REFERENCES

1. Haynes B, Haines A. Barriers and bridges to evidence based clinical practice. BMJ 1998;317:273.
2. Connor EM, Sperling RS, Gelber R, et al. Reduction of maternal-infant transmission of human immunodeficiency virus type 1 with zidovudine treatment. N Engl J Med 1994;331(18):1173–80.
3. Whitmore SK, Patel-Larson A, Espinoza L, et al. Missed opportunities to prevent perinatal human immunodeficiency virus transmission in 15 jurisdictions in the United States during 2005–2008. Women Health 2010;50:414–25.
4. Tang J, Nour NM. HIV and pregnancy in resource poor settings. Rev Obstet Gynecol 2010;3:66–71.
5. CDC. Subpopulation Estimates from the HIV Incidence Surveillance System—United States, 2006. MMWR 2008;57(36):985–9.
6. Ramachandrappa A, Jain L. Health issues of the late preterm infant. Pediatr Clin North Am 2009;56:565–77.

Preface

Perinatal HIV Infection

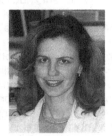 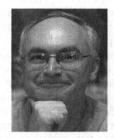

Athena P. Kourtis, MD, PhD, MPH   Marc Bulterys, MD, PhD
Guest Editors

These are exciting times in the prevention of perinatal (mother-to-child) transmission of HIV and the clinical care and treatment of pregnant HIV-positive women and their children. Since the first cases of AIDS in infants and young children were described in the United States in the early 1980s, tremendous progress has been made in the prevention and care of HIV infection in infants and children. The Centers for Disease Control and Prevention reports a more than 90% decline in the number of perinatally acquired AIDS cases in children in the United States during the past 16 years and potent new antiretroviral regimens are highly effective in preventing progression of disease and improving the quality of life. The December 2010 issue of *Clinics in Perinatology* entitled "Perinatal HIV Infection" is a comprehensive review of the biology, epidemiology, and prevention of perinatal HIV transmission as well as the clinical care and optimal management of the pregnant mother and her exposed or infected infant.

The first article in this volume provides an overview of perinatal HIV/AIDS in the United States and worldwide and describes progress that has been made in recent years towards an HIV-free generation of infants. The second article outlines the biology of perinatal HIV transmission and deals with timing and known virologic and immunologic risk factors. Article 3 serves as a comprehensive introduction to viral sequencing from HIV-infected mothers and their infants and the molecular evolution and diversity that exists in mother-infant HIV transmission. Article 4 covers the diagnosis of perinatally acquired HIV infection. Articles 5 through 7 include the latest information on antiretroviral drug strategies, the role of Caesarean section, and immune-based approaches to reduce mother-to-child transmission of HIV. Article 8 reviews the biology of breastfeeding and HIV transmission and incorporates the most recent research advances in the prevention of postnatal HIV transmission. Article 9 focuses on HIV drug resistance and perinatal HIV transmission and the reasons drug resistance should be assiduously avoided, whenever possible. Article 10 summarizes the compelling epidemiologic data on the risks and benefits of various infant feeding practices for

Clin Perinatol 37 (2010) xix–xxi
doi:10.1016/j.clp.2010.09.001
0095-5108/10/$ – see front matter © 2010 Elsevier Inc. All rights reserved.

perinatology.theclinics.com

HIV-infected mothers living in different resource environments. Article 11 provides a contemporary view on the clinical care of the HIV-exposed infant, while article 12 reviews the recommendations and evidence for initiating antiretroviral therapy and other clinical care interventions in HIV-infected infants. Article 13 focuses on the complex challenge of prematurity and HIV. The final article reviews current knowledge of the pharmacology of antiretroviral drugs during pregnancy and in the newborn period, highlighting those pharmacologic issues critical to the safe and effective use of these drugs in the perinatal period.

Significant progress has been made in the global scale-up of prevention of mother-to-child transmission of HIV, including in many resource-poor settings. However, it is critically important to use the best evidence-based interventions to reduce the risk of mother-to-child transmission while also providing appropriate care and treatment for the HIV-infected mother and her newborn child. We need to recognize that the HIV epidemic has impacted especially the most vulnerable populations of women (in Africa, often the young and the poor are especially impacted; in the United States, minority women; and in China and other parts of Asia, female sex workers, injecting drug users, and ethnic minority women). An effective perinatal HIV prevention program, then, relies on universal access to health care services, availability, and acceptance of HIV testing (throughout pregnancy and lactation), adherence to antiretroviral drug prophylaxis and other interventions, and culturally sensitive care and follow-up of the mother and child. The most effective programs will be integrated with HIV prevention and include promoting maternal and child health, preventing HIV in women of childbearing age, and preventing unwanted pregnancies.

This volume has a remarkable group of talented authors who are experts in this field. We would like to thank all of them for their excellent contributions and their willingness to make often substantial revisions in order to benefit the whole rather than the part. We owe a great deal of thanks to Ms Carla Holloway and the rest of the publishing staff at the *Clinics*, for sage advice and timely nudging during the preparation of this issue. Some omissions are inevitable in a volume of this type. We apologize for any such occurrences and wish that the articles in this issue will stimulate further refined thinking and enthusiasm for improving the care of HIV-infected women and their infants worldwide. We wish you an illuminating and enjoyable read.

Athena P. Kourtis, MD, PhD, MPH
Division of Reproductive Health
National Center for Chronic Disease Prevention and Health Promotion
Centers for Disease Control and Prevention
Atlanta, GA, USA

Department of Pediatrics
Emory University School of Medicine
4770 Buford Highway
NE, MSK34 Atlanta
GA 30341, USA

Department of Obstetrics and Gynecology
Eastern Virginia Medical School
825 Fairfax Avenue
Norfolk, VA 23507, USA

Marc Bulterys, MD, PhD
Division of HIV/AIDS, Center for Global Health
Centers for Disease Control and Prevention (CDC)
Atlanta, GA 30333

CDC Global AIDS Program
China, Suite #403, Dongwai Diplomatic Office
23 Dongzhimenwai Dajie
Beijing, China

E-mail addresses:
apk3@cdc.gov (A.P. Kourtis)
zbe2@cdc.gov (M. Bulterys)

Perinatal HIV and Its Prevention: Progress Toward an HIV-free Generation

Mary Glenn Fowler, MD, MPH[a,b,*], Alicia R. Gable, MPH[a],
Margaret A. Lampe, RN, MPH[c], Monica Etima, MBChB, MMed[b],
Maxensia Owor, MBChB, MMed[b]

KEYWORDS

- Mother-to-child transmission of HIV-1
- Epidemiology of perinatal HIV infections • Early infant diagnosis
- United States • Resource-limited settings

Since the first cases of infant HIV infection were described in the early 1980s, significant progress has been made in our understanding of risk factors for mother-to-child transmission (MTCT) of HIV as well as effective interventions to prevent transmission. MTCT of the human immunodeficiency virus type-1 (HIV-1) can occur during pregnancy particularly in the third trimester, during the intrapartum period, and for infants exposed to HIV, who are breastfed, throughout the period of lactation.[1] Before the availability of antiretroviral and obstetric interventions, about 1 in 4 infants born to women infected with HIV became infected. Among these infected infants, 50% to 60% of transmission occurred around the time of labor or delivery based on newborn infants exposed to HIV having negative cord blood or newborn polymerase chain reaction (PCR) tests that subsequently became positive within the first weeks of life.[2] Among HIV-infected breastfeeding populations, about 20% to 25% of infections occurred in utero based on positive PCRs at birth; 35% to 50% intrapartum; and another 25% to 35% of infants negative at birth and in the first 6 weeks became infected later, presumably as a result of transmission through breast milk.[1]

The authors have no conflicts of interest.
a Department of Pathology, The Johns Hopkins University School of Medicine, 600 North Wolfe Street, Baltimore, MD 21224, USA
b Makerere University-Johns Hopkins University Research Collaboration, Upper Mulago Hill Road, Kampala, Uganda
c Division of HIV/AIDS Prevention, Epidemiology Branch, National Center for HIV/AIDS, Viral Hepatitis, STD and TB Prevention, Centers for Disease Control and Prevention, 1600 Clifton Road, MS E-45, Atlanta, GA 30333, USA
* Corresponding author. Makerere University-Johns Hopkins University Research Collaboration, Upper Mulago Hill Road, Kampala, Uganda.
E-mail address: mgfowler@mujhu.org

Clin Perinatol 37 (2010) 699–719
doi:10.1016/j.clp.2010.09.002
0095-5108/10/$ – see front matter © 2010 Elsevier Inc. All rights reserved.
perinatology.theclinics.com

Since the initial US Pediatric AIDS Clinical Trials Group Protocol (PACTG) 076 clinical trial results[3] were announced in 1994, which showed that giving pregnant women infected with HIV oral zidovudine from 14 weeks, intravenously at labor and delivery, and followed by 6 weeks of zidovudine prophylaxis to their newborns, could reduce transmission by two-thirds, significant progress has been made in resource-rich settings such as the United States and Europe, where combination antiretroviral drugs are routinely given during pregnancy and at labor, and where breast milk substitutes can be safely used and provided by government programs. Current transmission rates are estimated at less than 2% with the use of triple anti-retroviral drugs during pregnancy.[4,5] International trials aimed at reducing transmission among women infected with HIV in resource-limited settings using simpler deliverable regimens have also been conducted and shown to be efficacious.[6-8] Recent studies[9-11] have focused on ways to make breastfeeding safer given the high risk of mortality from other causes among infants exposed to HIV who are not breastfed.

Despite this progress, researchers still have limited understanding of the exact mechanisms of transmission; including the maternal and infant host factors that either protect or increase the risk of transmission; whether mucosal exposure is the primary route of transmission during labor, or occurs by microtransfusions across the placenta during contractions; whether transmission through breast milk is primarily caused by cell-associated or cell-free virus; and how the virus is transported across the infant gastrointestinal mucosa.

This update focuses primarily on the epidemiology of MTCT of HIV-1 in the United States, briefly summarizes what is known about the timing and mechanisms of MTCT, and describes current efforts in the United States to eliminate new cases of mother-to-child HIV-1 transmission, including innovative national and state strategies. Updates on the epidemiology of the global MTCT epidemic, current prevention of mother-to-child transmission (PMTCT) strategies in international settings, as well as challenges, and future research directions in PMTCT of HIV are provided.

TIMING AND MECHANISMS OF TRANSMISSION
In Utero Infection

The placenta has proved an effective barrier to HIV transmission during pregnancy given that even before effective interventions only about 1 in 4 infants who were exposed to HIV became infected. Based on the timing of positivity, only about 20% to 25% of infections occurred in utero[1] and PCR analyses of aborted fetuses and early miscarriages indicated almost no transmission in the first trimester[12] or during the second trimester based on amniocentesis.[13] However, in the third trimester, the vascular integrity of the placenta begins to break down and statistical modeling data[14] suggest that most in utero transmissions probably occur in the last few weeks before delivery. It has been postulated that this may be caused by microtransfusions across the maternal-fetal placenta circulation during late pregnancy.[15,16] Intrauterine contractions during labor/delivery could also increase the risk of intrapartum transmission.

Intrapartum Infection

Other mechanisms that can contribute to intrapartum transmission are infant mucosal exposure to maternal blood and other HIV-infected secretions as the baby goes through the birth canal. The protective effect of scheduled cesarean delivery before labor onset with a 50% reduction in transmission risk[17-19] is potentially due to preventing both microtransfusions during active labor and avoidance of infant gut and conjunctival exposure to HIV, which can occur during vaginal delivery. Inflammation of the placenta such as seen with malaria has also been associated with increased risk of HIV transmission in some malarial placenta studies[20,21] but not all such studies among pregnant women infected with HIV.[22,23]

Late Infection Through Breastfeeding

The exact mechanisms of transmission during breastfeeding have not yet been determined. It has been postulated that the transmission may occur via transfer across the infant gut by attachment to immature dendritic cells in the gut mucosa, which then transport the virus to lymph nodes (Peyer patches) from where HIV is then transmitted to CD4+ cells.[24] The first several days of life may be a particularly vulnerable period because of lack of acidic gastric fluid, which can inactivate HIV, and ingestion by the infant of HIV-infected macrophages present in colostrum. However, despite continual exposure to HIV in breast milk, the risk of infant infection by mouth is low (0.6%–0.8%) but cumulative for the duration of breastfeeding.[25]

There are several maternal factors in breast milk that may provide some protection against transmission including CD8+ cytotoxic T lymphocytes, secretory leukocyte protease inhibitor, other innate factors, and HIV-specific IgG and IgA immunoglobulins present in breast milk.[26] Specific IgA secretory natural antibodies in breast milk, which include anti-DC-SIGN antibodies, have been shown to prevent HIV attachment to dendritic cell membranes in vitro as well as to inhibit transfer of the HIV virus to CD4+ lymphocytes.[27] The relative contribution of cell-free versus cell-associated virus to MTCT through breast milk ingestion is not known. Early mixed feeding compared with exclusive breastfeeding during the first 3 months of life has been associated with increased risk of HIV infection among breastfed infants exposed to HIV,[28] whereas exclusive breastfeeding is associated with lowered risk.[29] Possible mechanisms of increased transmission with mixed feeding include damage to the integrity of the infant intestinal mucosa and local inflammation, which enhance the transfer of the HIV virus across the infant gut lumen.[26]

Maternal immunologic and clinical host factors also modulate the risk of transmission with documentation from several United States and European longitudinal perinatal cohorts that maternal CD4 less than 200 cells/mm^3 was a clear risk factor for transmission as was clinical AIDS.[30,31] Maternal-infant HLA incompatibility seems to afford a protective effect against transmission based on studies from Kenya.[32] In addition, clinical mastitis, breast abscess,[33] as well as subclinical mastitis based on increased sodium levels[34] are associated with increased risk of transmission during lactation.

However, the overriding risk factor for transmission during pregnancy, intrapartum, and during breastfeeding remains increased maternal viral load in plasma or breast milk.[35–37] This risk can be sharply reduced with use of combination antiretrovirals. In the United States, there is a less than 2% risk of MTCT among women infected with HIV with very low (<1000 RNA copies/mL) or undetectable viral loads, which has been achieved using potent combination antiretroviral prophylaxis during pregnancy and intrapartum.[4,5] In resource-limited international settings, low rates of MTCT among women infected with HIV who breastfeed have also been achieved in clinical trials with use of prophylaxis during pregnancy and continued during prolonged breastfeeding.[10,11]

CURRENT EPIDEMIOLOGY OF MTCT OF HIV IN THE UNITED STATES

The annual number of children less than 13 years of age with AIDS has declined by more than 96%[38] in the United States (**Fig. 1**). Estimates of the annual number of perinatal HIV infections peaked in 1992 at 1650,[39] declined to an estimated low of 96 to 186 cases in 2004,[40] and were estimated at 215 to 370 for 2005,[41] representing an approximate 92% decline overall in perinatally acquired HIV infection. These reductions are largely attributed to routine HIV screening of women during pregnancy, the use of antiretroviral (ARV) drugs for maternal treatment and perinatal prophylaxis, the use of elective cesarean delivery when appropriate and avoidance of breastfeeding. Transmission rates of less than 1% have been achieved in some settings where pregnant women have received highly active antiretroviral therapy (HAART) and successfully suppressed their HIV viral load to undetectable levels.[42–44]

In the United States, the estimated perinatal HIV transmission rate in 2005 was 1.1% to 2.8% among infants born to women infected with HIV that year in the 15 sites conducting Enhanced Perinatal HIV Surveillance,[41] however, the substantial racial/ethnic disparities that have been observed since the early days of the US HIV/AIDS epidemic persist.[45] From 2004 to 2007, the average annual overall rate of diagnoses of perinatal HIV infection was 2.7 per 100,000 infants age 1 year or less in 34 states with name-based HIV reporting. During this same time period, the average rate of diagnoses of perinatal HIV infection was 12.3 per 100,000 among blacks, 2.1 per 100,000 among Hispanics and 0.5 per 100,000 among whites. The rates for black and Hispanic children were 23 and 4 times the rate for white children, respectively. However, from 2004 to 2007, the racial/ethnic disparity narrowed, as the annual rate of diagnoses of perinatal HIV infection for black children decreased from 14.8 to 10.2 per 100,000 (P = .003), and the rate for Hispanic children decreased from 2.9 to 1.7 per 100,000 (P = .04) (**Fig. 2**).

Further reductions in perinatal HIV transmission are achievable in the United States, toward an elimination goal of less than 1% among infants born to women

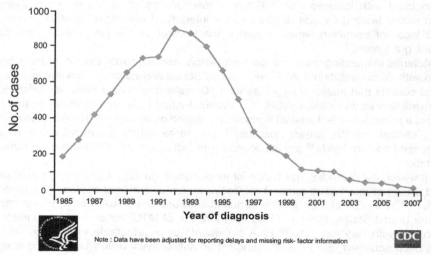

Note : Data have been adjusted for reporting delays and missing risk- factor information

Fig. 1. Estimated numbers of perinatally acquired AIDS cases by year of diagnosis, 1985 to 2007, United States and Dependent Areas. (*From* Centers for Disease Control and Prevention. HIV/AIDS surveillance slide sets. Available at: http://www.cdc.gov/hiv/topics/surveillance/resources/slides/pediatric/index.htm.)

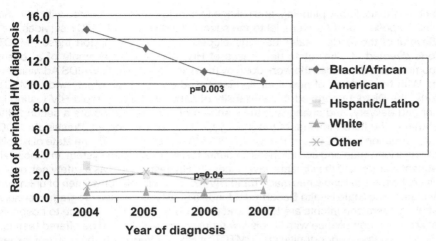

Fig. 2. Annual rate of diagnoses of perinatal HIV infection per 100,000 infants aged 1 year or less, by race/ethnicity, 34 states, 2004 to 2007. (*Data from* Centers for Disease Control and Prevention (CDC). Racial/ethnic disparities among children with diagnoses of perinatal HIV infection – 34 states, 2004–2007. CDC. MMWR Morb Mortal Wkly Rep 2010:59(4):97–101.)

infected with HIV and less than 1 transmission per 100,000 live births.[45] The Centers for Disease Control and Prevention (CDC) collaborated with 4 national organizations and published recommendations to eliminate perinatal HIV transmission in the United States.[46] The *National Organizations' Collaborative to Eliminate Perinatal HIV in the United States* recommended that to maintain the gains in PMTCT and to reach the goal of eliminating perinatal HIV in the United States, 3 strategies are needed: standardize and solidify medical interventions and policy changes that support PMTCT; institute HIV screening as part of routine health care so that HIV infection can be identified in women before pregnancy; and, most critically, focus attention and resources on the primary prevention of HIV infection in women. In addition, the investigators concluded that health care providers should incorporate HIV prevention education and routine HIV screening into women's primary health care, and public health leaders should support and fund prevention strategies directed to young women. An estimated 8700 (8663–8921) women infected with HIV gave birth to live infants in 2006,[47] representing an approximate 30% increase from the estimate of 6075 to 6422 in 2000.[48] With stable annual incidence of HIV among women,[49] and with treatment advances affording longer survival and improved quality of life, it is likely that the number of births to women infected with HIV will continue to increase. Therefore, ongoing vigilance for PMTCT in the United States will continue to be important.

HIGH-PREVALENCE STATES AND NEW STRATEGIES TO ELIMINATE PERINATAL HIV TRANSMISSION IN THE UNITED STATES

In 1999, the US Congress provided specific funding for perinatal HIV prevention. These funds were targeted at states with high prevalence to support the cascade of services needed to maximize PMTCT efforts. These include strategies to encourage routine opt-out HIV screening of all pregnant women, encourage rapid HIV testing at labor/delivery for women whose HIV status is still unknown,[50,51] and support PMTCT interventions for women found to be infected with HIV. After delivery, early infant diagnosis, family planning, and linkage to care for mothers infected with HIV and infants exposed to HIV are crucial to the successful delivery of PMTCT services.

Several of the funded states have developed strategies to support these PMTCT efforts directed at eliminating new cases of HIV infection. An example of a recent accomplishment includes the work done by the Washington, DC HIV/AIDS Administration. With the addition of new staff and increased coordination of city-wide PMTCT efforts, the District improved the availability of early HIV testing, rapid HIV testing in labor and delivery, and changes in the standard of care to incorporate a second HIV test during the third trimester of pregnancy for all pregnant women. Washington, DC saw a reduction in MTCT from 10 cases in 2005 to 1 case in 2007.[52] The state of Illinois also has a long-standing comprehensive perinatal HIV prevention system. In Illinois, all pregnant women and their infants have access to HIV testing, and as a safety net, every delivery hospital in Illinois has made rapid HIV testing available for women of unknown HIV status. The State Health Department funds a quality assurance program to ensure that all mothers and infants are tested and provides technical assistance to hospitals that are not in compliance with Illinois law requiring that all women be offered testing.

Because missed opportunities for PMTCT of HIV are frequently the result of issues with local systems, CDC has worked with CityMatCH, the American College of Obstetricians and Gynecologists, and the National Fetal and Infant Mortality Review (FIMR) Program to develop a community-based, continuous quality improvement protocol called the FIMR-HIV Prevention Methodology (FHPM). This methodology is modeled on the FIMR program and was demonstrated to be an effective tool to improve perinatal HIV prevention systems in 3 pilot communities.[53] CDC has since supported a National Resource Center for the FHPM[54] and 9 communities are currently using the methodology. The FHPM is based on the premise that all cases of perinatal HIV infection in the United States are sentinel events that warrant full review. By collecting comprehensive quantitative and qualitative data about the pregnancy experiences of women with HIV infection through maternal interviews and medical record abstraction, the methodology provides an in-depth look at the systems that result in perinatal HIV exposure or transmission. This examination allows communities to identify system strengths, missed opportunities for prevention and, more rarely, failures of interventions to prevent perinatal transmission. Communities can then develop and implement improvements to systems of care for women with HIV infection and their infants. Subsequent case reviews identify any additional or ongoing systems issues that may not have been fully addressed by the community action team so that further action can be taken.

Because the clinical management of women infected with HIV and their children is complex, the Federal Health Resources and Services Administration funds the Perinatal Hotline (888-448-8765) at the National HIV/AIDS Clinicians Consultation Center in San Francisco, CA.[55] The Perinatal Hotline provides around-the-clock advice to health care providers on indications and interpretations of standard and rapid HIV testing in pregnancy, as well as consultation on antiretroviral use in pregnancy, labor and delivery, and the postpartum period. The Perinatal HIV Consultation and Referral Service also links women with HIV infection with appropriate local health care in all states.

The US Federal Government in collaboration with other key PMTCT stakeholders is considering new coordinated approaches to eliminate perinatal HIV transmission that build on the successes and proven strategies already established.

US PUBLIC HEALTH SERVICE PMTCT RECOMMENDATIONS

In 1994, following the dramatic results of the PACTG 076 trial[3] with ZDV for PMTCT, the US government created a taskforce to work with states to rapidly implement effective and proven interventions. The Department of Health and Human Services (DHHS) Panel on Treatment of HIV-Infected Pregnant Women and Prevention of Perinatal Transmission includes obstetric and pediatric clinician experts as well as US government experts from the National Institutes of Health (NIH), the CDC, and the US Food and Drug and Administration, and community representatives. The panel reviews and updates recommendations based on new clinical trial data, safety updates, as well as clinical practice information on use of new agents. On May 24, 2010, updated guidelines[56] were issued, which included the following key recommendations for PMTCT:

- Combined antepartum, intrapartum, and infant ARV prophylaxis are recommended for maximal PMTCT
- Combination antepartum ARV regimens containing at least 3 drugs are recommended rather than single-drug regimens
- Combined ARV prophylaxis is recommended for all pregnant women infected with HIV regardless of plasma HIV RNA copy number or CD4 cell count
- Initiating ARV prophylaxis after the first trimester, but ideally no later than 28 weeks, is recommended for pregnant women infected with who do not require ARV for their own health
- Intrapartum prophylaxis and infant ARV prophylaxis are recommended for women who do not receive antepartum ARV to reduce risk of perinatal transmission
- The addition of single-dose intrapartum/newborn nevirapine (NVP) to standard antepartum combination therapy is not recommended because of the potential risk for development of NVP resistance and lack of added efficacy based on trial results
- A 6-week ZDV chemoprophylaxis regimen is recommended for all neonates exposed to HIV and should be started as close to time of birth as possible, preferably within 6 to 12 h of delivery
- Early diagnosis of HIV infection in infants remains a priority
- Decisions regarding use of additional ARV drugs in infants exposed to HIV depends on multiple factors and should be resolved with input from a pediatric HIV specialist
- In the United States, breastfeeding should be completely avoided given the increased risk of HIV transmission to the infant and availability of safe formula replacement feeding.

The DHHS Perinatal Panel also provides guidance on preconceptual counseling, specific ARV prophylactic regimens for pregnant women based on ARV history, ARV drug resistance testing, screening for and management of pregnant women coinfected with hepatitis B and C, postnatal management of HIV-exposed neonates and those born to mothers with unknown HIV status, and long-term follow-up of infants exposed to ARV drugs.

These guidelines are generally in harmony with the Adult DHHS guidelines issued in December 1, 2009, by the DHHS Panel on the Use of Antiretroviral Agents in HIV-1 Infected Adults and Adolescents.[57] However, the perinatal recommendations differed from the adult guidelines by not generally recommending continued lifetime triple combination ARVs for women with CD4 greater than 350 cells/mm^3 who took these drugs during pregnancy solely for the purpose of perinatal prophylaxis.[56]

Important questions remain, however, about the risks and benefits of stopping or continuing ARV treatment of women infected with HIV who initiate combination ARV drugs solely for PMTCT who do not need it for their own health. Several randomized clinical trials are underway to provide more definitive data on these issues. The NIH-funded International Maternal Adolescent and Pediatric Clinical Trials Group is conducting a large multicenter, randomized clinical trial, PROMISE (Promoting Maternal and Infant Survival Everywhere) HAART standard version in areas where antepartum HAART is the standard of care. This study will answer outstanding questions regarding the effect on maternal health by randomizing women with high CD4 cell counts to stop or continue HAART after delivery. In addition, the NIH-funded International Network for Strategic Initiatives in Global HIV Trials (INSIGHT) network is conducting the START trial (Strategic Timing of AntiRetroviral Treatment), which is a randomized, international multicenter trial that will determine whether the immediate initiation of antiretroviral treatment in treatment-naive individuals infected with HIV with CD4 counts greater than 500 cells/mm^3 is superior, in terms of morbidity and mortality, to deferral of treatment until the CD4 count declines to less than 350 cells/mm^3. It is critical that these trials continue to enroll so that definitive evidence regarding appropriate CD4 cell count for initiation of lifelong antiretroviral treatment (ART) can be gathered.

MEASURING SUCCESS: EARLY DIAGNOSIS OF INFANT HIV

Given that the primary goal of PMTCT interventions is to prevent infants exposed to HIV from acquiring HIV infection, it is critical to be able to monitor the success of interventions both for the individual infant and overall rates of MTCT transmission. In the United States and in international settings, early infant diagnosis (EID) is crucial for timely initiation of essential ART in infected infants given that approximately one-third of children infected with HIV die by age 1 year and more than half by age 2 years without treatment.[58] Early diagnosis and initiation of ART can reduce early mortality and HIV disease progression among infants infected with HIV by 75%.[59]

Since the early 1990s, significant progress has been made in early diagnosis of infant HIV by using nucleic acid tests (eg, PCR testing) that can directly detect the HIV virus. This is necessary because antibody tests cannot be used to diagnose HIV infection in children less than 18 months of age because of passive transfer of maternal anti-HIV antibodies. Virologic assays that can be used in children include HIV DNA assays, HIV RNA assays, and p24 antigen assays. The progress in early infant diagnosis in the United States and internationally are described in the article by Palumbo and colleagues in this issue.

INTERNATIONAL SETTINGS: GLOBAL EPIDEMIOLOGY OF MTCT OF HIV

In 2008, an estimated 430,000 new HIV infections occurred among children less than 15 years of age, most of which were caused by MTCT during pregnancy, birth, or breastfeeding.[60] In the United States, western Europe, and other resource-advantaged areas, as described earlier, MTCT has been nearly eliminated as a result of a combination of highly effective interventions including combination antiretroviral prophylaxis, elective cesarean section for women with more than 1000 copies/mm^3, and exclusive formula feeding of infants born to mother infected with HIV.[19,56] However, the incidence of MTCT in many resource-limited countries remains high because of high prevalence of HIV in women of child-bearing age, lack of universal access to antiretroviral prophylaxis, and lack of acceptable, feasible, affordable, sustainable, safe alternatives to breastfeeding. Sub-Saharan Africa has the highest burden of HIV disease overall and for MTCT, accounting for 91% (390,000) of new infections among children less that 15 years old (**Fig. 3**).[60] The region also accounted for 86% (1.8 million) of children living with HIV and the most AIDS-related deaths in children in 2008 (**Table 1**).[60]

In 2008, an estimated 1.4 million pregnant women were living with HIV; 90% were living in 19 countries in sub-Saharan Africa and India.[61] HIV seroprevalence rates in antenatal clinics vary from less than 5% in some countries to more than one-third of pregnant women in some high-prevalence countries.[62] Sentinel surveillance at antenatal clinics in southern Africa shows extremely high rates of HIV seroprevalence among pregnant women. In some clinics in South Africa, Swaziland, Lesotho, and Botswana, HIV prevalence in pregnant women exceeds 35%.[62] HIV/AIDS is also the leading cause of mortality among women of reproductive age worldwide and is the leading cause of maternal mortality in some high-prevalence countries.[60]

Coverage of PMTCT services in low- and middle-income countries has improved in recent years. In 2008, 45% of pregnant women infected with HIV received some antiretroviral drugs either for their own health or to prevent transmission to their newborns compared with 10% in 2004.[61] Coverage of antiretroviral prophylaxis for infants born to mothers infected with HIV increased to 32% from 6% during the same time period.[61] However, there is considerable inter- and intraregional variation in coverage among low- and middle-income countries (**Fig. 4**). For example, the percentage of pregnant women infected with HIV receiving ARVs for PMTCT was 59% in eastern and southern Africa versus only 16% in western and central African countries in 2008. Regimens for PMTCT also vary considerably across countries with many women still receiving a single ARV versus more effective combination ARV regimens.[61] Data published in 2009 from the Elizabeth Glaser Pediatric AIDS Foundation and affiliated programs in 22 countries have shown some increased uptake and efficiency of PMTCT services through the use of routine opt-out testing, and by supplying ARV prophylaxis for the mother as well as for her newborn at the time of HIV diagnosis.[63] These data underscore the continued global epidemic of MTCT of HIV. Africa carries the heaviest burden but Asia and India also have a significant burden of HIV infection among infants and children.

Given the international mother-to-child epidemic, there have been intensive research efforts to find feasible cost-effective strategies to reduce MTCT of HIV. These began in the mid-1990s with interventions aimed at the intrapartum period with short-course ZDV and ZDV/lamivudine (3TC) trials from 34 to 36 weeks through to labor, and

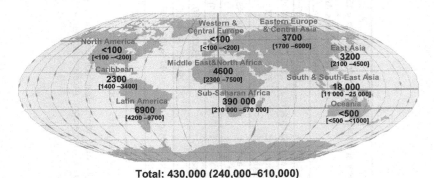

Total: 430,000 (240,000–610,000)

Fig. 3. Estimated number of children (<15 years) newly infected with HIV, 2008. (*Data from* World Health Organization, UNAIDS. AIDS epidemic update 2009. Geneva: World Health Organization. Available at: http://www.unaids.org/en/KnowledgeCentre/HIVData/EpiUpdate/EpiUpdArchive/2009/default.asp. Accessed July 12, 2010.)

Table 1
Regional HIV and AIDS statistics for children < 15 years old

Region	New Infections Among Children <15 Years (2001)	New Infections Among Children <15 Years (2008)	Children <15 Years Living with HIV (2008)	AIDS-related Deaths Among Children <15 Years (2008)
Sub-Saharan Africa	460,000 (260,000–640,000)	390,000 (210,000–570,000)	1.8 million (1.0–2.5 million)	230,000 (120,000–350,000)
Middle East and North Africa	3,800 (1900–64000)	4,600 (2300–7500)	15,000 (7600–24,000)	3300 (1600–5300)
Eastern Europe and Central Asia	3000 (1600–4300)	3700 (1700–6000)	20,000 (12,000–28,000)	1400 (<500–2700)
South, East, and South-east Asia	33,000 (18,000–49,000)	21,200 (13,100–29,500)	156,000 (102,000–223,000)	17,500 (5900–19,300)
Oceania	<500 (<200–<500)	<500 (<500–<1000)	1500 (<1000–2600)	<100 (<100–<500)
Latin America	6200 (3800–9100)	6900 (4200–9700)	31,000 (22,000–40,000)	3900 (2100–5700)
Caribbean	2800 (1700–4000)	2300 (1400–3400)	11,000 (7400–16,000)	1300 (<1000–2100)
North America, Western and Central Europe	<500 (<200–<500)	<500 (<200–<500)	5900 (<5000–7600)	<200 (<200–<400)
Total	510,000 (290,000–772,000)	430,000 (240,000–610,000)	2.1 million (1.2 –2.9 million)	280,000* (150,000–410,000)

* Rounded total estimates reported by UNAIDS.
Refs.[61,80]

Data from UNAIDS, World Health Organization. Epidemiology core slides - AIDS epidemic update 2009. Available at: http://data.unaids.org/pub/EPIslides/2009/2009_epiupdate_core_en.ppt. Accessed September 26, 2010.

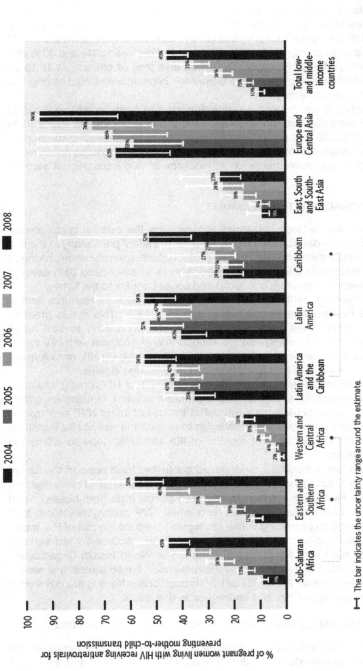

Fig. 4. Percentage of pregnant women with HIV receiving antiretrovirals for preventing mother-to-child transmission of HIV in low- and middle-income countries by region, 2004–2008. (*From* World Health Organization, UNAIDS and UNICEF. Towards universal access: scaling up priority HIV/AIDS interventions in the health sector. Progress report. 2009; Geneva (Switzerland): World Health Organization; 2009. p. 99; with permission. Available at: http://www.who.int/hiv/pub/2009progressreport/en/.)

infant prophylaxis. These randomized trials were performed in a nonbreastfeeding population in Thailand,[64] and in Africa among breastfeeding women.[6,7,65–67] In addition, in Uganda, investigators conducted a trial that focused on the peripartum period; a single tablet of NVP was given to mothers at labor onset and to their newborns.[8,68,69] Those interventions were encouraging and demonstrated between 33% and 43% efficacy compared with placebo. However, there was also loss of efficacy at 18 to 24 months for all the studies except the single-dose NVP intervention related to ongoing transmission during breastfeeding.

More recent studies have focused on antiretroviral and immune interventions to reduce the risk of transmission during breastfeeding and allow infants exposed to HIV to have the nutritional and immunologic protection of breastfeeding to improve child survival. The results of these more recent trials are quite encouraging although translation into policy and implementation in resource-limited international settings continues to lag.

RECENT INTERNATIONAL PMTCT TRIAL RESULTS

In most resource-limited settings, breastfeeding remains the cultural norm among mothers. Breast milk provides ideal nutritional food for the infant particularly in the first year of life and contains antiinfective factors that protect infants from common childhood illnesses such as pneumonia and diarrhea. In addition to its safety and birth-spacing properties, breastfeeding also offers economic and social benefits to the family.

However, breastfeeding, which is crucial to infant survival in resource-limited settings, accounts for one-third to one-half of MTCT of HIV.[1] This risk is greatest during the first 6 weeks of life and increases to an estimated 30% to 50% of all MTCT with prolonged breastfeeding into the second year.[70] Mothers with HIV therefore face a dilemma: to breastfeed their babies and risk passing on HIV or to formula feed and increase the risk of diarrhea, malnutrition, and related deaths.

Finding new strategies that can reduce the risk of MTCT of HIV among infants in settings where breastfeeding is critical to overall infant survival remains an urgent public health priority. Several trials have evaluated the use of infant NVP prophylaxis and maternal triple ARV prophylaxis as strategies to reduce the risk of HIV transmission via breastfeeding during the first months of life and offer hope to women in resource-limited settings.

Data from recent trials, including 2 randomized controlled trials support the use of infant NVP prophylaxis during the first months of life to reduce the risk of breastfeeding HIV transmission.[9,71] Results from 2 new randomized clinical trials from Malawi[10] and Botswana[11] support both maternal HAART and infant NVP prophylaxis for 6 to 7 months of breastfeeding as promising viable strategies to reduce the risk of HIV transmission among breastfeeding women infected with HIV in resource-limited settings who do not require treatment for their own health. The World Health Organization (WHO) now recommends the use of 1 of the 2 strategies.[72] These clinical trial results and the current state-of-the-art in PMTCT of HIV through breastfeeding are covered in more detail in an article by Kourtis and colleagues in this issue.

WHO STRATEGIES FOR PMTCT AND RELATED RAPID ADVICE AND GUIDELINES

Based on these and other findings on HIV prevention, the WHO in 2009 made several Rapid Advice recommendations for adult HIV treatment,[73] PMTCT,[72] and feeding of infants exposed to HIV.[74] These rapid advice reports were followed by more complete guidance released in 2010.[75–77] For PMTCT, the WHO issued a 4-pronged strategy to reduce PMTCT in low- and middle-income countries: "primary prevention of HIV infection among women of child-bearing age; preventing unintended pregnancies among women living with HIV; preventing HIV transmission from a woman living with HIV to her infant; and providing appropriate treatment, care and support to mothers living with HIV and their children and families."[(p6)78] The general guidance from the 2009 rapid advice/2010 guidelines is listed in **Table 2** along with changes from the 2006 WHO recommendations.

The recommendations were accompanied by suggested implementation strategies including

- Universal routine voluntary HIV testing and counseling for all pregnant women
- Availability of CD4 testing and ARVs at primary care level and antenatal facilities where maternal-child health care takes place, not just in specialized centers
- Improved follow-up of pregnant women antenatally and of mothers and infants exposed to HIV after birth
- Promotion and provision of ARV prophylaxis to the mother or baby throughout breastfeeding, as well as infant feeding counseling and support
- Provision of appropriately trained staff in PMTCT.

The 2009 WHO Rapid Advice and 2010 guidelines recommendations are being carefully reviewed by national Ministries of Health and policy makers in resource-limited settings. Because several of the recommendations were based on strong expert opinion but low or moderate quality of evidence, there is still a need for further research to corroborate and strengthen the recommendations. In addition, there is an urgent need for operational research to test strategies to support rapid implementation of proven effective interventions.

CHALLENGES, GAPS, AND FUTURE RESEARCH

Although progress toward elimination of MTCT of HIV in the United States and other resource-rich settings has been steady, there are still major challenges to prevent transmission and reduce the burden of pediatric HIV infection in most of the world. Some are related to crumbling health care infrastructure in settings such as Africa, which include constrained health care staffing, limited access to training, limited numbers of laboratories, and poor health care infrastructure. In addition, logistics of delivery of ARV interventions, drug stock outs, and delivery of early infant HIV diagnostics are ever present.

Other challenges include fear of stigma and lack of disclosure among pregnant women to their partners, which can lead to poor adherence to completion of more complex PMTCT regimens even if they are available. Further challenges include cultural traditions that discourage exclusive breastfeeding for the first 6 months of life, even though exclusive breastfeeding has been demonstrated to reduce the risk of HIV transmission among mothers infected with HIV in resource-limited settings compared with early mixed feeding.

Research gaps include limited clinical trial safety or efficacy data on using anti-retrovirals for prevention of transmission during breastfeeding beyond the first 6 months of life and whether maternal triple prophylaxis or infant prophylaxis is most efficacious, has fewer side effects, and is most cost-effective during prolonged breastfeeding up to 12 months. The recent BAN trial presents some information on using these strategies up to 6 months; and a new clinical trial (IMPAACT PROMISE) will address these questions in a large multisite study. Other gaps are in the area of operational research on how best to implement WHO

Table 2
WHO guidelines and rapid advice on PMTCT, ART treatment of pregnant women, and infant feeding for resource-limited settings

Status	WHO Guidelines 2006[79,80]	WHO Rapid Advice November 2009[72-74] and 2010 Guidelines[75-77]
1. HIV pregnant woman CD4 at or less than 350 cells/mm^3 regardless of symptoms, or WHO stage 3 or 4 regardless of CD4 count		Lifelong ART irrespective of gestational age using AZT+3TC NVP/EFV TDF+3TC /(FTC)+NVP/EFV (avoid EFV during first trimester) Infant 　Breastfeeding infant daily: NVP from birth to 6 weeks 　Nonbreastfeeding infant: AZT or NVP for 6 weeks
2. HIV pregnant woman CD4 more than 350 cells/mm^3, WHO stage 1 or 2	Provision of antiretroviral prophylaxis (AZT) from 28 weeks and single-dose NVP at onset of labor with 1 week tail of AZT/3TC to prevent resistance Infant 　Breastfeeding or nonbreastfeeding: combination antiretroviral prophylaxis replaced single-dose nevirapine. 　Single-dose NVP + AZT	Provision of antiretroviral prophylaxis from 14 weeks' gestation to 1 week after all exposure to breast milk Option A: maternal daily AZT from as early as 14 weeks' gestation and continued during labor; single-dose NVP at labor onset, AZT/3TC during labor and for 1 week Infant 　Breastfeeding infant: daily NVP from birth until 1 week after all exposure to breast milk has ended 　Nonbreastfeeding infant: 6 weeks daily AZT or NVP Option B: maternal triple ARV prophylaxis regimens from as early as 14 weeks 　AZT+3TC+LPV/r 　AZT +3TC + ABC 　AZT + 3TC + EFV 　TDF+FTC +EFV Labor: continue dosing Continue through duration of breastfeeding and for 1 week after Infant 　Breastfeeding infant, daily NVP from birth to 6 weeks
3. HIV-positive mother and baby	Breastfeed for 2 years	Breastfed for 2 years

Abbreviations: 3TC, lamivudine; AZT, zidovudine; EFV, efavirenz; FTC, emtricitabine; LPV/r, lopinavir/ritonavir; NVP, nevirapine; TDF, tenofovir.

guidance at a country and district level, particularly in rural settings with already constrained medical services.

Given these gaps, several research questions remain to be addressed:

- Is it better to provide infant prophylaxis or maternal triple ARV prophylaxis to prevent transmission during breastfeeding for women infected with HIV in resource-limited settings, considering both maternal disease progression and infant health and survival?
- Which strategy is most cost-effective in the short-term and in the long-term?
- What are the resistance patterns seen for mother-infant pairs exposed to long-term triple ARV interventions?
- Is it safer to stop or to continue triple ARVs used solely for PMTCT once started in 1 pregnancy among women who do not yet require treatment for their own care?
- Are there late adverse effects on physical growth, hematologic parameters, and cognitive development of infants and children exposed to PMTCT combination antiretrovirals in utero and for up to 18 months or more of breastfeeding?

Remaining key operational research questions include

- How to best integrate PMTCT efforts within the general maternal-child health framework so that it is not a vertical program operating in isolation
- How to use PMTCT funds to help support overall infant and maternal survival in resource-limited settings
- How to expand rapid development of inexpensive point-of-care early infant diagnostic testing, CD4 and viral load testing
- How to simplify ARV regimens (eg, as fixed dose once-a-day regimens) to promote adherence
- How to improve long-term adherence once individuals are feeling well
- How to set up monitoring systems to assess both short-term and long-term adverse effects of use of antiretroviral drugs for PMTCT.

SUMMARY

The progress in PMTCT has been one of the major successes in the US HIV epidemic with a greater than 96% reduction in perinatal AIDS cases from 1992 to the present. Perinatal HIV transmission rates are now less than 2% in most university medical settings where pregnant women infected with HIV receive combination antiretrovirals, scheduled cesarean delivery if they still have detectable viral load near delivery, and can safely avoid breastfeeding. The rapid implementation of effective interventions has been the result of strong collaboration and coordination between federal, state, and local agencies, dissemination of interventions, education of health care providers, and targeted funding to help support perinatal HIV prevention programs. However, the drive toward the elimination of MTCT in the United States is hampered by new incident infections among adolescents and women, late identification of their infection status leading to suboptimal late interventions among some pregnant women infected with HIV.

Internationally, clinical trial research has also shown slow but incremental progress in reducing transmission risk among women infected with HIV particularly antepartum, during labor and delivery, and during the first 6 months of breastfeeding. Finding feasible strategies to prevent transmission during more extended periods of breastfeeding remains a challenge. Current studies are addressing the use of either maternal triple ARV prophylaxis or infant ARV prophylaxis extending into the second year of life;

and assessing whether stopping of maternal ARVs may be harmful for mothers infected with HIV who do not yet meet treatment criteria. In resource-limited settings, the translation of PMTCT clinical trial findings into practice has been slow, given poor maternal-child health care infrastructure, lack of integration, and limitations on funding. In addition, primary prevention efforts to date have fallen short, with adolescents and women of child-bearing age remaining at high risk for acquiring HIV and passing it on to their infants.

An effective HIV vaccine which could be given to newborns and infants during breastfeeding; as well as to adolescents and sexually active adults would ideally be the best long-term solution to the global HIV epidemic and would eliminate new cases of MTCT. However, the quest for an efficacious vaccine remains elusive despite 30 years of intensive basic and clinical trial research. In the interim, advances in PMTCT are continuing based on research efforts and international programmatic support.

REFERENCES

1. De Cock KM, Fowler MG, Mercier E, et al. Prevention of mother-to-child HIV transmission in resource-poor countries: translating research into policy and practice. JAMA 2000;283(9):1175–82.
2. Simonon A, Lepage P, Karita E, et al. An assessment of the timing of mother-to-child transmission of human immunodeficiency virus type 1 by means of polymerase chain reaction. J Acquir Immune Defic Syndr 1994;7(9):952–7.
3. Connor EM, Sperling RS, Gelber R, et al. Reduction of maternal-infant transmission of human immunodeficiency virus type 1 with zidovudine treatment. Pediatric AIDS Clinical Trials Group Protocol 076 Study Group. N Engl J Med 1994;331(18): 1173–80.
4. Dorenbaum A, Cunningham CK, Gelber RD, et al. Two-dose intrapartum/newborn nevirapine and standard antiretroviral therapy to reduce perinatal HIV transmission: a randomized trial. JAMA 2002;288(2):189–98.
5. Cooper ER, Charurat M, Mofenson L, et al. Combination antiretroviral strategies for the treatment of pregnant HIV-1-infected women and prevention of perinatal HIV-1 transmission. J Acquir Immune Defic Syndr 2002;29(5):484–94.
6. Wiktor SZ, Ekpini E, Karon JM, et al. Short-course oral zidovudine for prevention of mother-to-child transmission of HIV-1 in Abidjan, Cote d'Ivoire: a randomised trial. Lancet 1999;353(9155):781–5.
7. PETRA Study Team. Efficacy of three short-course regimens of zidovudine and lamivudine in preventing early and late transmission of HIV-1 from mother to child in Tanzania, South Africa, and Uganda (PETRA study): a randomised, double-blind, placebo-controlled trial. Lancet 2002;359(9313):1178–86.
8. Jackson JB, Musoke P, Fleming T, et al. Intrapartum and neonatal single-dose nevirapine compared with zidovudine for prevention of mother-to-child transmission of HIV-1 in Kampala, Uganda: 18-month follow-up of the HIVNET 012 randomised trial. Lancet 2003;362(9387):859–68.
9. Six Week Extended-Dose Nevirapine (SWEN) Study Team, Bedri A, Gudetta B, et al. Extended-dose nevirapine to 6 weeks of age for infants to prevent HIV transmission via breastfeeding in Ethiopia, India, and Uganda: an analysis of three randomised controlled trials. Lancet 2008;372(9635):300–13.
10. Chasela CS, Hudgens MG, Jamieson DJ, et al. Maternal or infant antiretroviral drugs to reduce HIV-1 transmission. N Engl J Med 2010;362(24):2271–81.
11. Shapiro RL, Hughes MD, Ogwu A, et al. Antiretroviral regimens in pregnancy and breast-feeding in Botswana. N Engl J Med 2010;362(24):2282–94.

12. Brossard Y, Aubin JT, Mandelbrot L, et al. Frequency of early in utero HIV-1 infection: a blind DNA polymerase chain reaction study on 100 fetal thymuses. AIDS 1995;9(4):359–66.

13. Van Dyke RB, Korber BT, Popek E, et al. The Ariel Project: a prospective cohort study of maternal-child transmission of human immunodeficiency virus type 1 in the era of maternal antiretroviral therapy. J Infect Dis 1999;179(2):319–28.

14. Kourtis AP, Lee FK, Abrams EJ, et al. Mother-to-child transmission of HIV-1: timing and implications for prevention. Lancet Infect Dis 2006;6(11):726–32.

15. Lin HH, Kao JH, Hsu HY, et al. Least microtransfusion from mother to fetus in elective cesarean delivery. Obstet Gynecol 1996;87(2):244–8.

16. Kaneda T, Shiraki K, Hirano K, et al. Detection of maternofetal transfusion by placental alkaline phosphatase levels. J Pediatr 1997;130(5):730–5.

17. European Mode of Delivery Collaboration. Elective caesarean-section versus vaginal delivery in prevention of vertical HIV-1 transmission: a randomised clinical trial. Lancet 1999;353(9158):1035–9.

18. The International Perinatal HIV Group. The mode of delivery and the risk of vertical transmission of human immunodeficiency virus type 1–a meta-analysis of 15 prospective cohort studies. N Engl J Med 1999;340(13):977–87.

19. Boer K, England K, Godfried MH, et al. Mode of delivery in HIV-infected pregnant women and prevention of mother-to-child transmission: changing practices in western Europe. HIV Med 2010;11(6):368–78.

20. Ayisi JG, van Eijk AM, Newman RD, et al. Maternal malaria and perinatal HIV transmission, western Kenya. Emerg Infect Dis 2004;10(4):643–52.

21. Brahmbhatt H, Sullivan D, Kigozi G, et al. Association of HIV and malaria with mother-to-child transmission, birth outcomes, and child mortality. J Acquir Immune Defic Syndr 2008;47(4):472–6.

22. Inion I, Mwanyumba F, Gaillard P, et al. Placental malaria and perinatal transmission of human immunodeficiency virus type 1. J Infect Dis 2003;188(11): 1675–8.

23. Mwapasa V, Rogerson SJ, Molyneux ME, et al. The effect of Plasmodium falciparum malaria on peripheral and placental HIV-1 RNA concentrations in pregnant Malawian women. AIDS 2004;18(7):1051–9.

24. Belyakov IM, Berzofsky JA. Immunobiology of mucosal HIV infection and the basis for development of a new generation of mucosal AIDS vaccines. Immunity 2004;20(3):247–53.

25. Miotti PG, Taha TE, Kumwenda NI, et al. HIV transmission through breastfeeding: a study in Malawi. JAMA 1999;282(8):744–9.

26. Kourtis AP, Jamieson DJ, de Vincenzi I, et al. Prevention of human immunodeficiency virus-1 transmission to the infant through breastfeeding: new developments. Am J Obstet Gynecol 2007;197(Suppl 3):S113–22.

27. Requena M, Bouhlal H, Nasreddine N, et al. Inhibition of HIV-1 transmission in trans from dendritic cells to CD4+ T lymphocytes by natural antibodies to the CRD domain of DC-SIGN purified from breast milk and intravenous immunoglobulins. Immunology 2008;123(4):508–18.

28. Coutsoudis A, Pillay K, Spooner E, et al. Randomized trial testing the effect of vitamin A supplementation on pregnancy outcomes and early mother-to-child HIV-1 transmission in Durban, South Africa. South African Vitamin A Study Group. AIDS 1999;13(12):1517–24.

29. Iliff PJ, Piwoz EG, Tavengwa NV, et al. Early exclusive breastfeeding reduces the risk of postnatal HIV-1 transmission and increases HIV-free survival. AIDS 2005; 19(7):699–708.

30. Pitt J, Brambilla D, Reichelderfer P, et al. Maternal immunologic and virologic risk factors for infant human immunodeficiency virus type 1 infection: findings from the women and infants transmission study. J Infect Dis 1997;175(3):567–75.
31. European Collaborative Study. HIV-infected pregnant women and vertical transmission in Europe since 1986. AIDS 2001;15(6):761–70.
32. Mackelprang RD, John-Stewart G, Carrington M, et al. Maternal HLA homozygosity and mother-child HLA concordance increase the risk of vertical transmission of HIV-1. J Infect Dis 2008;197(8):1156–61.
33. Embree JE, Njenga S, Datta P, et al. Risk factors for postnatal mother-child transmission of HIV-1. AIDS 2000;14(16):2535–41.
34. Semba RD, Kumwenda N, Hoover DR, et al. Human immunodeficiency virus load in breast milk, mastitis, and mother-to-child transmission of human immunodeficiency virus type 1. J Infect Dis 1999;180(1):93–8.
35. Sperling RS, Shapiro DE, Coombs RW, et al. Maternal viral load, zidovudine treatment, and the risk of transmission of human immunodeficiency virus type 1 from mother to infant. Pediatric AIDS Clinical Trials Group Protocol 076 Study Group. N Engl J Med 1996;335(22):1621–9.
36. Shaffer N, Roongpisuthipong A, Siriwasin W, et al. Maternal virus load and perinatal human immunodeficiency virus type 1 subtype E transmission, Thailand. Bangkok Collaborative Perinatal HIV Transmission Study Group. J Infect Dis 1999;179(3):590–9.
37. Semrau K, Ghosh M, Kankasa C, et al. Temporal and lateral dynamics of HIV shedding and elevated sodium in breast milk among HIV-positive mothers during the first 4 months of breast-feeding. J Acquir Immune Defic Syndr 2008;47(3):320–8.
38. Centers for Disease Control and Prevention (CDC). HIV/AIDS surveillance report, 2007, vol. 19. Atlanta (GA): US Department of Health and Human Services, Centers for Disease Control and Prevention; 2009. Available at: http://www.cdc.gov/hiv/topics/surveillance/resources/reports/. Accessed June 16, 2010.
39. Lindegren ML, Byers RH Jr, Thomas P, et al. Trends in perinatal transmission of HIV/AIDS in the United States. JAMA 1999;282(6):531–8.
40. McKenna MT, Hu X. Recent trends in the incidence and morbidity that are associated with perinatal human immunodeficiency virus infection in the United States. Am J Obstet Gynecol 2007;197(Suppl 3):S10–6.
41. Zhang X, Rhodes P, Blair J. Estimated number of perinatal HIV infections in the United States, 2005–2009. In: Programs and abstracts of the National HIV Prevention Conference 2009. Atlanta (GA), August 23–29, 2009.
42. Naver L, Lindgren S, Belfrage E, et al. Children born to HIV-1-infected women in Sweden in 1982–2003: trends in epidemiology and vertical transmission. J Acquir Immune Defic Syndr 2006;42(4):484–9.
43. Townsend CL, Cortina-Borja M, Peckham CS, et al. Low rates of mother-to-child transmission of HIV following effective pregnancy interventions in the United Kingdom and Ireland, 2000–2006. AIDS 2008;22(8):973–81.
44. Warszawski J, Tubiana R, Le Chenadec J, et al. Mother-to-child HIV transmission despite antiretroviral therapy in the ANRS French perinatal cohort. AIDS 2008; 22(2):289–99.
45. Centers for Disease Control and Prevention (CDC). Racial/ethnic disparities among children with diagnoses of perinatal HIV infection –34 states, 2004–2007. MMWR Morb Mortal Wkly Rep 2010;59(4):97–101.
46. Burr CK, Lampe MA, Corle S, et al. An end to perinatal HIV: success in the US requires ongoing and innovative efforts that should expand globally. J Public Health Policy 2007;28(2):249–60.

47. Whitmore SK, Zhang X, Taylor AW, et al. Estimated number of infants born to HIV-infected women in the United States and five dependent areas 2006 [abstract 924]. In: Program and abstracts of the 16th Conference on Retroviruses and Opportunistic Infections. Montréal (Canada), February 8–11, 2009.
48. Fleming P, Lindegren M, Byers R, et al. Estimated number of perinatal HIV infections, U.S., 2000. The XIV International AIDS Conference. Barcelona (Spain), July 11–16, 2002.
49. Hall HI, Song R, Rhodes P, et al. Estimation of HIV incidence in the United States. JAMA 2008;300(5):520–9.
50. Jamieson DJ, Cohen MH, Maupin R, et al. Rapid human immunodeficiency virus-1 testing on labor and delivery in 17 US hospitals: the MIRIAD experience. Am J Obstet Gynecol 2007;197(Suppl 3):S72–82.
51. ACOG Committee on Obstetric Practice. ACOG committee opinion number 304, November 2004 Prenatal and perinatal human immunodeficiency virus testing: expanded recommendations. Obstet Gynecol 2004;104(5 Pt 1): 1119–24.
52. Government of the District of Columbia. Annual report 2009 update HIV/AIDS, hepatitis, STD and TB epidemiology. 2009. Available at: http://www.doh.dc.gov/hahsta. Accessed June 15, 2010.
53. Lampe MA, Thompson B, Carlson R, et al. All perinatal HIV transmission is local: using FIMR to identify and address missed prevention opportunities. abstract C16-1. In: National HIV Prevention Conference 2009. Atlanta (GA), August 23–29, 2009.
54. National Resource Center. FIMR-HIV prevention methodology. Available at: http://www.fimrhiv.org/. Accessed October 26, 2010.
55. American Academy of Pediatrics (AAP). Perinatal HIV hotline. AAP News 2008; 29(12):26.
56. Panel on Treatment of HIV-Infected Pregnant Women and Prevention of Perinatal Transmission. Recommendations for use of antiretroviral drugs in pregnant HIV-1-infected women for maternal health and interventions to reduce perinatal HIV transmission in the United States. May 24, 2010. p. 1–117. Available at: http://aidsinfo.nih.gov/ContentFiles/PerinatalGL.pdf. Accessed June 1, 2010.
57. Panel on Antiretroviral Guidelines for Adults and Adolescents. Guidelines for the use of antiretroviral agents in HIV-1-infected adults and adolescents. Department of Health and Human Services. 2009. p. 1–161. Available at: http://www.aidsinfo.nih.gov/ContentFiles/AdultandAdolescentGL.pdf. Accessed May 2, 2010.
58. Newell ML, Coovadia H, Cortina-Borja M, et al. Mortality of infected and uninfected infants born to HIV-infected mothers in Africa: a pooled analysis. Lancet 2004;364(9441):1236–43.
59. Violari A, Cotton MF, Gibb DM, et al. Early antiretroviral therapy and mortality among HIV-infected infants. N Engl J Med 2008;359(21):2233–44.
60. UNAIDS, World Health Organization. Epidemiology core slides - AIDS epidemic update 2009. Available at: http://data.unaids.org/pub/EPISlides/2009/2009_epiudate_core_cn.ppt. Accessed September 26, 2010.
61. World Health Organization, UNAIDS, UNICEF. Towards universal access: scaling up priority HIV/AIDS interventions in the health sector: Progress report 2009. Geneva (Switzerland): World Health Organization; 2009. Available at: http://data.unaids.org/pub/Report/2009/20090930_tuapr_2009_en.pdf. Accessed May 1, 2010.

62. US Census Bureau, Population Division, International Programs Center, Health Studies Branch. HIV/AIDS surveillance data base, Table 1: HIV1 seroprevalence. Available at: http://hivaidssurveillancedb.org/hivdb/MAP/tab1.htm. Accessed October 26, 2010.

63. Spensley A, Sripipatana T, Turner AN, et al. Preventing mother-to-child transmission of HIV in resource-limited settings: the Elizabeth Glaser Pediatric AIDS Foundation experience. Am J Public Health 2009;99(4):631–7.

64. Shaffer N, Chuachoowong R, Mock PA, et al. Short-course zidovudine for perinatal HIV-1 transmission in Bangkok, Thailand: a randomised controlled trial. Bangkok Collaborative Perinatal HIV Transmission Study Group. Lancet 1999; 353(9155):773–80.

65. Leroy V, Karon JM, Alioum A, et al. Twenty-four month efficacy of a maternal short-course zidovudine regimen to prevent mother-to-child transmission of HIV-1 in West Africa. AIDS 2002;16(4):631–41.

66. Gray GE, Urban M, Chersich MF, et al. A randomized trial of two postexposure prophylaxis regimens to reduce mother-to-child HIV-1 transmission in infants of untreated mothers. AIDS 2005;19(12):1289–97.

67. Dabis F, Msellati P, Meda N, et al. 6-month efficacy, tolerance, and acceptability of a short regimen of oral zidovudine to reduce vertical transmission of HIV in breastfed children in Cote D'ivoire and Burkina Faso: a double-blind placebo-controlled multicentre trial. DITRAME Study Group. Diminution de la Transmission Mere-Enfant. Lancet 1999;353(9155):786–92.

68. Guay LA, Musoke P, Fleming T, et al. Intrapartum and neonatal single-dose nevirapine compared with zidovudine for prevention of mother-to-child transmission of HIV-1 in Kampala, Uganda: HIVNET 012 randomised trial. Lancet 1999; 354(9181):795–802.

69. Guay LA, Hom DL, Kabengera SR, et al. HIV-1 ICD p24 antigen detection in Ugandan infants: use in early diagnosis of infection and as a marker of disease progression. J Med Virol 2000;62(4):426–34.

70. Nduati R. Breastfeeding and HIV-1 infection. A review of current literature. Adv Exp Med Biol 2000;478:201–10.

71. Kumwenda NI, Hoover DR, Mofenson LM, et al. Extended antiretroviral prophylaxis to reduce breast-milk HIV-1 transmission. N Engl J Med 2008;359(2): 119–29.

72. World Health Organization. Rapid advice: use of antiretroviral drugs for treating pregnant women and preventing HIV infection in infants. Geneva (Switzerland): World Health Organization; 2009. p. 1–23. Available at: http://www.searo.who. int/LinkFiles/HIV-AIDS_Rapid_Advice_MTCT%28web%29.pdf. Accessed May 20, 2010.

73. World Health Organization. Rapid advice: antiretroviral therapy for HIV infection in adults and adolescents. Geneva (Switzerland): World Health Organization; 2009. p. i–25. Available at: http://www.who.int/hiv/pub/arv/rapid_advice_art.pdf. Accessed May 20, 2010.

74. World Health Organization. Rapid advice: revised WHO principles and recommendations on infant feeding in the context of HIV. Geneva (Switzerland): World Health Organization; 2009. p. i–24. Available at: http://www.searo.who.int/ LinkFiles/HIV-AIDS_Rapid_Advice_Infant_feeding%28web%29.pdf. Accessed May 20, 2010.

75. World Health Organization. Antiretroviral therapy for HIV infection in adults and adolescents: recommendations for a public health approach. 2010 revision. Geneva (Switzerland): World Health Organization; 2010. p. 1–145.

Available at: http://whqlibdoc.who.int/publications/2010/9789241599764_eng.pdf. Accessed August 18, 2010.

76. World Health Organization. Guidelines on HIV and infant feeding. Principles and recommendations for infant feeding in the context of HIV and a summary of evidence. 2010. p. 1–49. Available at: http://whqlibdoc.who.int/publications/2010/9789241599535_eng.pdf. Accessed August 18, 2010.

77. World Health Organization. Antiretroviral drugs for treating pregnant women and preventing HIV infection in infants. Recommendations for a public health approach. Geneva (Switzerland): WHO; 2010. p. 1–105. Available at: http://whqlibdoc.who.int/publications/2010/9789241599818_eng.pdf. Accessed August 18, 2010.

78. World Health Organization. PMTCT strategic vision 2010–2015: preventing mother-to-child transmission of HIV to reach the UNGASS and millennium development goals. Geneva (Switzerland): World Health Organization; 2010.

79. World Health Organization. Antiretroviral drugs for treating pregnant women and preventing HIV infection in infant: towards universal access. Recommendations for a public health approach. Geneva (Switzerland): World Health Organization; 2006. p. 1–92. Available at: http://www.who.int/hiv/pub/mtct/antiretroviral/en/index.html. Accessed May 30, 2010.

80. World Health Organization, UNICEF, UNAIDS, UNFPA. HIV and infant feeding: updated based on the technical consultation held on behalf of the inter-agency team (IATT) on prevention of HIV infections in pregnant women, mothers and their infants. Geneva (Switzerland), October 25–27, 2006. Geneva (Switzerland): World Health Organization; 2007. Available at: http://www.who.int/child_adolescent_health/documents/9789241595964/en/index.html. Accessed August 18, 2010.

Mother-to-Child Transmission of HIV: Pathogenesis, Mechanisms and Pathways

Athena P. Kourtis, MD, PhD, MPH[a,b,*], Marc Bulterys, MD, PhD[c,d]

KEYWORDS
- Human immunodeficiency virus • Mother-to-child transmission
- Infant • Mechanisms

Without doubt, one of the greatest medical and public health achievements has been the significant reduction in mother-to-child transmission (MTCT) of human immunodeficiency virus (HIV), especially in the developed world. Transmission rates lower than 1% to 2% have been achieved,[1,2] even in some resource-limited settings,[3] compared with transmission rates of 14% to 42% without any intervention.[4] This has been achieved with the use of antiretroviral drug combinations during pregnancy, labor/delivery, and neonatal prophylaxis, as well as with elective caesarean delivery and avoidance of breast feeding. Modalities to prevent mother-to-child transmission of HIV are highly dependent on the timing and mechanisms of HIV transmission. The mechanisms and timing of MTCT of HIV, however, have not been fully elucidated, are likely multifactorial, and many of their aspects remain unclear.

The findings and conclusions in this article are those of the authors and do not necessarily represent the views of the Centers for Disease Control and Prevention.

[a] Division of Reproductive Health, National Center for Chronic Disease Prevention and Health Promotion, Centers for Disease Control and Prevention, 4770 Buford Highway, NE, MS-K34, Atlanta, GA 30341, USA

[b] Department of Pediatrics, Emory University School of Medicine, Atlanta, GA, USA

[c] Division of HIV/AIDS, Center for Global Health, Centers for Disease Control and Prevention, Atlanta, GA 30333, USA

[d] CDC Global AIDS Program, China, Suite #403, Dongwai Diplomatic Office, 23 Dongzhimenwai Dajie, Beijing, China

* Corresponding author. Division of Reproductive Health, National Center for Chronic Disease Prevention and Health Promotion, Centers for Disease Control and Prevention, 4770 Buford Highway, NE, MS-K34, Atlanta, GA 30341.
E-mail address: apk3@cdc.gov

Clin Perinatol 37 (2010) 721–737
doi:10.1016/j.clp.2010.08.004
0095-5108/10/$ – see front matter. Published by Elsevier Inc.

perinatology.theclinics.com

TIMING AND MECHANISMS OF MTCT OF HIV

MTCT can occur:

In utero by direct hematogenous transplacental spread or ascending infection of the amniotic membranes and fluid

At the time of delivery by mucocutaneous contact of the infant with maternal blood, amniotic fluid, and cervicovaginal secretions during passage through the birth canal; ascending infection from the cervix; or maternal–fetal transfusion from uterine contractions at labor and delivery

During breastfeeding.

There is not complete concurrence about the relative contribution of these different periods in transmission of HIV to the infant.[5] Approximately one-third of infant HIV infections in nonbreastfeeding populations are detected in the first 2 days of life, and two-thirds are detected after the first week of life and by 6 weeks of age, leading some to argue that one-third of transmission occurs during pregnancy and the remaining two thirds during labor in nonbreastfeeding populations.[6–8] Indeed, the working definition of in utero versus intrapartum HIV infection is based on virologic detection of infection in the infant's first 2 days of life versus after the first week.[6] By synthesizing results from many prevention studies using antiretroviral agents at various stages during pregnancy, as well as the preventive benefits of cesarean section when performed before the onset of labor,[9] the authors have argued that approximately one-half of MTCT of HIV occurs late in pregnancy, possibly in the days before delivery, as the placenta begins to separate from the uterine wall.[10] Only a small proportion of MTCT (<4%) seems to occur in the first trimester,[11] and less than 20% by 36 weeks of gestation.[10] Indeed, several studies using highly sensitive polymerase chain reaction PCR techniques have found very little or no HIV positivity in lymphoid tissues of first or second trimester human fetuses.[12–14] A large study with twins did not find that the birth order of twins was associated with risk for HIV-1 infection,[15] supporting the idea that birth canal exposure is not the major contributor to the baby's risk; the authors believe that about one-third of MTCT occurs during delivery.[10]

Postexposure infant prophylaxis, through administration of antiretroviral drugs to the infant within hours of birth, protects against cell-free or cell-associated virus that might have obtained access to the fetal/infant systemic circulation through maternal–fetal transfusion or through systemic dissemination of virus swallowed by the infant during passage through the birth canal.[16] This approach likely provides benefit when the virus remains unintegrated in quiescent cells.[17,18] With the use of a PCR that detects viral long terminal repeats (LTR) rather than gag, thus a partly reverse-transcribed HIV-1 genome, it was found that about 18% of uninfected infants born to HIV-1 infected mothers had evidence of unintegrated virus in their peripheral blood mononuclear cells.[18] The unintegrated viral intermediate is biologically active, but in the absence of appropriate activation it decays with time.[17] These findings support the notion that HIV-1 might enter a fetus, but in the absence of appropriately activated lymphocytes it might not integrate and establish infection until a later time, if at all. Support for the efficacy of infant postexposure prophylaxis also comes from studies in macaques.[19] If indeed HIV-1 cannot complete reverse transcription until cell activation occurs, then viral entry might not equal transmission, which arguably occurs only at the time of viral integration and thus the establishment of infection. Accepting this premise, most instances of MTCT must occur around the time of birth (when extensive lymphocyte activation starts to occur), even though viral entry could have occurred days or weeks earlier. Of interest, significant reduction in the in utero transmission rate of HIV-1 was shown when nevirapine at labor was added to a zidovudine regimen started at 28 weeks of gestation.[2] An explanation for this is that perinatal nevirapine may delay infant PCR positivity or even prevent infection from virus that entered the fetus during the last few weeks of gestation, a conclusion consistent with the hypothesis presented.

Breast feeding is also a time of major risk for MTCT of HIV in settings where safe feeding alternatives are not available. The postnatal transmission rate is estimated to be as high as 15% if women engage in prolonged breast feeding of about 2 years.[20–22] This represents a substantial proportion (over one-third) of MTCT of HIV, and indeed the period of highest risk if antiretroviral prophylaxis is given during pregnancy and peripartum.[5,23]

It is believed that the risk of breast feeding transmission of HIV to the infant is higher during early lactation because of increased breast milk viral load in colostrum. The risk, however, continues throughout breast feeding and is associated with low maternal CD4 count, longer duration of breast feeding, higher maternal viral load, mastitis, and mixed feeding.[24–28] The Breastfeeding and HIV International Transmission meta-analysis calculated the risk of postnatal HIV transmission after 4 weeks of age to be 8.9 transmissions per 100 child–years of breast feeding, with a generally constant rate of transmission between 1 and 18 months of infant age.[29] Maternal breast pathologies, such as mastitis (including subclinical mastitis, identified through elevated breast milk sodium levels), nipple lesions and breast abscess[26,29] and infant oral candidiasis[30] also have been identified as risk factors for MTCT of HIV in the breastfed infant.

FACTORS INFLUENCING MTCT OF HIV

Many factors may influence the risk of MTCT of HIV (**Box 1**). The risk of HIV transmission is higher for mothers with clinical and immunologic indicators of advanced disease, and with increased viral load.[31,32]

Viral Factors of MTCT of HIV

Amount of virus

A higher maternal viral RNA load in the peripheral blood is associated with a higher risk of MTCT for HIV,[1,33] with the risk increasing as viral load increases.[34–36] However, overlap in HIV RNA copy number has been observed in women who transmitted and those who did not transmit the virus to their infants. Although the risk of transmission of HIV from mothers with peripheral blood viral loads below the limit of detection is very low, no threshold of peripheral blood viral load has been identified below which transmission does not occur.[37] Receipt of highly active antiretroviral therapy by the mothers, which decreases viral load, has achieved very low MTCT rates. Antiretroviral drugs decrease maternal viral load in the blood and genital secretions when given antenatally. However, this is not the only mechanism by which they exert their benefit. Antiretroviral drugs have been shown to reduce the risk of transmission even among women with HIV RNA levels less than 1000 copies/mL.[38] Additionally, the level of HIV RNA at delivery and receipt of antenatal antiretroviral therapy are each independently associated with the risk of transmission, suggesting that antiretroviral prophylaxis does not work solely through its effects in viral load.[1,39] Primary maternal HIV infection during pregnancy or postpartum in the nursing mother, associated with higher viral load, is also associated with an increased risk of MTCT.[11,40] Indeed, the observed increase in MTCT of HIV when mothers had frequent unprotected sexual intercourse during pregnancy might be related to increased risk of primary HIV infection during

---

Box 1
Factors influencing mother-to-child transmission of HIV

Viral factors

Viral load in plasma, genitourinary tract, breast milk

Viral characteristics: genotype, phenotype, tropism, resistance to antiretroviral agents, capacity for immune escape

Host factors

Immunologic factors

Maternal CD4 count–stage of HIV disease

Maternal immune factors (such as neutralizing antibodies)

Breast milk immune factors

Fetal/neonatal immune response (such as cytotoxic lymphocyte [CTL] responses)

Genetic factors (fetal HLA type, maternal-fetal HLA concordance, single nucleotide polymorphisms [SNPs] for chemokines/chemokine receptors/innate immune factors)

Tissue/mucosal integrity

Chorioamnionitis/placental pathology/maturational stage

Maternal genitourinary (GU) lesions/sexually transmitted diseases (STDs)

Cracked or bleeding nipples/breast abscess/clinical or subclinical mastitis

Barrier integrity (neonatal skin and mucosal membranes)

Infant gastrointestinal (GI) maturity

Vitamin A/other micronutrient deficiency

Obstetric factors

Mode of delivery

Timing of delivery

Invasive monitoring/obstetric procedures

Duration of membrane rupture

---

pregnancy, or to the acquisition of other STDs increasing HIV viral load in those already infected with HIV.[41,42]

In addition to peripheral blood viral load, a higher maternal genital tract viral load is independently associated with a higher risk of MTCT of HIV.[29] However, intrapartum cleansing of the genital canal with virucidal agents such as benzalkonium chloride (evaluated in a small study in West Africa),[43] or 0.25% chlorhexidine (evaluated in Malawi),[44] and 0.2% and 0.4% chlorhexidine (evaluated in Kenya)[45,46] did not show a benefit in decreasing MTCT of HIV. A trial of 1% chlorhexidine, thought to be the highest tolerated concentration,[47] has been proposed. The viral load of HIV in the breast milk of the nursing mother is associated with risk of postnatal transmission to the infant.[24]

Type of virus

It is likely that transmitted HIV has an advantage in either crossing mucosal barriers, infecting or replicating in target cells, or evading immune responses compared with the nontransmitted variants.[48] Most evidence supports restricted viral heterogeneity in the blood near the time of infection in most infected infants, with only one or very few viral variants transmitted from mother to child.[49,50] However, transmission of multiple variants to infants also has been described.[51–53] Transmission at the time of delivery has been primarily associated with a single viral quasispecies,[53–55] usually a minor maternal variant,[53] whereas in utero transmitters were more likely to transmit single or multiple major maternal viral variants.[51,53,56] The authors recently compared the viral sequences from the blood and cervicovaginal fluid of three mothers who transmitted HIV to their infants with those in their infants. Results indicate the presence of more than one HIV variant in the neonate's plasma that are derived from the maternal blood and from the vaginal compartment, pointing to more than one episode of transmission with more than one viral strain from different maternal compartments.[57] The authors' findings also show transmission of cell-associated maternal virus. This result concurs with those of several other studies, where higher cell-associated HIV-1 DNA levels in blood and genital secretions or breast milk significantly increased risk of transmission to the infant.[24,29,39,58–60] Even though early studies of MTCT of HIV had identified plasma cell-free RNA viral load at delivery as the most significant predictor of transmission,[20,39,53] cell-free HIV-1 RNA in plasma may only be a surrogate marker for the source of virus that is transmitted. Taken together, the results of studies suggest that, in addition to levels of cell-free virus in blood and genital secretions, cell-associated virus can independently predict vertical transmission risk in utero, intrapartum, and via breast feeding.

HIV subtype differences in MTCT have been observed in some cohorts but not others.[48,60–64] Some have suggested that subtype C is preferentially transmitted in utero compared with subtypes A and D.[62] A predominance of CCR5 utilizing, macrophage-tropic, nonsyncytium-inducing viruses is noted in perinatal transmission.[65] Restricted N-linked glycosylation of the infant viral envelopes (Env) compared with the maternal Env is another characteristic of newly transmitted viruses.[65,66] Most studies have concentrated on the variable regions of the viral envelope surface protein gp120, as this region defines viral tropism and contains major targets of the neutralizing antibody response. A study recently reported, however, that the replication capacity of the polymerase gene from transmitting mothers was greater than that of nontransmitters, suggesting that factors outside of the envelope may play a role in transmission.[67]

Host Factors of MTCT of HIV

Immunologic factors
Innate immune parameters Chemokines, the natural ligands of viral coreceptors, may inhibit HIV-1 infection; the β-chemokines CCL3, CCL4, and CCL5 are natural ligands for CCR5, and their overexpression in exposed uninfected infants suggests a possible role in mediating inhibition of MTCT.[68] The role of a single strand polymorphism (or SNP) in the conserved 3′ untranslated region of the cell-derived factor −1 (SDF-1) gene, which encodes an α chemokine ligand of the CXCR4 viral coreceptor, is still unclear, as there are significant geographic and ethnic variations in the frequency distributions of α and β chemokines and chemokine receptor polymorphisms.[69–71]

Defensins are an important family of antimicrobial peptides in people, and they may play a role in protection from HIV infection. In an Italian study, SNP −44G/G of β defensin 1 seemed to protect against MTCT of HIV,[72] and in a Brazilian study where this SNP was rare, SNPs −52A/A and −20G/G were associated with a lower risk of MTCT.[73] Homozygosity for −550G/G, the SNP of mannose-binding protein MBL2, which plays a role in activation of the complement pathway and in phagocytosis, was associated with protection against MTCT of HIV.[74]

Adaptive immune parameters HIV-specific humoral and cellular immune responses may be important in influencing MTCT. Early studies had shown that higher levels of maternal HIV-specific immunoglobulin (Ig)-G did not protect against MTCT.[11] Such studies, however, did not measure neutralizing activity. Neutralizing antibodies in maternal serum have been correlated with protection from perinatal HIV transmission in some studies,[75–77] but not others.[77,78] Perinatally transmitted envelope variants were found to be neutralization-resistant but with relatively few glycosylation sites,[67] indicating that maternal neutralizing antibody imposes a selective pressure on the transmitted virus. Interestingly, a lack of maternal autologous neutralizing antibody has been associated with in utero but not intrapartum infection in some studies,[78,79] indicating that immune protection may differ by the route of infection.

HIV-specific CTL responses have been detected in uninfected, HIV-exposed individuals, including uninfected infants of HIV-infected mothers.[80,81] Their role in viral clearance and prevention of infection is not fully elucidated. HIV-specific immune responses among uninfected infants born to HIV-infected mothers have been detected in several cohorts, and in some of them they were associated with protection against transmission during delivery and breast feeding,[82,83] but the significance of these responses remains generally unclear.[48,84] One study suggested that higher levels of suppressive regulatory T cells were associated with HIV-specific immune responses among exposed uninfected infants.[85] Another study suggested that reduced maternal immune activation was associated with HIV-1 specific cellular immune responses among exposed uninfected children.[86] The authors have found that infants whose HIV PCR becomes positive after the first week of life have lower levels of plasma-soluble L-selectin, and thus immune activation levels,[87] suggesting that higher levels of immune activation in the fetus and newborn promote HIV replication. Thus, higher levels of immune activation may promote HIV transmission from mother to child.[48]

Breast milk contains a multitude of factors with antimicrobial and immunomodulatory properties, both innate and adaptive, that may modulate the risk of MTCT of HIV. Such factors include lactoferrin, lysozyme, epidermal growth factor, interleukins, defensins, chemokines, secretory leukocyte protease inhibitor, specific antibodies, as well as T lymphocytes, NK cells and macrophages that may provide protection to the infant via different mechanisms.[88]

Genetic factors

Strong associations between infant gender and in utero transmission have been reported in several cohorts.[11,89,90] Female infants have a two-fold increased risk of infection at birth when compared with male infants, perhaps because in utero mortality is higher for male HIV-1 infected infants or because the Y antigens, present in male but not female fetuses, activate maternal lymphocytes and either cause release of cytokines with anti-HIV effects or limit maternal HIV-infected lymphocyte survival in male infants.[90]

CCR5 is the coreceptor for R5-type isolates, predominantly transmitted from mother to child.[69] A 32 base pair deletion (Δ32) within the CCR5 coreceptor generates a truncated protein that is not expressed on the cell surface, and Δ32 homozygosity confers resistance to infection by R5-type HIV isolates.[91] Mothers who transmit infection to Δ32 heterozygous infants have a significantly higher viral load than mothers who transmit infection to wild-type homozygous infants.[92]

Antepartum transmission of HIV is unique in that it occurs in a setting where the child shares at least half of his or her major histocompatibility (MHC) genes with the mother, and while the mother tolerates the paternally-derived fetal histocompatibility molecules. Antepartum MTCT is potentially related to HLA class 1 alleles of the MHC because of their role both in determining maternal–infant compatibility and in regulating the CD8 T cell response to virally infected cells that results in either their killing or in the production of factors that interfere with viral replication. In addition, HLA class 1 molecules interact with natural killer cell receptors, a part of the innate immune system. The HLA region includes 128 genes, and has considerable allele variation among individuals. The breadth of HLA diversity is beneficial for the immunologic response.

The fetus or infant of an HIV-positive mother is exposed to both free HIV virions and HIV-infected cells that display maternal MHC. Either fetal or newborn anti-MHC antibodies or alloreactive T cell responses, resulting from HLA discordance, could protect against infection from the mother. A higher risk of transmission has been observed in infants whose class I HLA alleles more closely resembled their mothers', thus possibly limiting the effectiveness of infant immune responses against HIV with a history of immune escape in the mother.[48,78,93] In addition, maternal-infant HLA concordance has been associated with clinical disease progression in HIV–infected infants.[94]

Several studies suggest that HLA discordance and specific maternal HLA polymorphisms (such as B4901, B5301, A2/6802 and B18) are associated with a reduced risk of MTCT, while others are associated with increased such risk.[95–99] Certain polymorphisms in chemokine receptors (CCR5–59356-T)[100] and chemokine ligands (SDF1–3′A)[70] also have been associated with MTCT in African populations. The HLA-G molecule is of particular interest, as it is a nonclassical MHC class 1 molecule highly expressed in the placental trophoblasts at the maternal–fetal interface. HLA-G has several SNPs that have been associated with a decreased risk of perinatal HIV infection.[98] The field of host genomics and associations with susceptibility to HIV infection and with rate of disease progression is rapidly expanding as the means to study the human genome have been revolutionized.

Tissue and mucosal integrity: placenta, infant skin and GI tract, maternal GU tract and breast pathology

Detection of HIV in the placenta does not correlate with infant infection.[101,102] As placental morphology changes during gestation, it is possible that placental cells with different susceptibility to HIV infection may appear at different times, and thus the degree of risk of HIV infection of the placenta may differ throughout gestation. Virus transmission also might occur by passage of cell-free virus through the placental barrier. Maternal infections associated with chorioamnionitis could perturb the integrity of the placental barrier. If the placental membranes of an HIV-infected woman have a bacterial infection, maternal white blood cells infected with HIV could enter the amniotic fluid, resulting in chorioamnionitis. Chorioamnionitis and funisitis have been associated with an increased risk of MTCT.[103,104] A randomized, placebo-controlled trial of antibiotic treatment during pregnancy to prevent chorioamnionitis-associated MTCT of HIV was discontinued after interim analyses suggested no effect, however.[105] Chorioamnionitis also can mediate premature delivery and premature rupture of the membranes, both factors associated with a higher risk of MTCT of HIV.[106] A contributing factor in the case of a premature infant is the immaturity of his or her skin and mucosal membranes, resulting in higher permeability to HIV.

Inflammation of the maternal genital tract mucosa, as occurs in genital ulcer disease, has been shown to increase MTCT of HIV independent of maternal plasma HIV load,[29] and a clinical diagnosis of herpes simplex type 2 infection during pregnancy increased MTCT of HIV in several studies.[19,107,108] Genital lesions increase local inflammation and genital shedding of HIV.[11]

A study showed a marked correlation of maternal vitamin A deficiency with elevated risk of MTCT of HIV in Africa.[109] This observation led to a study investigating vitamin A supplementation to decrease MTCT of HIV. Four such studies have been completed.[110–113] Collectively, these studies showed no benefit of vitamin A supplementation in decreasing MTCT of HIV, with the study from Tanzania showing an increased risk.[112] Other data suggest that deficiencies of other micronutrients (such as selenium) may be associated with increased risk of MTCT, through increased genital shedding of HIV and mastitis.[114,115] A recent study from Tanzania indicated a higher risk of MTCT of HIV, perinatally and through breast feeding, in women with low vitamin D level.[116] Vitamin D has immunomodulatory properties and contributes to the development of the fetal immune system, mechanisms possibly mediating the observed effect.

With regards to breastfeeding transmission of HIV to the infant, integrity of the infant's GI mucosa may be an important factor in determining transmission, and breaches to such integrity when inflammation occurs may facilitate passage of HIV.[22] Similarly, oral candidiasis in the infant has been associated with increased risk of postnatal HIV transmission.[30] Mastitis and elevated sodium-to-potassium ratio in breast milk, thought to be a marker of subclinical mastitis, is associated with higher risk of HIV transmission to the infant, with an increased risk as the mother's plasma HIV load increases.[117]

Obstetric Factors

Although several studies have noted an increased rate of MTCT with preterm delivery, it remains unclear whether preterm delivery is a result or cause of HIV infection.[118–121] Prolonged rupture of the amniotic membranes before delivery can increase MTCT of HIV.[119,122–124] In an analysis of 4271 deliveries with duration of ruptured membranes of 24 hours of less (vaginal deliveries as well as cesarean deliveries after ruptured membranes or onset of labor), the risk of MTCT of HIV increased approximately 2% with an increase of 1 hour in the duration of ruptured membranes.[125] Amniocentesis is linked to increased risk of MTCT, as are use of scalp electrodes, forceps, and vacuum extractors during birth.[126,127]

Elective cesarean section prior to onset of labor and rupture of the amniotic membranes has been shown in clinical trials to decrease risk of MTCT of HIV.[9,34,128,129] Potential mechanisms include avoidance of microtransfusions of maternal blood to the fetus during labor contractions and of direct contact of the fetus's skin and mucosal membranes with infected secretions or blood in the maternal genital canal. An individual patient data meta-analysis incorporating data from 8533 mother–infant pairs showed that the likelihood of MTCT of HIV was approximately 87% lower if a cesarean section was performed before labor and delivery and if antiretroviral therapy was provided antepartum, intrapartum, and postpartum, as compared with other modes of delivery and the absence of such therapy.[125]

THE ROLE OF COINFECTIONS: CYTOMEGALOVIRUS, HUMAN HERPESVIRUS, HEPATITIS B AND C, MALARIA, TUBERCULOSIS

The role of other systemic maternal infections influencing MTCT of HIV is unclear. HIV-infected mothers seem to transmit human herpesvirus (HHV)-6, cytomegalovirus (CMV), and hepatitis B and C to their babies more frequently than uninfected women.[130–132] MTCT of HIV appears to be more frequent among newborns with congenital CMV infection.[133] A study of perinatally HIV-infected infants from Thailand showed that the rates of HHV-6 infection were lower in HIV-infected children, but that HHV-6 coinfection correlated with faster progression of HIV disease.[134]

Malaria infects the placenta and leads to adverse pregnancy outcomes.[135] This is especially true in primigravidae, among whom malaria tends to be more severe.[136,137] Several earlier studies have failed to reveal an interaction between malaria and MTCT of HIV.[135,138] More recent data, however, indicate that malaria increases HIV load, and treatment of malaria reduces HIV load.[139] A few recent studies have suggested an increased risk of MTCT of HIV in pregnant women with malaria,[140–142] while others have not shown a significantly increased risk.[137,143,144] In a study in Western Kenya of women who were dually infected with HIV-1 and malaria, higher parasitemia levels (>10,000 parasites/μL of blood) were associated with an increased risk of MTCT of HIV compared to lower levels of parasitemia.[145] Inconsistencies in study results may be due, at least in part, to the epidemiology of malaria in different settings, which could affect maternal immunity. Another very recent study suggested that maternal tuberculosis was associated with increased odds of MTCT of HIV independent of maternal HIV viral load and CD4 count or of antiretroviral therapy.[146]

CONCLUSIONS AND FUTURE DIRECTIONS

The accumulated evidence so far suggests that the most comprehensive antiretroviral regimens for preventing MTCT of HIV are those initiated early in pregnancy and continued throughout the first weeks of neonatal life and, in a breastfeeding mother, continued during breast feeding.[147,148] Early initiation of antiretroviral prophylaxis during pregnancy is important, as it takes several weeks for optimal HIV suppression. Neonatal prophylaxis is also important, both in the case the mother did not receive optimal prophylaxis during pregnancy, and when she did receive prophylaxis, as it might suppress low-level viremia; it is critical when the baby has to breast feed. Approaches aimed at targeting early steps of viral entry and integration, taking advantage of innate resistance to infection or a vaccine against HIV might provide future advances in preventing MTCT of HIV that would minimize antenatal exposure to multiple antiretroviral agents, the long-term effects of which on child health have yet to be fully identified.

REFERENCES

1. Cooper ER, Charurat M, Mofenson LM, et al. Combination antiretroviral strategies for the treatment of pregnant HIV-infected women and prevention of perinatal HIV-1 transmission. J Acquir Immune Defic Syndr Hum Retrovirol 2002; 29:484–94.
2. Lallemant M, Jourdain G, Le Coeur S, et al. Single-dose perinatal nevirapine plus standard zidovudine to prevent mother-to-child transmission of HIV-1 in Thailand. N Engl J Med 2004;351:217–28.
3. Zhou Z, Meyers K, Li X, et al. Prevention of mother-to-child transmission of HIV-1 using highly active antiretroviral therapy in rural Yunnan, China. J Acquir Immune Defic Syndr 2010;53:S15–22.
4. Kourtis AP, Duerr A. Prevention of perinatal HIV transmission: a review of novel strategies. Expert Opin Investig Drugs 2003;12:1–10.
5. Kourtis AP, Lee FK, Abrams EJ, et al. Mother-to-child transmission of HIV-1: timing and implications for prevention. Lancet Infect Dis 2006;6:726–32.
6. Bryson YY, Luzuriaga K, Sullivan JL, et al. Proposed definitions for in utero versus intrapartum transmission of HIV-1. N Engl J Med 1992;327:1246–7.
7. Kuhn L, Abrams EJ, Chincilla M, et al. New York City Perinatal HIV transmission collaborative study group. Sensitivity of HIV-1 DNA polymerase chain reaction in the neonatal period. AIDS 1996;10:1181–2.

8. Kalish LA, Pitt J, Lews J, et al. Defining the time of fetal or perinatal acquisition of HIV-1 infection on the basis of age at first positive culture. J Infect Dis 1997;175:712–5.
9. The European Mode of Delivery Collaboration. Elective caesarean section versus vaginal delivery in prevention of vertical HIV-1 transmission: a randomized clinical trial. Lancet 1999;353:1035–9.
10. Kourtis AP, Bulterys M, Nesheim SR, et al. Understanding the timing of HIV transmission from mother to infant. JAMA 2001;285:709–12.
11. Lehman DA, Farquhar C. Biological mechanisms of vertical HIV-1 transmission. Rev Med Virol 2007;17:381–403.
12. Papiernick M, Brossard Y, Mulliez N, et al. Thymic abnormalities in fetuses aborted from HIV-1 seropositive women. Pediatrics 1992;89:297–301.
13. Pascual A, Bruna I, Cerrolaza J, et al. Absence of maternal–fetal transmission of HIV-1 to second trimester fetuses. Am J Obstet Gynecol 2000;183:838–42.
14. Brossard Y, Aubin J, Mandelbrot L, et al. Frequency of early in utero HIV-1 infection: a blind DNA polymerase chain reaction study on 100 fetal thymuses. AIDS 1995;9:359–64.
15. Biggar RJ, Cassol S, Kumwenda N, et al. The risk of HIV-1 infection in twin pairs born to infected mothers in Africa. J Infect Dis 2003;188:850–5.
16. Mandelbrot L, Burgard M, Teglas JP, et al. Frequent detection of HIV-1 in the gastric aspirates of neonates born to HIV-infected mothers. AIDS 1999;13:2143–9.
17. Zack JA, Haislip AM, Krogstad P, et al. Incompletely reverse-transcribed HIV-1 genomes in quiescent cells can function as intermediates in the retroviral life cycle. J Virol 1992;66:1717–25.
18. Lee FK, Scinicariello F, Ou CY, et al. Partially reverse transcribed HIV genome in uninfected HIV-exposed infants. Presented at the 11th Conference on Retroviruses and Opportunistic Infections. San Francisco (CA), February 8–12, 2004.
19. Van Rompay KK, Miller MD, Marthas ML, et al. Prophylactic and therapeutic benefits of short-term PMPA administration to newborn macaques following oral inoculation with simian immunodeficiency virus with reduced susceptibility to PMPA. J Virol 2000;74:1767–74.
20. Fawzi W, Msamanga G, Spiegelman D, et al. Transmission of HIV-1 through breastfeeding among women in Dar es Salaam, Tanzania. J Acquir Immune Defic Syndr 2002;31:331–8.
21. Miotti PG, Taha TE, Kumwenda N, et al. HIV transmission during breastfeeding: a study in Malawi. JAMA 1999;282:744–9.
22. Kourtis AP, Butera ST, Ibegbu C, et al. Breast milk and HIV-1: vector of transmission or vehicle of protection? Lancet Infect Dis 2003;3:786–93.
23. Bulterys M, Wilfert CM. HAART during pregnancy and during breastfeeding among HIV-infected women in the developing world: has the time come? AIDS 2009;23:2473–7.
24. Rousseau CM, Nduati RW, Richardson BA, et al. Longitudinal analysis of HIV-1 RNA in breast milk and its relationship to infant infection and maternal disease. J Infect Dis 2003;187:741–7.
25. John G, Nduati R, Mbori-Ngacha D, et al. Correlates of mother to child HIV-1 transmission: association with maternal plasma HIV-1 RNA load, genital HIV-1 DNA shedding, and breast infections. J 63. Infect Dis 2001;182:206–12.
26. Semba RD, Kumwenda N, Hoover DR, et al. HIV-1 load in breast milk, mastitis, and mother to child transmission of HIV-1. J Infect Dis 1999;180:93–8.
27. Willumsen J, Filteau SM, Coutsoudis A, et al. Breastmilk RNA viral load in HIV-1 infected South African women: effects of subclinical mastitis and infant feeding. AIDS 2003;17(3):407–14.

28. Coutsoudis A, Pillay K, Kuhn L, et al. Method of feeding and transmission of HIV-1 from mothers to children by 15 months of age: prospective cohort study from Durban, South Africa. AIDS 2001;15:379–87.
29. The Breastfeeding and HIV International Transmission Study (BHITS) Group. Late postnatal transmission of HIV-1 in breast-fed children: an individual patient data meta-analysis. J Infect Dis 2004;189:2154–66.
30. Embree JE, Njenga D, Datta P, et al. Risk factors for postnatal mother–child transmission of HIV-1. AIDS 2000;14:2535–41.
31. Newell ML, Thorne C. The safety of antiretroviral drugs in pregnancy. Expert Opin Drug Saf 2005;4:323–35.
32. Mofenson LM, McIntyre JA. Advances and research directions in the prevention of mother to child HIV-1 transmission. Lancet 2000;355:2237–44.
33. Mayaux MJ, Dussaix E, Isopet J, et al. Maternal virus load during pregnancy and the mother to child transmission of HIV-1: the French Perinatal Cohort Studies. J Infect Dis 1997;175:172–5.
34. The European Collaborative Study. Maternal viral load and vertical transmission of HIV: an important factor but not the only one. AIDS 1999;13:1377–85.
35. Garcia PM, Kalish LA, Pitt J, et al. Maternal levels of plasma human immunodeficiency virus type 1 RNA and the risk of perinatal HIV transmission. N Engl J Med 1999;341:394–402.
36. Mofenson LM, Lambert JS, Stiehm ER, et al. Risk factors for perinatal transmission in HIV-infected women and infants receiving zidovudine prophylaxis. N Engl J Med 1999;341:385–93.
37. Read JS. Prevention of mother-to-child transmission of HIV. In: Zeichner S, Read J, editors. Textbook of pediatric HIV care. Cambridge (UK): Cambridge University Press; 2005. p. 111–33.
38. Ioannidis JP, Abrams EJ, Ammann A, et al. Perinatal transmission of HIV-1 by pregnant women with RNA viral loads <1000 copies/mL. J Infect Dis 2001; 183:539–45.
39. Sperling RS, Shapiro DE, Coombs RW, et al. Maternal viral load, zidovudine treatment, and the risk of transmission of HIV-1 from mother to infant. Pediatric AIDS Clinical Trials Group Protocol 076 Study Group. N Engl J Med 1996;335:1621–9.
40. Dunn D, Newell ML. Vertical transmission of HIV. Lancet 1992;339:364–5.
41. Bulterys M, Landesman S, Burns DN, et al. Sexual behavior and injection drug use during pregnancy and vertical transmission of HIV-1. J Acquir Immune Defic Syndr Hum Retrovirol 1997;15:76–82.
42. Matheson PB, Thomas PA, Abrams EJ, et al. Heterosexual behavior during pregnancy and perinatal transmission of HIV-1. AIDS 1996;10:1249–56.
43. Msellati P, Meda N, Leroy V, et al. Safety and acceptability of vaginal disinfection with benzalkonium chloride in HIV-infected pregnant women in West Africa: ANRS 049b phase II randomized, double-blinded placebo-controlled trial. Sex Transm Infect 1999;75:420–5.
44. Biggar R, Miotti P, Taha T, et al. Perinatal intervention trial in Africa: effect of a birth canal cleansing intervention to prevent HIV transmission. Lancet 1996; 347:1647–50.
45. Gaillard P, Mwanyumba F, Verhofstede C, et al. Vaginal lavage with chlorhexidine during labor to reduce mother-to-child HIV-1 transmission: clinical trial in Mombasa, Kenya. AIDS 2001;15:389–96.
46. Mandelbrot L, Msellati P, Meda N, et al. 15-month follow-up of African children following vaginal cleansing with benzalconium chloride of their HIV-1 infected mothers during late pregnancy and delivery. Sex Transm Infect 2002;78:267–70.

47. Wilson C, Gray G, Read J, et al. Tolerance and safety of different concentrations of chlorhexidine for peripartum vaginal and infant washes: HIVNET 025. J Acquir Immune Defic Syndr 2004;35:138–43.
48. Walter J, Kuhn L, Aldrovandi GM. Advances in basic science understanding of mother-to-child HIV-1 transmission. Curr Opin HIV AIDS 2008;3:146–50.
49. Kliks S, Cogtag CH, Corliss H, et al. Genetic analysis of viral variants selected in transmission of HIV to newborns. AIDS Res Hum Retroviruses 2000;16:1223–33.
50. Zhang H, Orti G, Du Q, et al. Phylogenetic and phenotypic analysis of HIV type 1 env gp120 in cases of subtype C mother-to-child transmission. AIDS Res Hum Retroviruses 2002;18:1415–23.
51. Renjifo B, Chung M, Gilbert P, et al. In utero transmission of quasispecies among HIV type 1 genotypes. Virology 2003;307:278–82.
52. Scarlatti G, Leitner T, Halapi E, et al. Comparison of variable region 3 sequences of HIV-1 from infected children with the RNA and DNA sequences of the virus population of their mothers. Proc Natl Acad Sci U S A 1993;90:1721–5.
53. Dickover RE, Garratty EM, Plaeger S, et al. Perinatal transmission of major, minor, and multiple maternal human immunodeficiency virus type 1 variants in utero and intrapartum. J Virol 2001;75:2194–203.
54. Wolinsky SM, Wike CM, Korber BT, et al. Selective transmission of HIV-1 variants from mothers to infants. Science 1992;255:1134–7.
55. Ahmad N, Baroudy BM, Baker RC, et al. Genetic analysis of HIV-1 envelope V3 region isolates from mothers and infants after perinatal transmission. J Virol 1995;69:1001–12.
56. Kwiek JJ, Russell ES, Dang KK, et al. The molecular epidemiology of HIV-1 envelope diversity during HIV-1 subtype C vertical transmission in Malawian mother–infant pairs. AIDS 2008;22:863–71.
57. Kourtis AP, Amedee AM, Bulterys M, et al. Various viral compartments in HIV-1-infected mothers contribute to in utero transmission of HIV-1. AIDS Res Hum Retrovir 2010, in press.
58. Montano M, Russell M, Gilbert P, et al. Comparative prediction of perinatal HIV-1 transmission using multiple virus load markers. J Infect Dis 2003;188:406–13.
59. Tuomala RE, O'Driscoll PT, Bremer JW, et al. Cell-associated genital tract virus and vertical transmission of HIV-1 in antiretroviral experienced women. J Infect Dis 2003;187:375–84.
60. Koulinska IN, Villamor E, Chaplin B, et al. Transmission of cell-free and cell-associated HIV-1 through breastfeeding. Virus Res 2006;120:191–8.
61. Eshleman SH, Church JD, Chen S, et al. Comparison of HIV-1 mother-to-child transmission after single-dose nevirapine prophylaxis among African women with subtypes A, C, and D. J Acquir Immune Defic Syndr 2006;42:518–21.
62. Renjifo B, Gilbert P, Chaplin B, et al. Preferential in utero transmission of HIV-1 subtype C as compared to HIV-1 subtype A or D. AIDS 2004;18:1629–36.
63. Yang C, Li M, Newman RD, et al. Genetic diversity of HIV-1 in western Kenya: subtype-specific differences in mother-to-child transmission. AIDS 2003;17:1667–74.
64. Eshleman SH, Becker-Pergola G, Deseyve M, et al. Impact of HIV-1 subtype on women receiving single-dose nevirapine prophylaxis to prevent HIV-1 vertical transmission (HIV network for prevention trials 012 study). J Infect Dis 2001;184:914–7.
65. Derdeyn CA, Hunter E. Viral Characteristics of transmitted HIV. Curr Opin HIV AIDS 2008;3:16–21.

66. Wu X, Parast AB, Richardson BA, et al. Neutralization escape variants of HIV-1 are transmitted from mother to infant. J Virol 2006;80:835–44.
67. Eshleman SH, Lie Y, Hoover DR, et al. Association between the replication capacity and mother-to-child transmission of HIV-1, in antiretroviral drug-naïve Malawian women. J Infect Dis 2006;193:1512–5.
68. DeRossi A. Virus–host interactions in paediatric HIV infection. Curr Opin HIV AIDS 2007;2:399–404.
69. John GC, Rousseau CM, Dong T, et al. Maternal SDF1-3'A polymorphism is associated with increased perinatal HIV-1 transmission. J Virol 2000;74:5736–9.
70. Tresoldi E, Romiti ML, Boniotto M, et al. Prognostic value of the stromal cell-derived factor 1 3'A mutation in pediatric HIV-1 infection. J Infect Dis 2002;185:696–700.
71. Gonzales E, Dhanda R, Bamshand M, et al. Global survey of genetic variation in CCR5, RANTES, and MIP-1alpha: impact of the epidemiology of HIV-1 pandemic. Proc Natl Acad Sci U S A 2001;98:5199–204.
72. Braida L, Boniotto M, Pontillo A, et al. A single nucleotide polymorphism in the human beta-defensin 1 gene is associated with HIV-1 infection in Italian children. AIDS 2004;18:1598–600.
73. Milanese M, Segat L, Pontillo A, et al. DEFB1 gene polymorphisms and increased risk of HIV-1 infection in Brazilian children. AIDS 2006;20:1673–5.
74. Boniotto M, Crovella S, Pirulli D, et al. Polymorphisms in the MBL2 promoter correlated with risk of HIV-1 transmission and AIDS progression. Genes Immun 2000;1:346–8.
75. Kliks SC, Wara DW, Landers DV, et al. Features of HIV-1 that could influence maternal–child transmission. JAMA 1994;272:467–74.
76. Scarlatti G, Albert J, Rossi V, et al. Mother to child transmission of HIV-1: correlation with neutralizing antibodies against primary isolates. J Infect Dis 1993;168:207–10.
77. Tranchat C, Van de Perre P, Simonon-Sorel A, et al. Maternal humoral factors associated with perinatal HIV-1 transmission in a cohort from Kigali, Rwanda, 1988–94. J Infect 1999;39:213–20.
78. Hengel RL, Kennedy MS, Steketee RW, et al. Neutralizing antibody and perinatal transmission of HIV-1. New York City Perinatal HIV Transmission Collaborative Study Group. AIDS Res Hum Retroviruses 1998;14:475–81.
79. Dickover R, Garratty E, Yusim K, et al. Role of maternal autologous neutralizing antibody in selective perinatal transmission of HIV-1 escape variants. J Virol 2006;80:6525–33.
80. DeMaria A, Cirrilo C, Moretta L. Occurrence of HIV-1 specific cytolytic T cell activity in apparently uninfected children born to HIV-1 infected mothers. J Infect Dis 1994;170:1296–9.
81. Rowland-Jones S, Nixon DR, Aldhous MC, et al. HIV-1 specific cytotoxic T cell activity in an HIV-exposed but uninfected infant. Lancet 1993;341:860–1.
82. Clerici M, Sison AV, Berzovsky JA, et al. Cellular immune factors associated with mother-to-infant transmission of HIV. AIDS 1993;7:1427–33.
83. Kuhn L, Coutsoudis A, Moodley D, et al. T-helper cell responses to HIV envelope peptides in cord blood: protection against intrapartum and breastfeeding transmission. AIDS 2001;15:1–9.
84. Farquhar C, John-Stewart G. The role of infant immune responses and genetic factors in preventing HIV-1 acquisition and disease progression. Clin Exp Immunol 2003;134:367–77.

85. Legrand FA, Nixon DF, Loo CP, et al. Strong HIV-1 specific T cell responses in HIV-1 exposed uninfected infants and neonates revealed after regulatory T cell removal. PLoS One 2006;1:e102.

86. Schramm DB, Meddows-Taylor S, Gray GE, et al. Low maternal viral loads and reduced granulocyte–macrophage colony-stimulating factor levels characterize exposed, uninfected infants who develop protective HIV-1 specific responses. Clin Vaccine Immunol 2007;14:348–54.

87. Kourtis AP, Nesheim S, Thea D, et al. Correlation of virus load and soluble L-selectin, a marker of immune activation, in pediatric HIV infection. AIDS 2000;14: 2429–36.

88. Kuhn L. Milk mysteries: why are women who exclusively breastfeed less likely to transmit HIV during breastfeeding? Clin Infect Dis 2010;50:770–2.

89. Taha TE, Nour S, Kumwenda NI, et al. Gender differences in perinatal HIV acquisition among African infants. Pediatrics 2005;115:e167–72.

90. Biggar RJ, Taha TE, Hoover DR, et al. Higher in utero and perinatal HIV infection risk in girls than boys. J Acquir Immune Defic syndr 2006;41:509–13.

91. Liu R, Paxton WA, Choe S, et al. Homozygous defect in HIV-1 coreceptor accounts for resistance of some multiply exposed individuals to HIV-1 infection. Cell 1996;86:367–77.

92. Ometto L, Zanchetta M, Mainardi M, et al. Co-receptor usage of HIV-1 primary isolates, viral burden, and CCR5 genotype in mother-to-child HIV-1 transmission. AIDS 2000;14:1721–9.

93. MacDonald KS, Embree J, Njenga S, et al. Mother–child class I HLA concordance increases perinatal HIV-1 transmission. J Infect Dis 1998;177:551–6.

94. Kuhn L, Abrams EJ, Palumbo P, et al. Maternal versus paternal inheritance of HLA class I alleles among HIV-infected children: consequences for clinical disease progression. AIDS 2004;18:1281–9.

95. MacDonald KS, Embree J, Nagelkerke NJ, et al. The HLA A2/6802 supertype is associated with reduced risk of perinatal HIV-1 transmission. J Infect Dis 2001; 183:503–6.

96. Winchester R, Chen Y, Rose S, et al. Transmission of HIV-1 from an infected woman to her offspring during gestation and delivery was found to be influenced by the infant's major histocompatibility complex class II DRB1 alleles. Proc Natl Acad Sci U S A 1995;92:12371–8.

97. Winchester R, Pitt J, Charurat M, et al. Mother to child transmission of HIV-1: strong association with certain maternal HLA-B alleles independent of viral load implicates innate immune mechanisms. J Acquir Immune Defic Syndr 2004;36:659–70.

98. Aikhionbare FO, Hodge T, Kuhn L, et al. Mother-to-child discordance in HLA-G exon 2 is associated with a reduced risk of perinatal HIV-1 transmission. AIDS 2001;15:2196–8.

99. Farquhar C, Rowland-Jones S, Mbori-Ngacha D, et al. Human leukocyte antigen (HLA) B*18 and protection against mother-to-child HIV type 1 transmission. AIDS Res Hum Retroviruses 2004;20:692–7.

100. Kostrikis LG, Neumann AU, Thompson B, et al. A polymorphism in the regulatory region of the CC-chemokine receptor 5 gene influences perinatal transmission of HIV-1 to African-American infants. J Virol 1999;73:10264–71.

101. Mattern CF, Murray K, Jensen A, et al. Localization of HIV core antigen in term human placentas. Pediatrics 1992;89:207–9.

102. Spector SA. Mother-to-infant transmission of HIV-1: the placenta fights back. J Clin Invest 2001;107:267–9.

103. St Louis M, Kamenga M, Brown C, et al. Risk of perinatal HIV-1 transmission according to maternal immunologic, virologic, and placental factors. J Am Med Assoc 1993;269:2853–9.
104. Wabwire-Mangen F, Gray R, Mmiro F, et al. Placental membrane inflammation and risks of maternal to child transmission of HIV-1 in Uganda. J Acquir Immune Defic Syndr 1992;22:379–85.
105. Taha TE, Brown ER, Hoffman IF, et al. A phase III clinical trial of antibiotics to reduce chorioamnionitis-related perinatal HIV-1 transmission. AIDS 2006;20:1313–21.
106. Taha TE, Gray RH. Genital tract infections and perinatal transmission of HIV. Ann N Y Acad Sci 2000;918:84–98.
107. Chen KT, Segu M, Lumey LH, et al. Genital herpes simplex virus infection and perinatal transmission of HIV. Obstet Gynecol 2005;106:1341–8.
108. Drake AL, John-Stewart GC, Wald A, et al. Herpes simplex virus type 2 and risk of intrapartum HIV transmission. Obstet Gynecol 2007;109:403–9.
109. Semba RD, Miotti P, Chiphangwi J, et al. Maternal vitamin A deficiency and mother-to-child transmission of HIV-1. Lancet 1994;343:1593–7.
110. Kumwenda N, Miotti P, Taha T, et al. Antenatal vitamin A supplementation increases birthweight and decreases anemia, but does not prevent HIV transmission or decrease mortality in infants born to HIV-infected women in Malawi. Clin Infect Dis 2002;35:618–24.
111. Coutsoudis A, Pillay K, Spooner E, et al. Randomized trial testing the effect of vitamin A supplementation on pregnancy outcomes and early mother-to-child transmission in Durban, South Africa. AIDS 1999;13:1517–24.
112. Fawzi W, Msamanga G, Hunter D, et al. Randomized trial of vitamin supplements in relation to transmission of HIV-1 through breastfeeding and early child mortality. AIDS 2002;16:1935–44.
113. Humphrey JH, Iliff PJ, Marinda ET, et al. Effects of a single large dose of vitamin A, given during the postpartum period to HIV-positive women and their infants, on child HIV infection, HIV-free survival, and mortality. J Infect Dis 2006;193:860–71.
114. Baeten J, Mostad S, Hughes M, et al. Selenium deficiency is associated with shedding of HIV-1 infected cells in the female genital tract. J Acquir Immune Defic Syndr 2001;26:360–4.
115. Kupka R, Garland M, Msamanga G, et al. Selenium status, pregnancy outcomes, and mother-to-child transmission of HIV-1. J Acquir Immune Defic Syndr 2005;29:201–10.
116. Mehta S, Hunter DJ, Mugusi FM, et al. Perinatal outcomes, including mother-to-child transmission of HIV, and child mortality and their association with maternal vitamin D status in Tanzania. J Infect Dis 2009;200:1022–30.
117. Lunney KM, Iliff P, Mutasa K, et al. Associations between breast milk viral load, mastitis, exclusive breast-feeding, and postnatal transmission of HIV. Clin Infect Dis 2010;50:762–9.
118. Kuhn L, Steketee RW, Weedon J, et al. Distinct risk factors for intrauterine and intrapartum HIV transmission and consequences for disease progression in infected children. Perinatal AIDS Collaborative Transmission Study. J Infect Dis 1999;179:52–8.
119. Landesman SH, Kalish SA, Burns DN, et al. Obstetrical factors and the transmission of HIV-1 from mother to child. N Engl J Med 1996;334:1617–23.
120. Pitt J, Schluchter M, Jenson H, et al. Maternal and perinatal factors related to maternal–infant transmission of HIV-1 in the P2C2 HIV Study. The role of EBV

shedding Pediatric Pulmonary and Cardiovascular Complications of Vertically Transmitted HIV-1 infection (P2C2 HIV) Study Group. J Acquir Immune Defic Syndr Hum Retrovirol 1998;19:462–70.

121. Simonds RJ, Steketee R, Nesheim S, et al. Impact of zidovudine use on risk and risk factors for perinatal transmission of HIV Perinatal AIDS Collaborative Transmission Studies. AIDS 1998;12:301–8.

122. International Perinatal HIV Group. Duration of ruptured membranes and vertical transmission of HIV-1: a meta-analysis from fifteen prospective cohort studies. AIDS 2001;15:357–68.

123. Mandelbrot L, Mayaux M, Bongain A, et al. Obstetric factors and mother-to-child transmission of HIV-1: the French perinatal cohorts. Am J Obstet Gynecol 1996; 175:661–7.

124. Kuhn L, Abrams E, Matheson P, et al. Timing of maternal–infant HIV transmission: association between intrapartum factors and early polymerase chain reaction results. AIDS 1997;11:429–35.

125. The International Perinatal HIV Group. The mode of delivery and the risk of vertical transmission of HIV-1. N Engl J Med 1999;340:977–87.

126. European Collaborative Study. Risk factors for mother-to-child transmission of HIV-1. Lancet 1992;339:1007–12.

127. Van Dyke RB, Korber BT, Popek E, et al. The Ariel project. A prospective cohort study of maternal–child transmission of HIV-1 in the era of maternal antiretroviral therapy. J Infect Dis 1999;179:319–28.

128. Mandelbrot L, LeChenadec J, Berrebi A, et al. Perinatal HIV-1 transmission: interaction between zidovudine prophylaxis and mode of delivery in the French Perinatal Cohort. JAMA 1998;280:55–60.

129. Kind C, Rudin C, Siegrist CA, et al. Prevention of vertical HIV transmission: additive protective effect of elective cesarean section and zidovudine prophylaxis. AIDS 1998;12:205–10.

130. D'Agaro P, Burgnich P, Comar M, et al. HHV-6 is frequently detected in dried cord blood spots from babies born to HIV-positive mothers. Curr HIV Res 2008;6:441–6.

131. Pembrey L, Newell ML, Tovo PA, et al. The management of HCV-infected pregnant women and their children. J Hepatol 2005;43:515–25.

132. Thio C, Locarnini S. Treatment of HIV/HBV coinfection: clinical and virologic issues. AIDS Rev 2007;9:40–53.

133. Kovaks A, Schluchter M, Easley K, et al. Cytomegalovirus infection and HIV-1 disease progression in infants born to HIV-1 infected women. Pediatric Pulmonary and Cardiovascular Complications of Vertically Transmitted HIV Infection Study Group. N Engl J Med 1999;341:77–84.

134. Kositanont U, Wasi C, Wanprapar N, et al. Primary infection of human herpesvirus 6 in children with vertical infection of HIV-1. J Infect Dis 1999;180:50–5.

135. Taha TE, Canner JK, Dallabetta GA, et al. Childhood malaria parasitaemia and HIV infection in Malawi. Trans R Soc Trop Med Hyg 1994;88:164–5.

136. Steketee RW, Wirima JJ, Bloland PB, et al. Impairment of a pregnant woman's acquired ability to limit *Plasmodium falciparum* by infection with human immunodeficiency virus type 1. Am J Trop Med Hyg 1996;55:42–9.

137. Msamanga GI, Taha TE, Young AM, et al. Placental malaria and mother-to-child transmission of human immunodeficiency virus-1. Am J Trop Med Hyg 2009;80: 508–15.

138. Greenberg AE, Nsa W, Ryder RW, et al. *Plasmodium falciparum* malaria and perinatally acquired HIV-1 infection in Kinshasa, Zaire. N Engl J Med 1991;325:105–9.

139. Hoffman IF, Jere C, Taylor T, et al. The effect of *Plasmodium falciparum* malaria on HIV-1 RNA blood plasma concentration. AIDS 1999;13:487–94.

140. Ayouba A, Badaut C, Kfutwah A, et al. Specific stimulation of HIV-1 replication in human placental trophoblasts by an antigen of *Plasmodium falciparum*. AIDS 2008;30:785–7.

141. Brahmbhatt H, Kigozi G, Wabwire-Mangen F, et al. The effects of placental malaria on mother-to-child HIV transmission in Rakai, Uganda. AIDS 2003;17:2539–41.

142. Brahmbhatt H, Sullivan D, Kigozi G, et al. Association of HIV and malaria with mother-to-child transmission birth outcomes and child mortality. AIDS 2008;47:472–6, 145.

143. Inion I, Mwanyumba F, Gaillard P, et al. Placental malaria and perinatal transmission of human immunodeficiency virus type 1. J Infect Dis 2003;188:1675–8.

144. Mwapasa V, Rogerson SJ, Molyneux ME, et al. The effect of *Plasmodium falciparum* malaria on peripheral and placental HIV-1 RNA concentrations in pregnant Malawian women. AIDS 2004;18:1051–9.

145. Ayisi JG, van Eijk AM, Newman RD, et al. Maternal malaria and perinatal HIV transmission, western Kenya. Emerg Infect Dis 2004;10:643–52.

146. Gupta A, Gupte N, Patil S, et al. Maternal TB is associated with increased risk of HIV mother-to-child transmission. Presented at the 17th Conference for Retroviruses and Opportunistic Infections 2010. San Francisco (CA), February 16–19, 2010.

147. Public Health Service Task Force. Recommendations for use of antiretroviral drugs in pregnant HIV-infected women for maternal health and interventions to reduce perinatal HIV transmission in the United States. Available at: http://aidsinfo.nih.gov/ContentFiles/PerinatalGL.pdf. Accessed May 2, 2010.

148. Bulterys M, Fowler MG. Prevention of HIV infection in children. Pediatr Clin North Am 2000;47:241–60.

Viral Sequence Analysis from HIV-Infected Mothers and Infants: Molecular Evolution, Diversity, and Risk Factors for Mother-To-Child Transmission

Philip L. Bulterys, BSc[a,b], Sudeb C. Dalai, MSc[c,d],
David A. Katzenstein, MD[c],*

KEYWORDS

- HIV • Mother-to-child transmission • Sequence
- Molecular evolution • Diversity • Risk factor

In most wealthy or industrialized countries, the frequency of mother-to-child transmission (MTCT) of HIV type 1 (HIV-1) has been reduced to less than 2% as a result of prevention strategies, including access to highly active antiretroviral therapy (HAART), replacement of breastfeeding, elective cesarean section, or a combination thereof.[1] In many resource-limited countries with high levels of endemic infection, however, transmission of HIV-1 from mother to child is recognized as a leading cause of infant and child mortality, where in the absence of antiretroviral treatment (ART) and prophylaxis, more than 25% of infants born to HIV-positive women become infected with HIV.[2,3]

SCD is supported by the Howard Hughes Medical Institute, the California HIV Research Program, and the Paul and Daisy Soros Fellowship for New Americans. PLB is supported by the UCLA-Caltech Medical Scientist Training Program.

[a] Department of Biology, Stanford University, 371 Serra Mall, Stanford, CA 94305-4200, USA
[b] Medical Scientist Training Program, David Geffen School of Medicine, University of California Los Angeles, 10833 Le Conte Avenue, Los Angeles, CA 90095, USA
[c] Division of Infectious Disease, Stanford University Medical Center, Stanford University School of Medicine, S-141 Grant Building, 300 Pasteur Drive, Stanford, CA 94305, USA
[d] Division of Epidemiology, University of California-Berkeley, School of Public Health, 101 Haviland Hall, Berkeley, CA 94720-7358, USA
* Corresponding author.
E-mail address: davidkk@stanford.edu

Clin Perinatol 37 (2010) 739–750
doi:10.1016/j.clp.2010.08.003
0095-5108/10/$ – see front matter © 2010 Elsevier Inc. All rights reserved.

MTCT may be influenced by several maternal characteristics, including high plasma viral load, low CD4+ T-lymphocyte count, other cervicovaginal infections at delivery, and concentration of virus in breast milk.[4–6] In settings where prolonged breastfeeding is practiced, infection rates may rise to nearly 40%. Social/behavioral risk factors for MTCT include lack of access to prevention of MTCT services and high-risk sexual behavior or injection drug use during the second and third trimesters of pregnancy.[7]

Consensus conventions adopted to classify the presumed timing of transmission distinguish between in utero, intrapartum/early postpartum, and late postpartum acquisition of infant infection. Infants are classified as having acquired in utero infection on the basis of polymerase chain reaction (PCR) detection of HIV-1 RNA or DNA from samples obtained within 72 hours of birth. Infants negative by PCR at birth but in whom infection is detectable by 2 to 6 weeks are regarded as cases of intrapartum or early postpartum transmission. In these infants, transmission of virus is thought to have occurred during late gestation, labor, or delivery, potentially through oral and mucosal exposure to maternal virus in blood, cervical secretions, or colostrum via early breastfeeding. Infants with undetectable infection by screening assays within 6 to 8 weeks of birth who later acquire infection are deemed to have late postpartum infection presumed to be transmitted through breastfeeding.[8,9]

Whether or not cell-associated provirus or viral RNA from blood, cervical secretions, or breast milk is the primary source of infection in each of these settings is not well understood. The early observation that the first-born twin of an HIV-infected mother is more likely to acquire infection than the subsequently born twin supported the idea that trauma and contact with maternal blood and secretions is important in MTCT,[10] although a more recent study did not corroborate this finding.[11] When maternal ART is initiated in the second trimester at 24 to 28 weeks, less than 2% of infants acquire HIV infection, suggesting that early infection in utero occurs less frequently than infection in later stages.[12] The most striking reductions in MTCT are seen when HIV RNA is suppressed by ART and postpartum prophylaxis is given to the newborn. Without ART, there is more than a twofold increase in transmission for every log increase in maternal virus load.[13] Transmission from mothers with fewer than 1000 copies/mL of plasma HIV RNA is unusual.[14] Similarly, there is an independent association of higher maternal CD4 cell numbers with reduced transmission, suggesting that the maternal immune response plays a role in limiting MTCT.[15]

It is hypothesized that infant infection acquired at different stages may result from distinct modes of viral transmission associated with unique virus subpopulations, or quasispecies, derived from the diversity of viruses present during chronic infection in the mother. The extent to which viral genetic and evolutionary characteristics influence the risk of MTCT of HIV remains unclear. Investigation of the genetic composition and evolution of HIV in the context of MTCT may elucidate viral risk factors for transmission, infection, and disease progression. As HIV sequence data become more widely available, analysis of these data will provide a more complete understanding of the factors influencing MTCT and enable development of additional prevention strategies.

SELECTION AND BOTTLENECKS IN MTCT OF HIV

Cases of MTCT represent an opportunity to identify the virologic characteristics associated with transmission. Some studies have investigated specific characteristics of viral genes, whereas others have analyzed the diversity of HIV-1 quasispecies, comparing the range of virus diversity in maternal samples to those obtained from the infant. These studies suggest that infection in infants is usually initiated by a single or limited number of maternal viruses, indicating the presence of a bottleneck in vertical HIV transmission.[16] Such a bottleneck may provide an opportunity for intervention strategies in MTCT and transmission in general.

The extensive diversity of viruses present in prolonged HIV-1 infection within individuals, including pregnant women, is the result of continuing viral expansion, selection, and evolution in the face of immune and/or drug pressures. In chronic infection, up to 10^{12} new virions are produced each day in an infected individual,[17] with a high rate of evolutionary change driven primarily by the poor fidelity of both reverse transcriptase and RNA polymerase. The rate of erroneous nucleotide substitution during reverse transcription is approximately one nucleotide per 10^5 base pairs.[18] This is accompanied by the absence of missense correction mechanisms in the reverse transcription and synthesis of the viral genome.

The viral diversity generated by mutation, nucleotide substitution and point mutation, insertion/deletions, and duplication is acted on by selective pressure from the host humoral and cellular immune systems, and, when present, antiretroviral drug therapy. In addition, the phenomenon of strand switching, in which the viral reverse transcriptase switches within or between viral RNA template strands in synthesizing a DNA transcript, enables frequent recombination events. A robust host immune response exerts a strong selective force on the viral population, and patients with longer asymptomatic phases typically show evidence of greater positive selection,[19,20] defined by a per-site rate of nonsynonymous mutation (d_N) exceeding that of synonymous mutation (d_S).[19,21,22] Vertical HIV transmission events are shaped by extensive diversity in maternal virus, genetic bottlenecks in MTCT, and potential founder effects in infected infants, resulting in a relatively homogeneous viral population in early infant infection, although the extent of diversity may vary by mode of transmission.[16,23] MTCT may result in the transmission of a minor subset of maternal viruses with subsequently limited viral diversity in infant viral sequences compared with the maternal sequences.[24–26] In some settings, there is evidence that infection in utero may involve transmission of a greater diversity of maternal viral variants compared with transmission at delivery.[24,27]

The associations between the strength of positive selection, progression of maternal disease, and HIV transmission are not well defined. Many small studies suggest that viral variants transmitted from mother to child are derived from a minority virus population which has effectively escaped the maternal immune response.[24,26,28–32] Transmitted viruses may also originate from the major maternal variant in compartments, including blood, placenta, or cervical secretions in the birth canal. Differences between maternal and infant immunogenetics, in particular, HLA specificity in the recognition of cytotoxic T-lymphocyte epitopes by maternal and infant immune responses, likely play a role in selection. Additionally, some transmitted viruses may have a replication advantage in infants and may, therefore, be naturally selected.[33] Alternatively, success of a particular variant may result from stochastic effects unrelated to selection.[34] In a phylogenetic analysis of maternal and infant C2V3 envelope sequences, Ceballos and colleagues[34] found that during early pregnancy a single minor viral variant was transmitted to the infant followed by subsequent evolution, suggesting either a selection process or a stochastic event, whereas in later maternal infection (during the final trimester or via breast feeding), maternal and infant sequences were intermingled, suggesting repeated transmission of multiple viral variants. This analysis did not detect positive selection ($d_N/d_S > 1$) in the maternal and infant sequences, suggesting that stochastic effects accounted for the viral quasispecies that were successfully transmitted.

ROLE OF VIRAL RECOMBINATION AND DIVERSITY IN MTCT OF HIV

HIV has an estimated recombination rate of three events per genome per replication, one of the highest rates of all organisms.[35] Recombination occurs as a result of host cell coinfection by distinct viruses.[36-38] Inter- and intrasubtype recombinations are major driving forces of HIV genetic diversity[39,40] and have resulted in a wide distribution of circulating recombinant forms, which contribute significantly to the global pandemic (accounting for >25% of infections in some areas).[39,41-43] Recombination events allow viruses to escape immune pressure, avoid accumulation of deleterious mutations, or jump between adaptive peaks.[44-47] Recombinant viruses may also have fitness and/or transmission advantages, potentially enhancing observed rates of MTCT.[48] Quan and colleagues[49] reported that defective HIV provirus with a lethal mutation in env can be rescued by superinfection with either a wild-type virion or a second replication-defective virus with a lethally mutated capsid protein. These findings suggest that noninfectious HIV-1 variants may constitute a large proportion of in vivo HIV populations (9 out of 10 clones isolated from infected brain, for example) and that the rescue of such defective variants may be attributable to recombination events.[50]

Within geographic settings where multiple HIV subtypes circulate and recombine, subtype-specific differences have been observed in timing and rate of transmission. It has been suggested that geographic differences in rates of MTCT may be related to the genetic diversity of HIV in different settings.[51,52] HIV-1 subtypes and recombinant forms may have functional and phenotypic differences, including chemokine coreceptor usage, replication efficiency, and viral load, that may lead to differences in rates of vertical transmission.[53-62] Studies examining the rate of MTCT by maternal subtype or recombinant infection have yielded discrepant findings. Pádua and colleagues[52] were unable to detect specific genetic forms in env or nef sequences associated with MTCT or a significant difference in RNA viral load by viral subtype but found a greater diversity of genetic forms among nontransmitting mothers. The latter suggests that increased maternal immune pressure may limit transmission. Renjifo and colleagues[62] found that MTCT was more common among Tanzanian mothers infected with viruses that included a subtype C envelope, compared with viruses with subtype A or D (or A/D recombinant) envelope. In Kenya, Yang and colleagues[63] found MTCT more common among mothers infected with subtype D or A/D recombinant viruses compared with subtype A. In a separate study based on the C2-C5 envelope and 5'long terminal repeat regions, Koulinska and colleagues[6] found that some intersubtype recombinant viruses are preferentially transmitted during breastfeeding.

Whether and how recombinant viruses have a transmission advantage in MTCT warrants further investigation, particularly with the increasing prevalence of circulating recombinant forms of HIV-1. Studies interpreting the effect of viral genotype on the risk of MTCT may be enhanced by increased sample sizes, measurement of and adjustment for confounding variables, and improved detection of recombinants on a population level.[6,60-65] Paradoxically, the success of ART and prevention limits the potential of MTCT studies as infant infection becomes less frequent in study populations.

PHYLOGENETICS AND COMPARTMENTALIZATION IN MTCT OF HIV

Phylogenetic analyses of HIV genetic sequences provide insight into the genetic relatedness of multiple virus variants within or between individuals and across populations. These analyses can uncover trends within an epidemic and also provide insight into the origins, timing, and demographic history of transmitted viruses.[66–68] Phylogenetic comparisons of infant and maternal sequences from various compartments are crucial to understanding the viral evolution in these tissues and their respective contributions to the risk of MTCT.

Compartmentalization of HIV infection involves the formation of distinct genetic populations in specific organs, cells, or tissues. Compartments of special importance to MTCT are the maternal genital tract, placenta, and breast milk. Multiple studies have shown that HIV variants from the genital tract appear distinct from the blood,[69–81] although HIV-1 viral load is typically lower in these compartments compared with plasma.[82–84] Localized inflammation, coinfections, physical and cellular barriers, incomplete penetration of antiretroviral drugs into the genital tract, or local immune responses may account for independent and divergent evolution within the maternal genital tract compared with plasma.[70–72,85,86]

Bull and colleagues[83] analyzed HIV-1 RNA and cell-associated HIV-1 DNA (*env*) from the blood and genital tract of women with chronic HIV-infection and reported low diversity of genital tract–specific phylogenetic clades, particularly from the cervix, consistent with bursts of viral replication or the proliferation of infected cells in compartments. The absence of tissue-specific genetic features and the phylogenetic overlap of genital tract HIV clades with those from the blood suggest, however, that HIV-1 flow is not restricted between the genital tract and blood and that viral evolution may not occur independently within the two compartments.[83]

HIV compartmentalization between blood and breast milk is also not well understood. Breast milk transmission is a major source of pediatric HIV infection,[87,88] yet the few studies of viral compartmentalization in breast milk provide contradictory results.[89–92] In the absence of antiretroviral therapy, HIV-1 viral load is 10- to 100-fold lower in breast milk than in plasma.[82] Whether or not this indicates limited exchange of virus between the two compartments or is instead a consequence of differential immune selection remains unclear. Immunologic elements, such as HIV-specific T-cells, antibodies, cytokines, and chemokines, seem highly compartmentalized in breast milk.[93–95] For example, Becquart and colleagues[96] detected compartmentalization of the humoral IgG response to HIV in the mammary gland. Despite these seemingly unique immunologic environments, Heath and colleagues[97] recently examined the compartmentalization of HIV-1 between breast milk and blood in envelope sequences from 13 breastfeeding women and uncovered substantial genetic overlap. Specifically, genetic compartmentalization in breast milk was only detected in one of six subjects with contemporaneously collected samples available. The investigators suggest that virologic selection in breast milk does not account for the genetic bottleneck associated with MTCT.[97] Further studies will clarify the extent to which potential tissue-specific virologic divergence may influence the risk of transmission or the characteristics of the transmitted variant.

IMPLICATIONS FOR DRUG RESISTANCE AND VACCINE DESIGN IN MTCT OF HIV

The ability of HIV to accumulate and exchange drug resistance via single-nucleotide mutations and recombination presents a clinical dilemma in the use of ART, in particular single-dose nevirapine, to prevent MTCT. Once drug resistance has been selected, it may persist in circulating viral RNA and within latent reservoirs of proviral DNA.[47] The persistence of maternal drug resistance mutations after drug exposure during pregnancy presents significant challenges to the design of optimal antiretroviral regimens that prevent MTCT without compromising the efficacy of HAART for mothers.[98] Short-course peripartum regimens in resource-poor settings, including maternal single-dose nevirapine and short-course zidovudine, significantly reduce MTCT (37%–50% compared with no intervention).[99–105] Up to two-thirds of mothers treated with these regimens, however, develop viral resistance to non-nucleoside reverse transcriptase inhibitor drugs.[106] Universal HAART, already a mainstay of maternal HIV treatment in developed or resource-rich countries, could mitigate some of the burden of drug resistance associated with peripartum regimens and has been recommended for pregnant and breastfeeding mothers in resource-poor settings.[98]

Consideration of HIV molecular evolution and diversity is also important in the design of HIV vaccine strategies.[22] There is compelling rationale to develop a preventive HIV vaccine for use in infants to prevent vertical transmission via breast milk and provide a foundation for lifelong immunity.[107] Several recent advances including the partial protection imparted by the ALVAC-AIDSVAX vaccine in Thailand,[108] identification of a novel HIV-1 vaccine target expressed on envelope protein,[109] and vaccine-induced control of simian immunodeficiency virus in rhesus monkeys,[110] have given momentum to renewed efforts to develop an HIV vaccine. The genetic bottlenecks observed in MTCT provide a model for selective transmission, which may inform the design of vaccines, the identification of target antigens, and, potentially, the inclusion of infants and pregnant women in preventive vaccine trials.

CONCLUSIONS AND FUTURE DIRECTIONS

Great progress has been made in understanding the evolution of HIV and the factors influencing the risk of MTCT. Translation of these scientific advances, primarily in the use of antiretroviral drugs to prevent MTCT of HIV, has led to successful interventions and significant reductions in infant infection where preventive strategies have been made widely available. Many questions regarding the impact of molecular evolution and extensive genetic diversity of HIV on MTCT remain unanswered, however. Studies of viral characteristics that contribute to the risk of vertical transmission may inform drug and vaccine prevention efforts. Further research to identify the selective factors governing which variants are transmitted, how the compartmentalization of HIV in different cells and tissues contributes to transmission, and the influence of viral diversity and recombination on the risk of MTCT may provide insight into new therapeutic and preventive strategies.

ACKNOWLEDGMENTS

The authors would like to thank Athena Kourtis, Marc Bulterys, and Keyan Salari for their helpful comments and critical reading of the manuscript. PLB would like to thank Dmitri Petrov and members of the Petrov molecular evolution laboratory at the Stanford Department of Biology for helpful discussion, guidance, and insight.

REFERENCES

1. Newell ML, Coovadia H, Cortina-Borja M, et al. Mortality of infected and uninfected infants born to HIV-infected mothers in Africa: a pooled analysis. Lancet 2004;364:1236–43.
2. Mofenson LM. Prevention in neglected subpopulations: prevention of mother-to-child transmission of HIV infection. Clin Infect Dis 2010;50:130–48.
3. Bulterys M, Wilfert CM. HAART during pregnancy and during breast feeding among HIV-infected women in the developing world: has the time come? AIDS 2009;23:2473–7.

4. Garcia PM, Kalish LA, Pitt J, et al. Maternal levels of plasma human immunodeficiency virus type 1 RNA and the risk of perinatal transmission. Women and Infants Transmission Study Group. N Engl J Med 1999;341:394–402.
5. Mofenson LM, Lambert JS, Stiehm ER, et al. Risk factors for perinatal transmission of human immunodeficiency virus type 1 in women treated with zidovudine. Pediatric AIDS Clinical Trials Group Study 185 Team. N Engl J Med 1999;341:385–93.
6. Koulinska IN, Villamor E, Msamanga G, et al. Risk of HIV-1 transmission by breastfeeding among mothers infected with recombinant and non-recombinant HIV-1 genotypes. Virus Res 2006;120:191–8.
7. Bulterys M, Landesman S, Burns D, et al. Sexual behavior and injection drug use during pregnancy and vertical transmission of HIV-1. J Acquir Immune Defic Syndr Hum Retrovirol 1997;15:76–82.
8. Kourtis AP, Bulterys M, Nesheim S, et al. Understanding the timing of HIV transmission from mother to infant. JAMA 2001;285:709–12.
9. Kourtis AP, Lee FK, Jamieson DJ, et al. Mother-to-child transmission of HIV-1: timing and implications for prevention. Lancet Infect Dis 2006;6:726–32.
10. Goedert JJ, Duliege AM, Amos CI, et al. High risk of HIV-1 infection for first-born twins. The International Registry of HIV-Exposed Twins. Lancet 1991;338:1471–5.
11. Biggar RJ, Cassol S, Kumwenda N, et al. The risk of human immunodeficiency virus–1 infection in twin pairs born to infected mothers in Africa. J Infect Dis 2003;188:850–5.
12. Connor EM, Sperling RS, Gelber R, et al. Reduction of maternal-infant transmission of human immunodeficiency virus type-1 with zidovudine treatment. N Engl J Med 1994;331:1173–80.
13. Guevara H, Casseb J, Zijenah LS, et al. Maternal HIV-1 antibody and vertical transmission in subtype C virus infection. J Acquir Immune Defic Syndr 2002;29:435–40.
14. Ioannidis J, Abrams E, Ammann A, et al. Perinatal transmission of human immunodeficiency virus type 1 by pregnant women with RNA virus loads <1000 copies/mL. J Infect Dis 2001;183:539–45.
15. Leroy V, Karon JM, Alioum A, et al. Twenty-four month efficacy of a maternal short-course zidovudine regimen to prevent mother-to-child transmission of HIV-1 in West Africa. AIDS 2002;16:631–41.
16. Delwart E, Magierowska M, Royz M, et al. Homogeneous quasispecies in 16 out of 17 individuals during very early HIV-1 primary infection. AIDS 2002;16:189–95.
17. Perelson AS, Neumann A, Markowitz M, et al. HIV-1 dynamics in vivo: virion clearance rate, infected cell life span, and viral generation time. Science 1996;271:1582–6.
18. Temin HM. Retrovirus variation and reverse transcription: abnormal strand transfers result in retrovirus genetic variation. Proc Natl Acad Sci U S A 1993;90:6900–3.
19. Ross HA, Rodrigo AG. Immune-mediated positive selection drives human immunodeficiency virus type 1 molecular variation and predicts disease duration. J Virol 2002;76:11715–20.
20. Williamson S. Adaptation in the env gene of HIV-1 and evolutionary theories of disease progression. Mol Biol Evol 2003;20:1318–25.
21. Bonhoeffer S, Holmes EC, Nowak MA. Causes of HIV diversity. Nature 1995;376:125.

22. Rambaut A, Posada D, Crandall KA, et al. The causes and consequences of HIV evolution. Nat Rev Genet 2004;5:52–61.
23. Zhu T, Mo H, Wang N, et al. Genotypic and phenotypic characterization of HIV-1 in patients with primary infection. Science 1993;261:1179–81.
24. Dickover RE, Garratty EM, Plaeger S, et al. Perinatal transmission of major, minor, and multiple maternal human immunodeficiency virus type 1 variants in utero and intrapartum. J Virol 2001;75:2194–203.
25. Wolinsky SM, Wike CM, Korber BT, et al. Selective transmission of human immunodeficiency virus type-1 variants from mothers to infants. Science 1992;255: 1134–7.
26. Ahmad N, Baroudy BM, Baker RC, et al. Genetic analysis of human immunodeficiency virus type 1 envelope V3 region isolates from mothers and infants after perinatal transmission. J Virol 1995;69:1001–12.
27. Renjifo B, Chung M, Gilbert P, et al. In-utero transmission of quasispecies among human immunodeficiency virus type 1 genotypes. Virology 2003;307:278–82.
28. Blish CA, Blay WM, Haigwood NL, et al. Transmission of HIV-1 in the face of neutralizing antibodies. Curr HIV Res 2007;5:578–87.
29. Kampinga GA, Simonon A, Van de Perre P, et al. Primary infections with HIV-1 of women and their offspring in Rwanda: findings of heterogeneity at seroconversion, coinfection, and recombinants of HIV-1 subtypes A and C. Virology 1997; 227:63–76.
30. Kliks S, Contag CH, Corliss H, et al. Genetic analysis of viral variants selected in transmission of human immunodeficiency viruses to newborns. AIDS Res Hum Retroviruses 2000;16:1223–33.
31. Verhofstede C, Demecheleer E, De Cabooter N, et al. Diversity of the human immunodeficiency virus type 1 (HIV-1) env sequence after vertical transmission in mother-child pairs infected with HIV-1 subtype A. J Virol 2003;77:3050–7.
32. Wu X, Parast AB, Richardson BA, et al. Neutralization escape variants of human immunodeficiency virus type 1 are transmitted from mother to infant. J Virol 2006;80:835–44.
33. Kuhn L, Abrams E, Palumbo P, et al. Maternal versus paternal inheritance of HLA class I alleles among HIV-infected children: consequences for clinical disease progression. AIDS 2004;18:1281–9.
34. Ceballos A, Andreani G, Ripamonti C, et al. Lack of viral selection in human immunodeficiency virus type 1 mother-to-child transmission with primary infection during late pregnancy and/or breastfeeding. J Gen Virol 2008;89:2773–82.
35. Zhuang J, Jetzt AE, Sun G, et al. Human immunodeficiency virus type 1 recombination: rate, fidelity, and putative hot spots. J Virol 2002;76:11273–82.
36. Jung A, Maier R, Vartanian JP, et al. Multiply infected spleen cells in HIV patients. Nature 2002;418:144.
37. Jost S, Bernard MC, Kaiser L, et al. A patient with HIV-1 superinfection. N Engl J Med 2002;347:731–6.
38. Koelsch KK, Smith DM, Little SJ, et al. Clade B HIV-1 superinfection with wild-type virus after primary infection with drug-resistant clade B virus. AIDS 2003;17:11–6.
39. Crandall KA, Templeton AR. The evolution of HIV . Baltimore (MD): The Johns Hopkins University Press; 1999. p. 153–76.
40. McVean G, Awadalla P, Fearnhead P. A coalescent-based method for detecting and estimating recombination from gene sequences. Genetics 2002;160: 1231–41.
41. Robertson DL, Sharp PM, McCutchan FE, et al. Recombination in HIV-1. Nature 1995;374:124–6.

42. Pandrea I, Robertson DL, Onanga R, et al. Analysis of partial pol and env sequences indicates a high prevalence of HIV type 1 recombinant strains circulating in Gabon. AIDS Res Hum Retroviruses 2002;18:1103–16.
43. Essex M, M'Boup S. Regional variation in the African epidemics. AIDS in Africa. 2nd edition. New York: Kluwer Academic/Plenum Publishers; 2002.
44. Liu SL, Mittler JE, Nickle DC, et al. Selection for human immunodeficiency virus type 1 recombinants in a patient with rapid progression to AIDS. J Virol 2002;76: 10674–84.
45. Nájera R, Delgado E, Pérez-Alvarez L, et al. Genetic recombination and its role in the development of the HIV-1 pandemic. AIDS 2002;16:3–16.
46. Kellam P, Larder BA. Retroviral recombination can lead to linkage of reverse transcriptase mutations that confer increased zidovudine resistance. J Virol 1995;69:669–74.
47. Morris A, Marsden M, Halcrow K, et al. Mosaic structure of the human immunodeficiency virus type 1 genome infecting lymphoid cells and the brain: evidence for frequent in vivo recombination events in the evolution of regional populations. J Virol 1999;73:8720–31.
48. Koulinska IN, Villamor E, Chaplin B, et al. Transmission of cell-free and cell-associated HIV-1 through breast-feeding. J Acquir Immune Defic Syndr 2006;41: 93–9.
49. Quan Y, Liang C, Brenner B, et al. Multidrug-resistant variants of HIV type 1 (HIV-1) can exist in cells as defective quasispecies and be rescued by superinfection with other defective HIV-1 variants. J Infect Dis 2009;9:1479–83.
50. Li Y, Kappes JC, Conway JA, et al. Molecular characterization of human immunodeficiency virus type 1 cloned directly from uncultured human brain tissue: identification of replication-competent and-defective viral genomes. J Virol 1991;65:3973–85.
51. Odaibo GN, Olaleye DO, Heyndrickx L, et al. Mother-to-child transmission of different HIV-1 subtypes among ARV naïve infected pregnant women in Nigeria. Rev Inst Med Trop Sao Paulo 2006;48:77–80.
52. Pádua E, Parreira R, Tendeiro R, et al. Potential impact of viral load and genetic makeup of HIV type 1 on mother-to-child transmission: characterization of env-C2V3C3 and nef sequences. AIDS Res Hum Retroviruses 2009;25:1171–7.
53. Bjorndal A, Sonnerborg A, Tscherning C, et al. Phenotypic characteristics of human immunodeficiency virus type 1 subtype C isolates of Ethiopian AIDS patients. AIDS 1999;15:647–53.
54. Hu DJ, Vanichseni S, Mastro TD, et al. Viral load differences in early infection with two HIV-1 subtypes. AIDS 2001;15:683–91.
55. Jeeninga RE, Hoogenkamp M, Armand-Ugon M, et al. Functional differences between the long terminal repeat transcriptional promoters of human immunodeficiency virus type 1 subtypes A through G. J Virol 2000;74:3740–51.
56. Kaleebu P, French N, Mahe C, et al. Effect of human immunodeficiency virus (HIV) type 1 envelope subtypes A and D on disease progression in a large cohort of HIV-1-positive persons in Uganda. J Infect Dis 2002;185:1244–50.
57. Kanki PJ, Hamel DJ, Sankale JL, et al. Human immunodeficiency virus type 1 subtypes differ in disease progression. J Infect Dis 1999;179:68–73.
58. Neilson JR, John GC, Carr JK, et al. Subtypes of human immunodeficiency virus type 1 and disease stage among women in Nairobi, Kenya. J Virol 1999;73: 4393–403.
59. Tscherning C, Alaeus A, Fredriksson R, et al. Differences in chemokine coreceptor usage between genetic subtypes of HIV-1. Virology 1998;241:181–8.

60. Blackard JT, Renjifo B, Chaplin B, et al. Diversity of the HIV-1 long terminal repeat following mother-to-child transmission. Virology 2000;274:402–11.

61. Renjifo B, Fawzi W, Mwakagile D, et al. Differences in perinatal transmission among human immunodeficiency virus type 1 genotypes. J Hum Virol 2001;4: 16–25.

62. Renjifo B, Gilbert P, Chaplin B, et al. Preferential in utero transmission of HIV-1 subtype C compared to subtype A or D. AIDS 2004;18:1629–36.

63. Yang C, Li M, Newman RD, et al. Genetic diversity of HIV-1 in western Kenya: subtype-specific differences in mother-to-child transmission. AIDS 2003;11: 1667–74.

64. Murray MC, Embree JE, Ramdahin SG, et al. Effect of human immunodeficiency virus (HIV) type 1 viral genotype on mother-to-child transmission of HIV-1. J Infect Dis 2000;181:746–9.

65. Tapia N, Franco S, Puig-Basagoiti F, et al. Influence of human immunodeficiency virus type 1 subtype on mother-to-child transmission. J Gen Virol 2003;84:607–13.

66. Dalai SC, de Oliveira T, Gordon W, et al. Evolution and molecular epidemiology of subtype C HIV-1 in Zimbabwe. AIDS 2009;23:2523–32.

67. Worobey M, Gemmel M, Teuwen DE, et al. Direct evidence of extensive diversity of HIV-1 in Kinshasa by 1960. Nature 2008;455:661–4.

68. Salemi M, de Oliveira T, Ciccozzi M, et al. High-resolution molecular epidemiology and evolutionary history of HIV-1 subtypes in Albania. PLoS One 2008;3: e1390.

69. Poss M, Martin HL, Kreiss JK, et al. Diversity in virus populations from genital secretions and peripheral blood from women recently infected with human immunodeficiency virus type 1. J Virol 1995;69:8118–22.

70. Poss M, Rodrigo AG, Gosink JJ, et al. Evolution of envelope sequences from the genital tract and peripheral blood of women infected with clade A human immunodeficiency virus type 1. J Virol 1998;72:8240–51.

71. Kovacs A, Wasserman SS, Burns D, et al. Determinants of HIV-1 shedding in the genital tract of women. Lancet 2001;358:1593–601.

72. Wright TC Jr, Subbarao S, Ellerbrock TV, et al. Human immunodeficiency virus 1 expression in the female genital tract in association with cervical inflammation and ulceration. Am J Obstet Gynecol 2001;184:279–85.

73. Ellerbrock TV, Lennox JL, Clancy KA, et al. Cellular replication of human immunodeficiency virus type 1 occurs in vaginal secretions. J Infect Dis 2001;184: 28–36.

74. Kemal KS, Foley B, Burger H, et al. HIV-1 in genital tract and plasma of women: compartmentalization of viral sequences, coreceptor usage, and glycosylation. Proc Natl Acad Sci U S A 2003;100:12972–7.

75. De Pasquale MP, Leigh Brown AJ, Uvin SC, et al. Differences in HIV-1 pol sequences from female genital tract and blood during antiretroviral therapy. J Acquir Immune Defic Syndr 2003;34:37–44.

76. Adal M, Ayele W, Wolday D, et al. Evidence of genetic variability of human immunodeficiency virus type 1 in plasma and cervicovaginal lavage in ethiopian women seeking care for sexually transmitted infections. AIDS Res Hum Retroviruses 2005;21:649–53.

77. Tirado G, Jove G, Reyes E, et al. Differential evolution of cell-associated virus in blood and genital tract of HIV-infected females undergoing HAART. Virology 2005;334:299–305.

78. Philpott S, Burger H, Tsoukas C, et al. Human immunodeficiency virus type 1 genomic RNA sequences in the female genital tract and blood: compartmentalization and intrapatient recombination. J Virol 2005;79:353–63.

79. Sullivan ST, Mandava U, Evans-Strickfaden T, et al. Diversity, divergence, and evolution of cell-free human immunodeficiency virus type 1 in vaginal secretions and blood of chronically infected women: associations with immune status. J Virol 2005;79:9799–809.
80. Andreoletti L, Skrabal K, Perrin V, et al. Genetic and phenotypic features of blood and genital viral populations of clinically asymptomatic and antiretroviral-treatment-naive clade a human immunodeficiency virus type 1-infected women. J Clin Microbiol 2007;45:1838–42.
81. Kemal KS, Burger H, Mayers D, et al. HIV-1 drug resistance in variants from the female genital tract and plasma. J Infect Dis 2007;195:535–45.
82. Semrau K, Ghosh M, Kankasa C, et al. Temporal and lateral dynamics of HIV shedding and elevated sodium in breast milk among HIV-positive mothers during the first 4 months of breast-feeding. J Acquir Immune Defic Syndr 2008;47:320–8.
83. Bull ME, Learn GH, McElhone S, et al. Monotypic human immunodeficiency virus type 1 genotypes across the uterine cervix and in blood suggest proliferation of cells with provirus. J Virol 2009;83:6020–8.
84. Dyer JR, Gilliam BL, Eron JJ Jr, et al. Quantitation of human immunodeficiency virus type 1 RNA in cell free seminal plasma: comparison of NASBA with Amplicor reverse transcription-PCR amplification and correlation with quantitative culture. J Virol Methods 1996;60:161–70.
85. Si-Mohamed A, Kazatchkine MD, Heard I, et al. Selection of drug-resistant variants in the female genital tract of human immunodeficiency virus type 1-infected women receiving antiretroviral therapy. J Infect Dis 2000;182:112–22.
86. Min SS, Corbett AH, Rezk N, et al. Protease Inhibitor and Nonnucleoside Reverse Transcriptase Inhibitor Concentrations in the Genital Tract of HIV-1-Infected Women. J Acquir Immune Defic Syndr 2004;37:1577–80.
87. Fowler MG, Lampe MA, Jamieson DJ, et al. Reducing the risk of mother-to-child human immunodeficiency virus transmission: past successes, current progress and challenges, and future directions. Am J Obstet Gynecol 2007;197:3–9.
88. Kuhn L, Aldrovandi GM, Sinkala M, et al. Effects of early, abrupt weaning for HIV-free survival of children in zambia. N Engl J Med 2008;359:1859.
89. Becquart P, Chomont N, Roques P, et al. Compartmentalization of HIV-1 between breast milk and blood of HIV-infected mothers. Virology 2002;300:109–17.
90. Becquart P, Courgnaud V, Willumsen J, et al. Diversity of HIV-1 RNA and DNA in breast milk from HIV-1-infected mothers. Virology 2007;363:256–60.
91. Henderson GJ, Hoffman NG, Ping LH, et al. HIV-1 populations in blood and breast milk are similar. Virology 2004;330:295–303.
92. Andreotti M, Galluzzo CM, Guidotti G, et al. Comparison of HIV type 1 sequences from plasma, cell-free breast milk, and cell-associated breast milk viral populations in treated and untreated women in Mozambique. AIDS Res Hum Retroviruses 2009;25:707–11.
93. Sabbaj S, Edwards BH, Ghosh MK, et al. Human immunodeficiency virus-specific CD8+ T cells in human breast milk. J Virol 2002;76:7365–73.
94. Sabbaj S, Ghosh MK, Edwards BH, et al. Breast milk-derived antigen-specific CD8+ T cells: an extralymphoid effector memory cell population in humans. J Immunol 2005;174:2951–6.
95. Nickle DC, Jensen MA, Shriner D, et al. Evolutionary indicators of human immunodeficiency virus type 1 reservoirs and compartments. J Virol 2003;77:5540–6.
96. Becquart P, Hakim H, Benoit G, et al. Compartmentalization of the IgG immune response to HIV-1 in breast milk. AIDS 1999;13:1323–31.

97. Heath L, Conway S, Jones L, et al. Restriction of HIV-1 genotypes in breast milk does not account for the population transmission genetic bottleneck that occurs following transmission. PLoS One 2010;5:e10213.

98. Becquet R, Ekouevi D, Arrive E, et al. Universal antiretroviral therapy for pregnant and breast-feeding HIV-1-infected women: towards the elimination of mother-to-child transmission of HIV-1 in resource-limited settings. Clin Infect Dis 2009;49:1936–45.

99. Dabis F, Msellati P, Meda N, et al. 6-month efficacy, tolerance, and acceptability of a short regimen of oral zidovudine to reduce vertical transmission of HIV in breastfed children in Cote d'Ivoire and Burkina Faso: a double-blind placebo-controlled multicentre trial. Lancet 1999;353:786–92.

100. Dabis F, Bequet L, Ekouevi DK, et al. Field efficacy of zidovudine, lamivudine and single-dose nevirapine to prevent peripartum transmission of HIV. The ANRS 1201/1202 Ditrame Plus study, Abidjan, Cote d'Ivoire. AIDS 2005;19: 309–18.

101. Guay LA, Musoke P, Fleming T, et al. Intrapartum and neonatal single-dose nevirapine compared with zidovudine for prevention of mother-to-child transmission of HIV-1 in Kampala, Uganda: HIVNET 012 randomised trial. Lancet 1999;354:795–802.

102. Lallemant M, Jourdain G, Le Coeur S, et al. Single-dose perinatal nevirapine plus standard zidovudine to prevent mother-to-child transmission of HIV-1 in Thailand. N Engl J Med 2004;351:217–28.

103. Petra study team. Efficacy of three short-course regimens of zidovudine and lamivudine in preventing early and late transmission of HIV-1 from mother to child in Tanzania, South Africa, and Uganda (Petra study): a randomised, double-blind, placebo-controlled trial. Lancet 2002;359:1178–86.

104. Shaffer N, Chuachoowong R, Mock PA, et al. Short-course zidovudine for perinatal HIV-1 transmission in Bangkok, Thailand: a randomised controlled trial. Lancet 1999;353:773–80.

105. Wiktor SZ, Ekpini E, Karon JM, et al. Short-course oral zidovudine for prevention of mother-to-child transmission of HIV-1 in Abidjan, Cote d'Ivoire: a randomised trial. Lancet 1999;353:781–5.

106. Arrive E, Newell ML, Ekouevi DK, et al. Prevalence of resistance to nevirapine in mothers and children after single-dose exposure to prevent vertical transmission of HIV-1: a meta-analysis. Int J Epidemiol 2007;36:1009–21.

107. Luzuriaga K, Dabis F, Excler JL, et al. Vaccines to prevent transmission of HIV-1 via breastmilk: scientific and logistical priorities. Lancet 2006;368:511–21.

108. Rerks-Ngarm S, Pitisuttithum P, Nitayaphan S, et al. Vaccination with ALVAC and AIDSVAX to Prevent HIV-1 Infection in Thailand. N Engl J Med 2009;361: 2209–20.

109. Walker L, Phogat S, Chan-Hui P, et al. Broad and potent neutralizing antibodies from an African donor reveal a new HIV-1 vaccine target. Science 2009;326: 285–9.

110. Hansen S, Vieville C, Whizin N, et al. Effector memory T cell responses are associated with protection of rhesus monkeys from mucosal simian immunodeficiency virus challenge. Nat Med 2009;15:293–9.

Diagnosis of HIV: Challenges and Strategies for HIV Prevention and Detection Among Pregnant Women and Their Infants

Margery Donovan, ND, APRN, PNP-BC, Paul Palumbo, MD*

KEYWORDS

- Human immunodeficiency virus • Perinatal HIV • Pregnancy
- Antiretroviral prophylaxis • HIV diagnostics

A new immunodeficiency syndrome that would become known as AIDS was first recognized in the early 1980s. Substantial progress on defining some of the clinical and epidemiologic features of AIDS occurred before identification of the underlying retrovirus, which was initially called lymphadenopathy-associated virus or human T-lymphotropic virus type III, and would subsequently be known as human immunodeficiency virus type 1 (HIV-1).[1,2] The first cases of AIDS in young infants were reported in 1983 to a somewhat disbelieving public and global medical community, widening the scope of HIV-1 infection to the perinatal setting.[3–5]

Today in the United States, with universal testing and appropriate treatment, the transmission of perinatally acquired HIV infection can be decreased to approximately 1%.[6] Perinatal infection rates have significantly declined since 1983, but in 2004 there were still approximately 138 (95% confidence interval, 96–186) infants born in the United States with HIV infection.[7]

An infant born with HIV represents a missed opportunity, and often more than one opportunity is missed throughout the continuum of care for the mother-infant pair. The Centers for Disease Control and Prevention (CDC) refer to these missed opportunities as the Perinatal Prevention Cascade (**Table 1**).[8] Prevention opportunities

Dartmouth-Hitchcock-Medical Center, Dartmouth Medical School, 1 Medical Center Drive, Lebanon, NH 03756, USA
* Corresponding author.
E-mail address: Paul.E.Palumbo@Dartmouth.edu

Clin Perinatol 37 (2010) 751–763
doi:10.1016/j.clp.2010.08.014
0095-5108/10/$ – see front matter © 2010 Elsevier Inc. All rights reserved.

perinatology.theclinics.com

Table 1	
The CDC's perinatal prevention cascade	
Missed Opportunities	**Prevention Opportunities**
HIV-infected woman	Primary HIV prevention for women
Pregnancy in HIV-infected woman	Prevention of unintended pregnancies in HIV-positive women
Inadequate prenatal care	Accessible prenatal care
No or late HIV test	Universal prenatal testing
No antiretroviral prophylaxis	Antiretroviral prophylaxis for all HIV-positive pregnant women and their exposed infants

Data from presentation by A.W. Taylor at the conference, Consultation on Prevention of Mother-to-Child HIV Transmission in the United States, Atlanta, Georgia, April 2008.

can occur throughout a succession of stages and include primary HIV prevention for women, prevention of unintended pregnancies in HIV-positive women, accessible prenatal care, universal prenatal testing, and antiretroviral prophylaxis for all HIV-positive pregnant women and their exposed newborns. When an infant is exposed to HIV, specialized testing is needed to diagnose perinatal infection. Sophisticated laboratory support is central to perinatal transmission prevention efforts, particularly in the form of HIV diagnostics that have evolved continuously during the last 3 decades (**Table 2**). Specific and unique HIV diagnostic and management challenges exist within both maternal and neonatal/infant populations, which are the focus of this article.

HISTORICAL PERSPECTIVE

With viral isolation in vitro by cell culture and subsequent identification of HIV-1 in 1983–1984,[1,2] diagnostic tests were developed that allowed for the detection of antibodies to HIV-1 in human blood specimens.[9,10] Progressive evolution of antibody detection assays occurred over the ensuing 2.5 decades, most using a 2-step screening and confirmation approach. This diagnostic approach is the preferred strategy for HIV diagnosis targeting pregnant women as well as adults and children older than 18 to 24 months. Additional improvements currently in the field or in development include point-of-care (POC) strategies as well as specimen flexibility (dried blood spots, saliva, and urine).

Infant diagnosis presented a unique challenge in that all infants born to HIV-infected mothers are born with transplacentally acquired maternal antibodies and thus test positive with traditional serologic, antibody-based assays regardless of their infection status. This situation naturally led to the search for and development of assays for the direct detection of HIV-1 within biologic specimens. The first of these was viral culture, achieved by the cocultivation of lymphocytes from a test subject with lymphocytes from an HIV-uninfected donor. This assay required many days to weeks, was conducted in sophisticated biologic containment, and was labor intensive. A simpler approach was soon developed, which detected an HIV protein—p24 from the viral gag protein—from blood samples using an enzyme immunoassay format (p24 antigen assay). With the advent of the polymerase chain reaction (PCR)[11] and other nucleic acid amplification techniques (NAATs) in the late 1980s, direct detection of amplified viral nucleic acids became possible and is currently the preferred approach for infant HIV diagnosis.[12,13]

Table 2	
Summary of currently used diagnostic tests in the perinatal setting	
Diagnostic Test	**Current Use in the Perinatal Setting**
Viral culture	Not currently in use
p24 antigen	Not routinely in use
Antibody-based assays (EIA/ELISA + WB/IFA)	Diagnosis of pregnant women, adults, and children >18 mo
First-generation (viral lysates)	Diagnosis of HIV-1 Window period 5 wk
Second-generation (DNA recombinant technology)	Diagnosis of HIV-1 and HIV-2 Window period 4 wk
Third-generation (detection of HIV-specific IgG and IgM antibodies)	Window period 3 wk
Fourth-generation (detection of both HIV antibody and p24 antigen)	Diagnosis of acute infection in pregnant women, adults, and children >2 y Window period 10–20 d
Nucleic Acid Amplification Tests	
Proviral DNA PCR	Diagnosis of neonate and infants <18 mo Done at birth or 14 d, and 1–4 mo, but wide variability with timing
Quantitative RNA PCR	Monitor viral load status in infected pregnant women, adults, children, and infants
Point-of-care Test	
EIA/ELISA based	Diagnosis of infection in prenatal clinics and in labor and delivery Positive results need laboratory confirmation
Nucleic acid amplification test technology	In development Diagnosis of infection in high prevalence, low resource settings

Abbreviations: EIA, enzyme immunoassay; ELISA, enzyme-linked immunosorbent assay; IFA, immunofluorescence assay; PCR, polymerase chain reaction; WB, Western blot.

ANTIBODY-BASED ASSAYS

Serologic assays for the diagnosis of HIV have evolved substantially over the years, a process that remains active. These assays have been grouped by their underlying principles into first through fourth generations. The earliest or first-generation assays employed crude viral lysates—HIV chemically and physically disrupted into its components—to bind and immobilize HIV antibody from a test subject's blood specimen. Viral lysates were fixed to the plastic surface of a well in a microtiter plate or to beads. A serum specimen was incubated with the prepared plate wells or beads and any HIV-specific antibody was allowed to bind to the fixed viral lysate. After extensive washing, the plate or beads were incubated with an antibody that specifically targeted human antibodies and that also had a chemically attached color marker for subsequent detection. The overall assay is referred to as an enzyme immunoassay (EIA) or enzyme-linked immunosorbent assay (ELISA).

Virus stocks used for the viral lysates in first-generation assays were generated in human cell culture, which resulted in the presence of some human antigens, such as human leukocyte antigen (HLA) and cluster differentiation (CD) antigens. This "contamination" may underscore the small but real incidence of false-positive reactions observed in individuals with autoimmune disorders, recent immunization, previous blood transfusions, and hematologic and liver diseases. Given the importance of establishing a rigorous diagnosis of infection or noninfection, a 2-step testing algorithm is mandated: an initial screening assay (EIA) often performed in duplicate followed by a supplemental or confirmatory assay, typically a Western blot (WB) or an immunofluorescence assay (IFA).[14,15] The WB employs distinct viral proteins electrophoretically separated by size on a nitrocellulose membrane as a binding substrate for HIV-specific antibodies in a test specimen. Secondary detection of viral protein antibody binding on the membrane by means of a second "antihuman" antibody results in a banding pattern. Discrete criteria for the number and types of viral protein bands required for positivity have been developed.[14,15]

Screening that requires repeatedly positive EIA duplicate tests has been documented to possess high sensitivity ($\geq$99.4%) and specificity ($\geq$98.5%).[15] Following repeatedly positive EIA tests, confirmatory WB or IFA rates vary with the population being tested, 70% or higher in populations at high infection risk but only 20% or less in groups with low infection risk. The 2-step screening algorithm has been optimized for diagnostic sensitivity (high probability of detecting an infected person—strength of screening EIA) and specificity (high probability of determining negative status—strength of confirmatory WB or IFA).

Additional progress was realized in the form of second-generation EIA assays, which featured the use of HIV proteins or peptides generated by DNA recombinant technology in place of crude viral lysates. These highly purified proteins were largely absent of contaminating human antigens, and resulted in higher sensitivity and specificity. In addition, this technology provided the opportunity to mix proteins from HIV-1 and HIV-2 for joint screening purposes. HIV-2 is primarily found in Western Africa where prevalence rates as high as 8% exist. Rates of HIV-2 infection in the United States have been very low and are generally found in individuals of West African ancestry.

Third- and fourth-generation EIA assays were developed to decrease the window period between HIV infection and subsequent detection time using standard antibody-based tests. Third-generation assays combine IgM and IgG detection whereas fourth-generation assays combine detection of HIV antigen and antibody (both discussed in subsequent sections).

PRIMARY HIV PREVENTION FOR WOMEN

With HIV serology available and improving over time, the implementation of testing for women of childbearing age and pregnant women in particular became a controversial focus. On the one hand, arguments in support of women's and infants' health and perinatal transmission prevention called for universal screening of women of childbearing age, pregnant women, and newborns. On the other hand, personal rights, confidentiality, and associated stigma led to the placing of limitations on testing and the general requirement for a complex pretest counseling and informed consent process. This debate played out across the United States and beyond, possibly no more visibly than in New York, which was home to some of the earliest legal mandates in favor of testing (The New York State Comprehensive Newborn Testing Program, February 1997; a similar program had been defeated in California in 1995). The time-honored approach supported by the CDC and most states encourages that HIV testing be offered to women in care in the context of HIV counseling.

In 2006 the CDC revised their HIV testing recommendations.[16] Testing is currently recommended for all adults and adolescents in a variety of health care settings using opt-out approaches and not requiring a separate written consent. Women who are at increased risk for HIV infection, such as individuals who inject drugs, exchange sex for drugs or money, or have partners who are infected with HIV, should be tested annually. Prevention counseling should not be linked to testing but should be offered to high-risk individuals. The objectives of these recommendations are to increase HIV testing, identify infection earlier, and link individuals to secondary prevention and treatment services. If women can be diagnosed during this stage, then they can make informed decisions about reproduction prior to pregnancy.

One of the barriers identified was that the recommendations were not consistent among all state HIV testing laws.[17] 34 state laws were consistent or neutral with the CDC recommendations, but 16 states were inconsistent. Since 2006, 9 of the 16 states have passed new legislation to align with the CDC recommendations.

PREVENTION OF UNINTENDED PREGNANCIES IN HIV-POSITIVE WOMEN

Comprehensive care for HIV-positive women includes preconception counseling that helps women make informed decisions regarding future pregnancies.[18] Focusing on behavioral change that improves women's health and reduces risk to future pregnancies is important and should address effective contraception, HIV risk reduction, and the elimination of alcohol, illicit drugs, and smoking. If a woman is on antiretroviral therapy, her medications need to be evaluated for efficacy and safety in case of unplanned pregnancy. If an HIV-positive woman wishes to become pregnant, she needs effective adherence counseling to attain a maximally suppressed virus. In the Women and Infants Transmission study (n = 2246), women who were at risk for repeat pregnancy were younger and had lower education status, higher CD4 counts, and lower viral loads than women who had only one pregnancy during the study.[19] Based on data from 1997 to 2004 from 28 states that collect perinatal HIV exposure data, 1183 births were reported in 1090 teens.[20] HIV status was known before pregnancy in about half of these teens, and most of the pregnancies (87%) were unplanned.

Another population in which repeat pregnancies are being seen is that of the immigrant and refugee communities.[21] In a descriptive study of West Africans who are HIV-positive and settled in the Providence, Rhode Island area, there was a high rate of pregnancies (20 among 14 women), and the median time from resettlement to first pregnancy was 16 months. These examples demonstrate the need for timely medical care that is both developmentally and culturally appropriate to prevent unintended pregnancies.

ACCESSIBLE PRENATAL CARE

A major missed opportunity in preventing perinatal HIV infection is a lack of prenatal care; women who do not get prenatal care are less likely to be offered HIV testing and prophylaxis if needed.[22,23] In the Mother-Infant Rapid Intervention at Delivery (MIRIAD) study of 18 hospitals in 6 United States cities, approximately 27% of the women who agreed to an interview (n = 667) reported no prenatal care before admission to labor and delivery.[24] Of infants born with HIV infection between 2001 and 2004 (n = 201), 16% of their mothers had no prenatal care.[25]

Maternal drug use has been significantly associated with lack of prenatal care.[22,24,26,27] In a special surveillance report of 16 perinatal HIV prevention programs, 20% of the HIV-infected women reported using illicit drugs during pregnancy.[28] The health beliefs of women who actively use drugs (n = 610) have been examined in order to learn more about their attitudes toward HIV testing.[29] Sixteen percent of women who injected drugs said that they would avoid prenatal care if HIV testing was mandatory during pregnancy. In addition, the majority of women interviewed believed that people who use drugs receive suboptimal care from health care providers. To eliminate the remaining cases of perinatal HIV infection, how health care is delivered to women at highest risk for HIV transmission needs to be evaluated and addressed.

UNIVERSAL PRENATAL TESTING

The CDC recommends that HIV screening during pregnancy be simplified and opportunities for women to learn their HIV status maximized.[16] All pregnant women should be offered HIV testing consistent with the recommendations for adults. HIV testing should be included in the routine panel of screening tests for pregnant women, and reasons for declining it should be explored and addressed. Screening should be offered early in pregnancy so that optimum HIV treatment can be offered.[30] A second test should be offered in the third trimester for women who decline the first test, are at high risk for infection, or live in areas where there is an increased incidence of HIV/AIDS. About half of the states meet this criterion in the United States.

Rapid bedside or clinic HIV testing provides substantial logistic benefits, for example, allowing timely intervention in labor and delivery, and minimizes the lost-to-follow-up variable in the sporadic clinical setting. In response to this need, manufacturers developed POC diagnostic devices that detect antibody without the need for a core referral laboratory in a 15- to 30-minute time frame. There are now many such assays, of which 6 are currently approved by the Food and Drug Administration (FDA). These assays have become widely used in the United States and other high-resource countries as well as in low-resource settings.[31,32]

The POC antibody detection assays all use a common theme: capture of HIV-specific antibody by antigen immobilized on a solid phase comprising either latex beads or thin membranes. Readout is determined by visualizing agglutination (latex beads) or color detection by addition of reagents that detect bound antibodies. The assays are thematically and logistically similar to the familiar home pregnancy tests. Sensitivity and specificity is equal to or superior to laboratory-based EIAs while they experience the same high false-positive rates in low HIV-prevalence populations. A current challenge is the development of testing algorithms for HIV POC assays that are robust and evidence-based. A common strategy is to use 2 distinct POC assays sequentially and, if both are reactive, a presumptive positive is declared that requires later laboratory-based confirmation.[33] POC assays that can use whole blood (obtained by finger-stick or venipuncture) or saliva have been developed.

Guidelines currently recommend that if HIV status is not documented at the time of labor, rapid testing should be offered using opt-out approaches. When a woman's HIV test result is still unknown at delivery, rapid testing should again be offered to either the woman or her newborn. If rapid testing is positive, then zidovudine (ZDV, AZT, Retrovir) should be initiated in the mother and/or infant before results of confirmatory testing. These guidelines have been adopted by the American College of Obstetrics and Gynecology (ACOG)[34] and the American Academy of Pediatrics.[30] In 2008, 10 states had mandatory HIV testing of newborns if the mothers' status was not known at delivery (Box 1).[35]

Investigation of translation to practice has demonstrated that perinatal providers have not fully adopted CDC recommendations for testing pregnant women. In one survey of ACOG fellows, 97% of the obstetricians that returned surveys (n = 582) reported that they recommend HIV testing to all pregnant patients, but only half of

---

Box 1
List of states with mandatory HIV testing of newborns when mother's status is not known at delivery, 2008

States with mandatory HIV testing of newborns

    Connecticut

    Illinois

    Mississippi

    Nevada

    New Jersey

    New York

    North Carolina

    South Carolina

    South Dakota

    Wisconsin

Data from Kaiser Family Foundation. HIV testing for mothers and newborns (February 2008). http://statehealthfacts.org. Accessed June 2010.

---

them said that they use opt-out approaches.[36] When prenatal providers from a low-incidence state were surveyed (n = 353), rural providers reported that they offer HIV testing to all pregnant patients, but they indicated that there is inadequate follow-up of patients who refuse testing.[37] Communication between prenatal and intrapartum providers has also been identified as a barrier to fully implementing the recommendations. The hospitals that participated in the MIRIAD study were required to document HIV status of pregnant women or their newborns at delivery.[38] Of the 653 women who did not have HIV status documented at the time of labor and delivery, 63% reported that they had an HIV test done at some point during their pregnancy, but results were not available to intrapartum providers.

HIV testing rates vary for pregnant women and are dependent on provider, method for offering test, and state law. Of infants born with HIV infection (n = 323), 26% of their mothers were diagnosed after delivery.[25] When women from 14 geographically diverse Ryan White funded clinics were surveyed (n = 853), 90% supported HIV testing as part of routine prenatal care using opt-out approaches.[39] Rescreening in the third trimester using rapid testing was not only accepted by pregnant women from an urban clinic (n = 75), but found to be less stressful than standard HIV testing.[40] However, low use of rapid testing in labor has been reported. In a New Jersey hospital, 18% of the women had unknown HIV status in labor (n = 403), but only 9% of those patients agreed to a rapid test.[41]

RECENT INFECTION

In high-risk HIV communities defined as an HIV incidence of greater than 1 in 1000 person-years, infection during pregnancy achieves a probability level that supports retesting late in pregnancy and/or at delivery. The challenge of detecting acute HIV infection has come under recent scrutiny. First-generation EIAs and WBs typically detect HIV antibody approximately 5 weeks after initiation of HIV infection while viral RNA first becomes detectable in a time frame of about 2 weeks postinfection.

The window period between detectable viral RNA and antibody is one of high virus levels and potential infectivity, and is also a critical period for blood donor screening. Second-, third-, and fourth-generation EIAs each cut an additional week off the 5-week first-generation detection period.

In an effort to increase detection rates early in the acute infection period, third-generation EIA assays introduced the simultaneous detection of HIV-specific IgG and IgM antibodies using a sandwich EIA format. Also targeting acute HIV infection, a fourth-generation EIA assay that combines HIV p24 antigen detection with HIV antibody detection was recently approved by the FDA in June 2010; it has been approved for use in adults, including pregnant women, and for children older than 2 years. This assay has not been approved for diagnosing infants because a positive result does not differentiate between infant antibody formation and maternal antibody acquired transplacentally. These assays have been useful for facilitating screening of the blood supply and for diagnosing acutely infected individuals (pregnant and nonpregnant), reducing the window to 10 to 20 days.

ANTIRETROVIRAL PROPHYLAXIS FOR ALL HIV-POSITIVE PREGNANT WOMEN AND THEIR EXPOSED INFANTS

The risk of perinatal infection can be decreased by intervening at any step along the continuum of care. Data were obtained from medical records of HIV-exposed infants (n = 3284) who were delivered at 6 sites from 1996 to 2000.[42] Perinatal HIV transmission was 3% when treatment included combination antiretroviral therapy, intrapartum and neonatal zidovudine (ZDV, AZT, Retrovir); 6% with prenatal, intrapartum, and neonatal ZDV; 8% with intrapartum and neonatal ZDV; 14% with neonatal ZDV alone started within 24 hours of birth; and 20% with no treatment. Today with highly active antiretroviral therapy (HAART or ART), maximally suppressed virus, intrapartum and neonatal ZDV, elective cesarean section, and no breastfeeding, the risk of transmission has been reported to be approximately 1%.[6] Treating HIV-positive women and their exposed infants with antiretroviral medications is addressed fully in another article in this issue.

NUCLEIC ACID AMPLIFICATION TESTS

The development of the PCR and related nucleic acid amplification assays in the 1980s was a boon to investigators searching for a sensitive viral detection assay for newborn and infant HIV diagnosis. Of note, infant HIV diagnosis was one of the first clinical applications of PCR, developed even before quantitative HIV PCR that has been used extensively over the past 15 years to monitor HIV disease status. Infant HIV diagnostic needs were immediate in the 1980s, whereas HIV treatment in the form of antiretroviral drugs and the need for disease monitoring had not yet arrived.

PCR is a disarmingly simple technique that enzymatically amplifies a targeted stretch of nucleic acids (eg, a segment of a gene), creating many millions of copies thus simplifying subsequent detection. Targeting is accomplished by generating an oligonucleotide primer—a short nucleic acid fragment that is 20 to 30 nucleotides in length—which is complementary to the targeted nucleic acid (HIV gene segment) and will bind specifically through DNA base pairing. An enzyme, Taq polymerase, extends the primer using the DNA target as template, resulting in a copy of the DNA target. A unique and essential property of Taq polymerase is its ideal operating temperature of 72°C and its tolerability of 100°C for brief periods of time. This property allows for temperature cycling with stops at 55°C for primer binding to target, 72°C for Taq polymerase synthesis of complementary DNA, and 95°C for dissociation (melting) of double-stranded DNA product. This cycle of 55-72-95°C is repeated 30 to 40 times, each cycle realizing a doubling of target DNA, resulting in 2^{30} copies in less than an hour.

NAATs, of which PCR is the most prevalent, have become the gold standard for infant HIV diagnosis in the developed world. Though it has been a struggle and has some way to go, it is also becoming widely available in resource-limited settings. PCR uses DNA as its template, and in the case of HIV diagnosis targets proviral HIV DNA that has integrated into a gene of an infected host cell. PCR is exquisitely sensitive in that it can detect as few as 1 to 10 infected cells within a sample. This sensitivity can also lead to false positives if extreme care is not taken to prevent even minute contamination with previously amplified material.

PCR and related NAATs have also been configured to quantify HIV viral RNA within plasma samples for the purposes of disease monitoring. In the case of PCR this is called "reverse transcriptase PCR" (RT-PCR) because viral RNA genetic material must first be reverse transcribed to double-stranded DNA before undergoing PCR amplification. Real-time monitoring of each PCR cycle allows rapid correlation of PCR product detection with the quantity of viral RNA in the original sample. Quantitative PCR/NAAT assays are widely available and have increasingly been used for infant diagnosis.

The timing of blood sampling for infant HIV diagnosis has been reasonably established, and also helps to inform the timing of maternal-to-child infection. Initial sample for NAAT-based diagnosis is recommended at birth (within 2 days of delivery) or at 14 days of age.[43] Infants whose birth sample is positive are felt to have been infected in utero, whereas those negative at birth but positive at 14 days or later have acquired infection during the peripartum period, assuming the infant is not breastfeeding.[44] Subsequent NAAT testing is done between 1 and 4 months of age and, while specific recommendations exist, wide variability in implementation has been documented.[45] A meta-analysis of early PCR-based diagnostic studies in infancy calculated a sensitivity of 93% by 14 days of age, which underscores the requirement for serial testing.[46] Most clinicians perform an antibody assay at 18 months of age, at which time greater than 98% of HIV-uninfected children will have metabolized maternally derived antibody to ensure noninfection status.

As with antibody-based diagnostics, there is a demand for POC accessibility for infant diagnosis employing NAAT technology, particularly in high-prevalence, low-resource settings. Many groups are attempting to address this by using microfluidic devices in a concept labeled Lab-on-a-Chip (LOC). Desirable performance characteristics are simplicity, low cost, mobility, temperature stability, and freedom from the electric power grid. Although no product is currently widely available, there are several promising candidates in development.

FAMILY CONCERNS

Diagnosis of perinatally acquired HIV infection can be a time of crisis and high anxiety for the infant's mother and family. If a woman is diagnosed before or early in pregnancy, then the woman has time to deal with her own diagnosis before addressing her infant's issues. However, if the diagnosis is made after the birth, the parents are not only dealing with their own diagnoses but also with the implications for their infant.

Initial reaction to a diagnosis of HIV can range from shock, disbelief, and anger to sadness, self blame, and denial. Some women acknowledge that they have been at risk for HIV due to their own or their partner's behavior, but have been unable or unwilling to seek out HIV testing. When HIV is suspected in an infant, the woman is forced to not only deal with her infant's health but her own.

Often a diagnosis of HIV uncovers individual and family secrets such as a sexual or drug abuse history. Once a woman is diagnosed, the risk to her partner(s) and other children need to be assessed and addressed. It is also not uncommon for a diagnosis of HIV to be associated with perceived losses: loss of the mother's health, a perfect infant, social support, and a future. Diagnosis of HIV occurs across all socioeconomic groups, but the hardest to reach are often women who are highly marginalized and stigmatized. These women may be dealing with drug addiction, poverty, or be a new refugee or immigrant, and have few resources and little support.

If a woman has been able to engage in obstetric and HIV care, and has taken ART with a high degree of adherence, the process of infant testing can be a hopeful time. If this has not occurred then fear and guilt may be triggered in the parents. Maternal uncertainty about her infant's HIV status has been demonstrated to be inversely related to social support and to decrease significantly over the testing process. If a mother had depressive symptoms during her pregnancy then she demonstrated more uncertainty during the testing process than mothers who were not depressed.[47]

Caring for HIV-exposed or HIV-positive infants and their families requires a team of skilled providers. A high degree of collaboration and coordination is needed between providers and among agencies to care for these complex family situations. A comprehensive team includes physicians, nurses, mental health providers, addiction counselors, peer counselors, and social service workers. There needs to be strong outreach that helps to identify women at risk for HIV and link them with testing and care as needed. Prenatal and obstetric providers need to communicate and coordinate care with HIV, mental health, addiction, and resettlement providers. Seamless processes between prenatal and intrapartum providers need to be established so that staff are aware of a woman's HIV status in labor and can quickly implement the required protocol as needed. This goal is easier to accomplish in high-incidence hospitals that have many HIV-exposed births than in those that may have only one such birth a year. Strong communication is also required between obstetric and pediatric providers so that exposed infants receive the required prophylaxis and testing.

Connecting with HIV-positive women during pregnancy is a unique opportunity because women often take care of their health issues better at this time than at other times. HIV providers need to meet families living with HIV, assess their emotional status, and establish relationships so that trust can be developed. Helping women engage in medical and psychosocial services during the perinatal process may have long-term effects on the family as women take positive steps to cope with their own disease.

REFERENCES

1. Barre-Sinoussi F, Chermann JC, Rey F, et al. Isolation of a T-lymphocyte retrovirus from a patient at risk for AIDS. Science 1983;220(4599):868–71.
2. Gallo RC, Salahuddin SZ, Popovic M, et al. Frequent detection and isolation of cytopathic retroviruses (HTLV-III) from patients with AIDS and at risk for AIDS. Science 1984;224(4648):500–3.
3. Oleske J, Minnefor A, Cooper R, et al. Immune deficiency syndrome in children. JAMA 1983;249:2345–9.
4. Rubinstein A, Sicklick M, Gupta A, et al. Acquired immunodeficiency with reversed T4/T8 ratios in infants born to promiscuous and drug addicted mothers. JAMA 1983;249:2350–6.

5. Scott GB, Buck BE, Letermann JG, et al. Acquired immunodeficiency syndrome in infants. N Engl J Med 1984;310:76–81.
6. Chou R, Smits AK, Huffman LH, et al. US Preventive Services Task Force. Prenatal screening for HIV: a review of the evidence for the U.S. preventive services task force. Ann Intern Med 2005;143(1):38–54.
7. McKenna MT, Hu X. Recent trends in the incidence and morbidity that are associated with perinatal human immunodeficiency virus infection in the United States. Am J Obstet Gynecol 2007;197(Suppl 3):S10–6.
8. Data for perinatal HIV prevention. Consultation on prevention of mother-to-child HIV transmission in the United States. April 1–3, 2008
9. Kalyanaraman VS, Cabradilla CD, Getchell JP, et al. Antibody to the core protein of lymphadenopathy-associated virus (LAV) in patients with AIDS. Science 1984; 225(4659):321–3.
10. Sarngadharan MG, Popovic M, Bruch L, et al. Antibodies reactive with human T-lymphotropic retrovirus (HTLV-III) in the serum of patients with AIDS. Science 1984;224(4648):506–8.
11. Mullis KB, Faloona FA, Scharf SJ, et al. Specific enzymatic amplification of DNA in vitro: the polymerase chain reaction. Cold Spring Harb Symp Quant Biol 1986;51:263–7.
12. Ou CY, Kwok S, Mitchell SW, et al. DNA amplification for direct detection of HIV-1 in DNA or peripheral blood mononuclear cells. Science 1988;239(4836):295–7.
13. Rogers M, Ou CY, Rayfield M, et al. Use of the polymerase chain reaction for early detection of the proviral sequences of human immunodeficiency virus in infants born to seropositive mothers. New York City collaborative study of maternal HIV transmission and Montefiore Medical Center HIV perinatal transmission study group. N Engl J Med 1989;320:1949–54.
14. CDC. Interpretation and use of the Western blot assay for serodiagnosis of human immunodeficiency virus type 1 infections. MMWR Morb Mortal Wkly Rep 1989;38:1–7.
15. CDC. Serologic testing for HIV-1 antibody—United States, 1988 and 1989. MMWR Morb Mortal Wkly Rep 1990;39(22):380–3.
16. Branson BM, Handsfield HH, Lampe MA, et al. Revised recommendations for HIV testing of adults, adolescents, and pregnant women in health-care settings. MMWR Recomm Rep 2006;55(RR-14):1–17.
17. Mahajan AP, Stemple L, Shapiro MF, et al. Consistency of state statues with the centers for disease control and prevention HIV testing recommendations for health care settings. Ann Intern Med 2009;150(4):263–9.
18. Panel on Treatment of HIV-Infected Pregnant Women and Prevention of Perinatal Transmission. Recommendations for the use of antiretroviral drugs in pregnant HIV-1 infected women for maternal health and interventions to reduce perinatal HIV transmission in the United States. May 24, 2010. p. 1–117. Available at: http://aidsinfo.nih.gov/ContentFiles/PerinatalGL.pdf. Accessed August 25, 2010.
19. Bryant AS, Leighty RM, Shen X, et al. Predictors of repeat pregnancy among HIV-1 infected women. J Acquir Immune Defic Syndr 2007;44(1):87–92.
20. Koenig LJ, Espinoza L, Hodge K, et al. Young, seropositive, and pregnant: epidemiologic and psychosocial perspectives on pregnant adolescents with human immunodeficiency virus infection. Am J Obstet Gynecol 2007;197(3):S123–31.
21. Blood E, Beckwith C, Bazerman L, et al. Pregnancy among HIV-infected refugees in Rhode Island. AIDS Care 2009;21(2):207–11.
22. Abatemarco DJ, Catov JM, Cross H, et al. Factors associated with zidovudine receipt and prenatal care among HIV-infected pregnant women in New Jersey. J Health Care Poor Underserved 2008;19(3):814–28.

23. Sarnquist CC, Cunningham SD, Sullivan B, et al. The effectiveness of state and national policy on the implementation of perinatal HIV prevention interventions. Am J Public Health 2007;97(6):1041–6.
24. Potter JE, Pereyra M, Lampe M, et al. Factors associated with prenatal care use among peripartum women in the mother-infant rapid intervention at delivery study. J Obstet Gynecol Neonatal Nurs 2009;38(5):534–43.
25. CDC. Achievements in public health: reduction in perinatal transmission of HIV infection—United States, 1985-2005. Morb Mortal Wkly Rep 2006;55(21): 592–7.
26. Cohen MH, Olszewski Y, Webber MP, et al. Women identified with HIV at labor and delivery: testing, disclosing and linking to care challenges. Matern Child Health J 2008;12(5):568–76.
27. Peters VB, Liu KL, Robinson LG, et al. Trends in perinatal HIV prevention in New York City, 1994-2003. Am J Public Health 2008;98(10):1857–64.
28. CDC. Enhanced perinatal surveillance—United States, 1999-2001. Atlanta (GA): U.S. Department of Health and Human Services; 2004. Report nr 4.
29. Fielder O, Altice FL. Attitudes toward and beliefs about prenatal HIV testing policies and mandatory HIV testing of newborns among drug users. AIDS Public Policy J 2005;20(3–4):74–91.
30. AAP Committee on Pediatric AIDS. HIV testing and prophylaxis to prevent mother-to-child transmission in the United States. Pediatrics 2008;122(5): 1127–34.
31. Pai NP, Tulsky JP, Cohan D, et al. Rapid point-of-care HIV testing in pregnant women: a systematic review and meta-analysis. Trop Med Int Health 2007;12: 162–73.
32. Rahangdale L, Sarnquist C, Feakins C, et al. Rapid HIV testing on labor and delivery. J Acquir Immune Defic Syndr 2007;46:376–8.
33. Association of Public Health Laboratories and CDC. HIV testing algorithms— a status report. Silver Spring (MD): Association of Public Health Laboratories; April 2009.
34. ACOG Committee on Obstetric Practice. ACOG committee opinion no. 418: prenatal and perinatal human immunodeficiency virus testing: expanded recommendations. Obstet Gynecol 2008;112(3):739–42.
35. HIV testing for mothers and newborns [Internet]; February 2008. Available at: http://statehealthfacts.org. Accessed July 2010.
36. Gray AD, Carlson R, Morgan MA, et al. Obstetrician gynecologists' knowledge and practice regarding human immunodeficiency virus screening. Obstet Gynecol 2007;110(5):1019–26.
37. Olges JR, Murphy BS, Caldwell GG, et al. Testing practices and knowledge of HIV among prenatal care providers in a low seroprevalence state. AIDS Patient Care STDS 2007;21(3):187–94.
38. Webber MP, Demas P, Blaney N, et al. Correlates of prenatal HIV testing in women with undocumented status at delivery. Matern Child Health J 2008; 12(4):427–34.
39. Podhurst LS, Storm DS, Dolgonos S. Women's opinions about routine HIV testing during pregnancy: implication for the opt-out approach. AIDS Patient Care STDS 2009;23(5):331–7.
40. Criniti SM, Aaron E, Levine AB. Using the rapid HIV test to rescreen women in the third trimester of pregnancy. J Midwifery Womens Health 2009;54(6):492–6.

41. Gaur S, Whitley-Williams P, Flash C, et al. Disparity in hospital utilization of rapid HIV-1 testing for women in labor with undocumented HIV status. Matern Child Health J 2010;14(2):268–73.
42. Peters V, Liu KL, Dominguez K, et al. Missed opportunities for perinatal HIV prevention among HIV exposed infants born 1996–2000, pediatric spectrum of disease cohort. Pediatrics 2003;111(5 Part 2):1186–91.
43. Havens PL, Mofenson LM. AAP Committee on Pediatric AIDS. Evaluation and management of the infant exposed to HIV-1 in the United States. Pediatrics 2009;123:175–87.
44. Bryson YJ, Luzuriaga K, Sullivan JL, et al. Proposed definitions for in utero versus intrapartum transmission of HIV-1. N Engl J Med 1992;327:1246–7.
45. Read JS, Brogly S, Basar M, et al. HIV diagnostic testing of infants at clinical sites in North America: 2002–2006. Pediatr Infect Dis J 2009;28:614–8.
46. Dunn DT, Brandt CD, Krivine A, et al. The sensitivity of HIV-1 DNA polymerase chain reaction in the neonatal period and the relative contributions of intra-uterine and intra-partum transmission. AIDS 1995;9:F7–11.
47. Shannon M, Lee KA. HIV-infected mothers' perceptions of uncertainty, stress, depression and social support during HIV viral testing of their infants. Arch Womens Ment Health 2008;11(4):259–67.

Prevention of Mother-to-Child Transmission of HIV: Antiretroviral Strategies

Jennifer S. Read, MD, MS, MPH, DTM&H

KEYWORDS

- Mother-to-child transmission • HIV-1 • Prevention
- Antiretrovirals

Prevention of mother-to-child transmission of human immunodeficiency virus type 1 (HIV) is just 1 component of the overall management of HIV-1–infected women and their children. Therefore, the use of antiretrovirals or other efficacious interventions for the prevention of mother-to-child transmission of HIV-1 (including cesarean section before labor and ruptured membranes, complete avoidance of breastfeeding) cannot be viewed in isolation from other components of optimal care for women of reproductive age, mothers, and children. The World Health Organization's[1] (WHO's) Strategic Approaches to the Prevention of HIV Infection in Infants includes 4 components: primary prevention of HIV-1 infection; prevention of unintended pregnancies among HIV-1–infected women; prevention of transmission of HIV-1 infection from mothers to children; and provision of ongoing support, care, and treatment to HIV-1–infected women and their families. Ideally, primary prevention of HIV-1 infection occurs, for example, an HIV-1–uninfected woman does not acquire HIV-1 infection either before or during pregnancy. To facilitate the prevention of acquisition of HIV-1 infection, individuals should know their own and their sexual partners' HIV-1 infection status, which is accomplished through the provision of and access to HIV-1 counseling and testing. Next, even if a woman acquires HIV-1 infection, prevention of unintended pregnancies is crucial. Antiretroviral therapy for women who need treatment of

The author has nothing to disclose.
Pediatric, Adolescent, and Maternal AIDS Branch, Center for Research for Mothers and Children, Eunice Kennedy Shriver National Institute of Child Health and Human Development, National Institutes of Health, Executive Building, Room 4B11C, 6100 Executive Boulevard, MSC 7510, Bethesda, MD 20892-7510, USA
E-mail address: JENNIFER_READ@NIH.GOV

Clin Perinatol 37 (2010) 765–776
doi:10.1016/j.clp.2010.08.007
0095-5108/10/$ – see front matter. Published by Elsevier Inc.

their HIV-1 infection, antiretroviral prophylaxis for women who do not yet need treatment, antiretroviral prophylaxis for infants of HIV-infected mothers, and other interventions to prevent mother-to-child transmission of HIV-1 should be available. Finally, HIV-1–infected women and their children need ongoing support, care, and treatment, including infant feeding, counseling, and support.

This review addresses antiretroviral strategies for the prevention of mother-to-child transmission of HIV-1 and is largely based on published US[2] and global[3] guidelines. Specifically, the review focuses on antiretrovirals for the secondary prevention of HIV-1 infection–prevention of HIV-1 transmission from a pregnant HIV-1–infected woman to her child. The review primarily addresses antiretroviral strategies for non-breastfeeding, HIV-1–infected women and their infants in resource-rich settings, such as the United States.[2] Antiretroviral strategies to prevent antepartum, intrapartum, and early postnatal transmission in resource-poor settings[3] are also addressed, albeit more briefly.

ANTIRETROVIRAL STRATEGIES TO PREVENT MOTHER-TO-CHILD TRANSMISSION OF HIV-1 IN THE UNITED STATES
Mechanisms of Action of Antiretrovirals in Preventing Mother-To-Child Transmission of HIV-1

Antiretrovirals prevent mother-to-child transmission of HIV-1 in 3 ways: decreasing the HIV-1 RNA concentration (viral load) in maternal blood and genital secretions[4,5]; infant pre-exposure prophylaxis; and infant post-exposure prophylaxis. The importance of maternal viral load as a risk factor for mother-to-child transmission has been clearly demonstrated.[4,6,7] However, the possibility of other mechanisms of action of antiretrovirals in preventing transmission besides simply lowering maternal viral load is suggested by several observations. First, there is no threshold maternal plasma viral load below which transmission does not occur; transmission has been observed at all maternal plasma viral loads.[4,7,8] Second, among women with low plasma viral loads (less than 1000 copies/mL), more intensive maternal antiretroviral regimens are associated with lower risks of transmission.[9] Also, maternal plasma load at delivery and antepartum antiretroviral use are each independent risk factors for transmission.[10] Preexposure infant prophylaxis can be achieved through the maternal administration of antiretrovirals that cross the placenta and result in adequate systemic drug concentrations in the infant. Postexposure infant prophylaxis can be accomplished through the administration of antiretrovirals to the infant after birth. In this situation, the antiretrovirals can protect the infant from acquiring infection from the virus transferred to the infant through maternal microtransfusions of blood during labor or swallowed by the infant during delivery. The efficacy of intrapartum or neonatal antiretroviral regimens for the prevention of mother-to-child transmission (ie, initiated too late to prevent transmission by decreasing maternal viral load)[11–17] lends further support to the concepts of infant pre- and postexposure prophylaxes.

Antiretrovirals for the Treatment of Maternal HIV-1 Infection and Prevention of Mother-To-Child Transmission of HIV-1

Guidelines for the administration of antiretrovirals in HIV-1–infected pregnant women in the United States have been developed to address antiretroviral treatment of women who meet criteria for treatment and antiretroviral prophylaxis for women who do not meet criteria for treatment.[2] Distinguishing between these 2 groups of women is accomplished by assessing the HIV-1 disease stage (clinical manifestations, plasma viral load, CD4 cell count) and has important implications with regard to when antiretroviral drugs are used during pregnancy, what drugs are given, and whether antiretrovirals are discontinued after delivery. Irrespective of whether or not antiretrovirals are given during pregnancy or whether antiretrovirals during pregnancy are given for treatment or prophylaxis, all infants of HIV-1–infected women should receive antiretroviral postexposure prophylaxis.

Antiretroviral therapy for HIV-1–infected pregnant women

In general, the indications for the initiation of antiretroviral therapy in women of reproductive age or in pregnant women are the same as those for other HIV-1–infected adults and adolescents.[18] According to these guidelines, antiretroviral therapy should be initiated in individuals with (1) a history of an AIDS-defining illness or with a CD4 cell count of less than 350 cells/mm^3, (2) HIV-1–associated nephropathy, and (3) hepatitis B virus coinfection when treatment of hepatitis B infection is indicated. Some experts recommend antiretroviral therapy for individuals with a CD4 cell count of 350 to 500 cells/mm^3. Once antiretroviral therapy is initiated, it is generally continued lifelong; antiretroviral therapy used during pregnancy should be continued through the intrapartum period (zidovudine administered as a continuous intravenous infusion during delivery and other antiretrovirals administered orally) and postpartum.

The choice of a specific antiretroviral treatment regimen during pregnancy is based on the antiretroviral history of the HIV-1–infected pregnant woman. Some women may already be receiving antiretroviral therapy for their own health when they become pregnant but others may initiate antiretroviral therapy after becoming pregnant. In general, if antiretroviral therapy is already being used when an HIV-1–infected woman becomes pregnant, this regimen should be continued if it is well tolerated and effectively suppressing the virus. However, because of the potential teratogenicity, it is generally recommended that efavirenz be avoided during the first trimester of pregnancy. Finally, a nevirapine-containing regimen should be continued, irrespective of the CD4 cell count, if the HIV-1–infected pregnant woman is tolerating the regimen and is virologically suppressed.

For those women who are not receiving antiretroviral therapy when they become pregnant but who meet the treatment criteria and initiate antiretroviral therapy during pregnancy, therapy should be started as soon as possible, even if the woman is in the first trimester of pregnancy. Antiretroviral resistance testing should be performed in all HIV-1–infected pregnant women before the initiation of antiretroviral therapy. This testing is especially important if there is detectable viremia or if the woman received antiretrovirals previously for prophylaxis or treatment. Nevirapine can be a component of the antiretroviral therapy regimen if the CD4 cell count is 250 cells/mm^3 or less. Because of an increased risk of hepatic toxicity at higher CD4 cell counts, it is recommended that nevirapine be included in the antiretroviral therapy regimen being initiated in pregnant women with higher CD4 cell counts only if the benefit clearly outweighs the risk.

HIV-1–infected pregnant women on antiretroviral therapy should use combination antiretroviral regimens including at least 3 antiretrovirals. A regimen including 2 nucleoside reverse transcriptase inhibitors (NRTIs) and either a non-NRTI (NNRTI) or a protease inhibitor (PI) should be used.

Based on clinical trials as well as a large amount of experience with use during pregnancy, zidovudine with lamivudine is the preferred NRTI regimen in pregnancy. Other NRTI regimens are used if the woman has a history of significant zidovudine toxicity (eg, severe anemia) or there is known zidovudine resistance. Zidovudine should be a component of any antiretroviral drug regimen used during pregnancy, if possible, because of its excellent transplacental passage. Of note, administering stavudine with didanosine should be avoided because of reports of hepatic failure and lactic acidosis among pregnant women who received this combination throughout pregnancy, and tenofovir (a preferred NRTI for nonpregnant women) should be given only in special circumstances (eg, zidovudine intolerance or resistance, chronic hepatitis B infection) because of potential fetal toxicity.

In terms of NNRTIs, efavirenz (a preferred NNRTI for nonpregnant women) is not recommended for use during the first trimester of pregnancy because of the potential for teratogenicity based on animal and human data. There are insufficient safety and pharmacokinetic data from pregnant women to recommend the administration of etravirine.

Based on efficacy data from adults and experience with use during pregnancy, lopinavir/ritonavir is the preferred PI in pregnant women. Of note, some PIs (eg, lopinavir/ritonavir) may require modification of dosing during pregnancy. Although experience with administration during pregnancy is more limited, alternative PIs for use in pregnant women are atazanavir/ritonavir, saquinavir, and indinavir. Saquinavir and indinavir may be less well tolerated. Data regarding administration during pregnancy are too limited to recommend darunavir, fosamprenavir, and tipranavir on a routine basis, although these drugs could be considered if other PIs are not tolerated.

Safety and pharmacokinetic data are too limited to recommend use of raltegravir (an integrase inhibitor) or enfuvirtide and maraviroc (entry inhibitors) during pregnancy. However, for those HIV-1–infected pregnant women in whom therapy with other classes of antiretrovirals has failed, these drugs could be considered in close consultation with obstetricians and others with appropriate expertise.

Antiretroviral prophylaxis for HIV-1–infected pregnant women

If an HIV-1–infected pregnant woman does not meet the criteria for antiretroviral therapy or chooses not to initiate antiretroviral therapy, use of antiretrovirals during pregnancy for the prevention of mother-to-child transmission should be considered. Antiretroviral prophylaxis is recommended for all HIV-1–infected pregnant women, irrespective of the plasma viral load. Unlike initiation of antiretroviral therapy, which is generally recommended as soon as possible (even during the first trimester), antiretroviral prophylaxis is generally initiated after the first trimester. Antiretroviral resistance testing should be performed in all HIV-1–infected pregnant women before the initiation of antiretroviral prophylaxis. This testing is especially important if the woman received antiretrovirals previously for transmission prophylaxis (ie, in a previous pregnancy).

In general, the same antiretroviral drug regimens used for treatment during pregnancy can be considered for use for transmission prophylaxis, but additional antiretroviral regimens also can be considered. For example, the combination of 3 NRTIs, zidovudine, lamivudine, and abacavir, can be considered for antiretroviral prophylaxis during pregnancy. If abacavir is given, testing for HLA-B*5701 should be performed to identify those at risk for hypersensitivity reactions.[19,20] Three-drug regimens including nelfinavir can be considered because of the large amount of experience with the use of nelfinavir during pregnancy. Because of the possibility of inadequate viral suppression and development of resistance, dual-NRTI regimens (ie, without a third antiretroviral) are not recommended.[21] US guidelines refer to the administration of zidovudine alone during pregnancy for transmission prophylaxis as controversial[2] but suggest considering zidovudine alone if the plasma viral load is less than 1000 copies/mL. However, British guidelines for the management of HIV-1–infected women recommend zidovudine alone beginning at 28 weeks as a valid option for women with plasma viral loads less than 10,000 copies/mL and wild-type virus, who do not require or do not want to use antiretroviral therapy during pregnancy, and who are willing to deliver by planned cesarean section.[22]

Although it is argued that, for prophylaxis, combination antiretroviral regimens of at least 3 drugs should be offered to all HIV-1–infected women in the United States,[2] new clinical trial data indicate that the risk of transmission among women with CD4 cell counts of 200 to 500 cells/mm^3 is indistinguishable whether a 3-drug antiretroviral regimen or a simpler antiretroviral prophylaxis regimen is used.[23] Specifically, women in the Kesho Bora trial were randomized to receive either zidovudine, lamivudine, and lopinavir/ritonavir or zidovudine (with a single dose of nevirapine at labor onset) beginning at 28 weeks' gestation. There was no statistically significant difference in the transmission rates at birth: 1.8% among women receiving the triple drug prophylaxis and 2.2% among women randomized to zidovudine with single-dose nevirapine. Thus, although the standard of care for antiretroviral prophylaxis among US women has been to give at least 3 antiretrovirals (based on observational data),[9,10] more complex antiretroviral regimens such as these do not definitively provide additional benefit in terms of transmission prevention.

In general, if antiretrovirals are being given only for transmission prophylaxis during pregnancy and not for treatment of the mother's own HIV-1 infection, the antiretrovirals are discontinued simultaneously after delivery. However, if planning to discontinue an NNRTI-containing regimen, it is important to consider continuation of the 2 NRTIs for a period (7–30 days) after stopping the NNRTI to reduce the risk of development of NNRTI resistance. If the woman used antiretrovirals during pregnancy for the prevention of mother-to-child transmission but subsequently (before discontinuation of the antiretrovirals after delivery) met the criteria for antiretroviral therapy, antiretrovirals for the treatment of her own HIV-1 infection would continue indefinitely (lifelong).

Intrapartum antiretroviral management of HIV-1–infected women
For those women who are known to be HIV-1–infected at the time of presentation for delivery, intravenous zidovudine during the intrapartum period is recommended (irrespective of receipt of antiretrovirals during pregnancy). If the woman was receiving a combination antiretroviral regimen during pregnancy, this regimen should be continued during the intrapartum period (with zidovudine being administered intravenously and other drugs administered orally).

For women of unknown HIV-1 infection status who present during labor, rapid HIV-1 antibody testing should be performed. If the result of the rapid test is positive, maternal (intravenous zidovudine) and infant antiretrovirals (see later discussion) should be initiated without waiting for the results of a confirmatory HIV-1 test. Some experts would add a single dose of maternal nevirapine (administered orally) to the maternal intravenous zidovudine regimen (see later discussion for infant management). If single-dose intrapartum/newborn nevirapine is administered, an antiretroviral tail should be used to decrease the risk of nevirapine resistance. The composition and duration of administration of this tail is not universally agreed on, but in the United States the use of maternal postpartum zidovudine/lamivudine for at least 7 days is suggested after intrapartum single-dose nevirapine.[2]

Antiretroviral management of infants born to HIV-1–infected women
Infants of HIV-1–infected women in the United States should receive 6 weeks of oral zidovudine, irrespective of maternal use of antiretrovirals during pregnancy and (if antiretrovirals used during pregnancy) the specific regimen. In the United Kingdom, a 4-week infant prophylaxis regimen is recommended,[22] and this shorter regimen could

be considered when there are concerns about adherence to the 6-week regimen or if significant toxicity is observed.

Other infant prophylaxis regimens have been evaluated in studies outside the United States, but such regimens have not been directly compared with the regimen comprising 6 weeks of oral zidovudine to the infant. HIV Prevention Trials Network (HPTN) 040/Pediatric AIDS Clinical Trials Group (PACTG) 1043 is an ongoing study evaluating the efficacy of different infant prophylaxis regimens in relationship to oral zidovudine for 6 weeks. Until the results of this or other studies are available, there are no data with which to make the decision to add drugs to the oral zidovudine infant prophylaxis regimen. However, some clinicians do administer additional antiretrovirals (besides oral zidovudine) to infants of HIV-1–infected women. For example, as noted earlier, some experts recommend addition of single-dose nevirapine (1 dose to the mother and 1 to the infant).

The timing of initiation of zidovudine prophylaxis for the infant is important. Zidovudine prophylaxis should begin as soon as possible after birth and preferably within the first 12 hours of life.[24] The dosing of zidovudine varies according to the gestational age of the infant (depending on whether the infant has a gestational age of<35 weeks or≥35 weeks).[2] This difference in dosing is because of the greater immaturity in hepatic metabolism with lower gestational ages.[25,26] In the United States, the administration of antiretrovirals other than zidovudine to preterm infants is not recommended because of the lack of pharmacokinetic and safety data.

MONITORING BEFORE, DURING, AND AFTER USE OF/EXPOSURE TO ANTIRETROVIRALS

The effectiveness of antiretroviral therapy in improving maternal CD4 cell counts and decreasing plasma viral load should be monitored carefully in any patient population, including HIV-1–infected pregnant women. In addition, the benefits of antiretrovirals for HIV-1–infected women and their infants (treatment of the mother's own HIV-1 infection, prevention of mother-to-child transmission of HIV-1) must be weighed against adverse events associated with these drugs.

Monitoring of HIV-1–Infected Pregnant Women Using Antiretrovirals

Response to therapy should be monitored by assessing the CD4 cell count at least every 3 months during pregnancy (and comparing these results to the those obtained at the initial antepartum visit). Similarly, the plasma viral load should be monitored at the initial antepartum visit, then 2 to 4 weeks after initiating or changing antiretroviral therapy, then monthly until the plasma viral load is undetectable, and then at least every 3 months during pregnancy. It is useful to obtain plasma viral load data at 34 to 36 weeks' gestation to make decisions regarding the mode of delivery (see the article by Legardy-Williams and colleagues elsewhere in this issue for further exploration of this topic).

As noted earlier, antiretroviral drug resistance testing should be performed for all women initiating antiretrovirals (either for treatment or for prophylaxis). Such testing should also be performed in pregnant women with suboptimal viral suppression after initiation of antiretroviral therapy (eg, failure to achieve a one log_{10} copies/mL decrease in plasma viral load after 30 days of therapy or failure to achieve a progressive decline to undetectable plasma viral load after 4 to 6 months of therapy) and in pregnant women with persistently detectable plasma viral loads despite having previously achieved undetectable plasma viral loads.

Laboratory monitoring to assess antiretroviral drug–related toxicities is based on known adverse events related to the drugs that the HIV-1–infected pregnant woman receives. For example, hepatic abnormalities have been associated with different classes of antiretrovirals: women (especially those with CD4 cell counts greater than 250 cells/mm^3) are at an increased risk of nevirapine-associated hepatotoxicity, PIs have been associated with hepatic dysfunction, and NRTIs are associated with hepatic steatosis and lactic acidosis. Another example is anemia associated with zidovudine. At a minimum, HIV-1–infected women receiving antiretrovirals during pregnancy should undergo a standard (1 hour, 50 g) glucose loading test at 24 to 28 weeks' gestation. Some experts recommend earlier glucose screening for women who initiated PI therapy before pregnancy.

Monitoring of HIV-1–Exposed Children with in Utero or Neonatal Exposure to Antiretrovirals

The first issue to consider in children of HIV-1–infected women who had in utero or neonatal exposure to antiretrovirals is drug toxicity. For example, zidovudine exposure is associated with anemia, and newborns with in utero and/or neonatal exposure to zidovudine should have a hematologic evaluation. Based on studies suggesting other laboratory abnormalities among infants with in utero or neonatal exposure to antiretrovirals,[27–33] some experts recommend more extensive laboratory assessments, such as a complete blood cell count with differential and hepatic transaminase assays.

In general studies to date evaluating in utero exposure to antiretrovirals, especially first trimester exposure, have not demonstrated significant associations between such antiretroviral exposure and infant congenital anomalies.[34–38] However, because of potential central nervous system abnormalities associated with first trimester exposure to efavirenz, use of this drug during the first trimester of pregnancy should be avoided. All cases of in utero antiretroviral drug exposure should be reported to the Antiretroviral Pregnancy Registry (http://www.APRegistry.com). (Note: some experts recommend that women who received antiretrovirals [especially efavirenz] during the first trimester of pregnancy undergo a second trimester ultrasonography to assess the fetal anatomy.)

The possibility of an association between the use of PIs during pregnancy (for treatment or prophylaxis) and infant preterm birth should be considered, although the data available at present are conflicting.[39–51] In general, however, the benefits of antiretrovirals for therapy and prophylaxis are thought to outweigh the small possible risk of preterm birth.

In utero exposure to NRTIs has been linked to mitochondrial dysfunction in French infants,[52,53] but other studies from the United States and Europe[28,54–59] have not corroborated the results of the French studies. Therefore, in the light of these conflicting data, further research in this area is needed. However, even if a clear association between in utero antiretroviral exposure and mitochondrial dysfunction is delineated, the absolute risk of severe mitochondrial dysfunction seems to be rare and is generally outweighed by the benefit of antiretrovirals in reducing the risk of mother-to-child transmission of HIV-1.

ANTIRETROVIRAL STRATEGIES TO PREVENT MOTHER-TO-CHILD TRANSMISSION OF HIV-1 IN RESOURCE-LIMITED SETTINGS

In November 2009, the WHO revised its guidelines regarding the use of antiretroviral drugs during pregnancy.[3] There were several key recommendations. The first set of recommendations addressed antiretroviral therapy for HIV-1–infected pregnant women and management of their infants. First, antiretroviral therapy is recommended for all HIV-1–infected pregnant women with CD4 cell counts of 350 cells/mm^3 or less, irrespective of the WHO clinical stage, and for all HIV-1–infected pregnant women in WHO clinical stage 3 or 4, irrespective of their CD4 cell count. Second, antiretroviral therapy, if indicated, should be initiated as soon as possible (even during the first trimester) and once initiated should be continued lifelong. Third, the preferred first-line therapeutic regimen should contain zidovudine and lamivudine, along with either nevirapine or efavirenz. Alternative regimens recommended include (1) tenofovir, with lamivudine or emtricitabine, and nevirapine or (2) tenofovir, with lamivudine or emtricitabine, and efavirenz. Fourth, infants of HIV-1–infected women receiving antiretroviral therapy should receive daily doses of nevirapine from birth until 6 weeks of age (breastfeeding infants) or daily doses of zidovudine or nevirapine from birth until 6 weeks of age (nonbreastfeeding infants).

The second set of recommendations addressed antiretroviral prophylaxis for HIV-1–infected pregnant women. First, all HIV-1–infected pregnant women who do not meet the criteria for antiretroviral therapy should receive antiretroviral prophylaxis. Such prophylaxis should be started as early as 14 weeks (second trimester), or as soon as possible if an HIV-1–infected woman presents late in pregnancy or during labor. Second, 2 different options for antiretroviral prophylaxis were recommended (Option A and Option B). Option A consists of daily zidovudine during the antepartum period, single-dose nevirapine at the onset of labor, and zidovudine with lamivudine during the intrapartum period and for 7 days after delivery. If zidovudine was used for more than 4 weeks during the antepartum period, then the other components of Option A (nevirapine and zidovudine/lamivudine) can be omitted. Breastfeeding infants of these women should receive daily nevirapine from birth until 1 week after complete cessation of breastfeeding. Nonbreastfeeding infants should receive daily zidovudine or nevirapine from birth until 6 weeks of age.

Option B consists of a 3-drug antiretroviral regimen, initiated as early as 14 weeks' gestation until 1 week after complete cessation of breastfeeding. The recommended regimens are: zidovudine, lamivudine, and lopinavir/ritonavir; zidovudine, lamivudine, and abacavir; zidovudine, lamivudine, and efavirenz; and tenofovir, lamivudine or emtricitabine, and efavirenz. Breastfeeding infants of these women should receive daily nevirapine from birth until 6 weeks of age. Nonbreastfeeding infants should receive daily zidovudine or nevirapine from birth until 6 weeks of age.

SUMMARY

Antiretrovirals for the secondary prevention of HIV-1 infection, prevention of HIV-1 transmission from an HIV-1–infected woman to her child, must be considered as part of an overall strategy for the prevention of pediatric HIV infection (primary prevention of HIV-1 infection; prevention of unintended pregnancies among HIV-1–infected women; prevention of transmission of HIV-1 infection from mothers to children; and provision of ongoing support, care, and treatment to HIV-1–infected women and their families). Antiretroviral strategies to prevent mother-to-child transmission of HIV-1 in nonbreastfeeding populations comprise antiretroviral treatment of HIV-1–infected pregnant women who need antiretrovirals for their own health, antiretroviral prophylaxis for HIV-1–infected pregnant women who do not yet meet the criteria for treatment, and antiretroviral prophylaxis for infants of HIV-1–infected mothers. Delineating between HIV-1–infected women who are eligible for antiretroviral treatment and other HIV-1–infected women who are not yet eligible for treatment and who should receive prophylaxis is essential. All infants of HIV-1–infected mothers should receive antiretroviral prophylaxis. The effectiveness of antiretrovirals during pregnancy should be monitored, and the benefits of antiretrovirals must be weighed against the adverse events associated with these drugs.

REFERENCES

1. World Health Organization. Strategies approaches to the prevention of HIV infection in infants: report of a WHO meeting, Morges (Switzerland) 2002. World Health Organization, 2003. Available at: http://www.who.int/hiv/pub/mtct/en/StrategicApproachesE.pdf. Accessed June 21, 2010.
2. Panel on Treatment of HIV-Infected Pregnant Women and Prevention of Perinatal Transmission. Recommendations for use of antiretroviral drugs in pregnant HIV-1-infected women for maternal health and interventions to reduce perinatal HIV transmission in the United States. May 24, 2010; p. 1–117. Available at: http://aidsinfo.nih.gov/ContentFiles/PerinatalGL.pdf. Accessed June 21, 2010.
3. World Health Organization. Rapid advice: use of antiretroviral drugs for treating pregnant women and preventing HIV infection in infants – November 2009. Geneva (Switzerland): World Health Organization, 2009. Available at: http://www.who.int/hiv/pub/mtct/rapid_advice_mtct.pdf. Accessed June 21, 2010.
4. Sperling RS, Shapiro DE, Coombs RW, et al. Maternal viral load, zidovudine treatment, and the risk of transmission of human immunodeficiency virus type 1 from mother to infant. Pediatric AIDS Clinical Trials Group Protocol 076 Study Group. N Engl J Med 1996;335(22):1621–9.
5. Chuachoowong R, Shaffer N, Siriwasin W, et al. Short-course antenatal zidovudine reduces both cervicovaginal human immunodeficiency virus type 1 RNA levels and risk of perinatal transmission. J Infect Dis 2000;181(1):99–106.
6. Dickover RE, Garratty EM, Herman SA, et al. Identification of levels of maternal HIV-1 RNA associated with risk of perinatal transmission: effect of maternal zidovudine treatment on viral load. JAMA 1996;275(8):599–605.
7. Shapiro DE, Sperling RS, Coombs RW. Effect of zidovudine on perinatal HIV-1 transmission and maternal viral load. Lancet 1999;354(9173):156.
8. Garcia PM, Kalish LA, Pitt J, et al. Maternal levels of plasma human immunodeficiency virus type 1 RNA and the risk of perinatal transmission. N Engl J Med 1999;341(6):394–402.
9. Ioannidis JP, Abrams EJ, Ammann A, et al. Perinatal transmission of human immunodeficiency virus type 1 by pregnant women with RNA virus loads < 1000 copies/mL. J Infect Dis 2001;183(4):539–45.
10. Cooper ER, Charurat M, Mofenson LM, et al. Combination antiretroviral strategies for the treatment of pregnant women and prevention of perinatal HIV-1 transmission. J Acquir Immune Defic Syndr Hum Retrovirol 2002;29(5):484–94.
11. Wade NA, Birkhead GS, Warren BL, et al. Abbreviated regimens of zidovudine prophylaxis and perinatal transmission of the human immunodeficiency virus. N Engl J Med 1998;339(20):1409–14.
12. Petra Study Team. Efficacy of three short-course regimens of zidovudine and lamivudine in preventing early and late transmission of HIV-1 from mother-to-child in Tanzania, South Africa, and Uganda (Petra study): a randomized, double-blind, placebo-controlled trial. Lancet 2002;359(9313):1178–86.
13. Jackson JB, Musoke P, Fleming T, et al. Intrapartum and neonatal single-dose nevirapine compared with zidovudine for prevention of mother-to-child transmission of HIV-1 in Kampala, Uganda: 18-month follow-up of the HIVNET 012 randomised trial. Lancet 2003;362(9387):859–68.

14. Moodley D, Moodley J, Coovadia H, et al. A multicenter randomized controlled trial of nevirapine versus a combination of zidovudine and lamivudine to reduce intrapartum and early postpartum mother-to-child transmission of human immunodeficiency virus type 1. J Infect Dis 2003;187(5):725–35.

15. Taha TE, Kumwenda NI, Gibbons A, et al. Short postexposure prophylaxis in newborn babies to reduce mother-to-child transmission of HIV-1: NVAZ randomised clinical trial. Lancet 2003;362(9391):1171–7.

16. Taha TE, Kumwenda NI, Hoover DR, et al. Nevirapine and zidovudine at birth to reduce perinatal transmission of HIV in an African setting: a randomized controlled trial. JAMA 2004;292(2):202–9.

17. Gray GE, Urban M, Chersich MF, et al. A randomized trial of two postexposure prophylaxis regimens to reduce mother-to-child HIV-1 transmission in infants of untreated mothers. AIDS 2005;19(12):1289–97.

18. Panel on Antiretroviral Guidelines for Adults and Adolescents. Guidelines for the use of antiretroviral agents in HIV-1-infected adults and adolescents. Department of Health and Human Services. 2009. p. 1–161. Available at: http://www.aidsinfo.nih.gov/ContentFiles/AdultandAdolescentGL.pdf. Accessed June 21, 2010.

19. Saag M, Balu R, Phillips E, et al. High sensitivity of human leukocyte antigen-b*5701 as a marker for immunologically confirmed abacavir hypersensitivity in white and black patients. Clin Infect Dis 2008;46(7):1111–8.

20. Mallal S, Phillips E, Carosi G, et al. HLA-B*5701 screening for hypersensitivity to abacavir. N Engl J Med 2008;568(6):568–79.

21. Clarke JR, Braganza R, Mirza A, et al. Rapid development of genotypic resistance to lamivudine when combined with zidovudine in pregnancy. J Med Virol 1999;59(3):364–8.

22. de Ruiter A, Mercey D, Anderson J, et al. British HIV Association and Children's HIV Association guidelines for the management of HIV infection in pregnant women 2008. HIV Med 2008;9:452–502.

23. de Vincenzi I, Kesho Bora Study Group. Triple-antiretroviral prophylaxis during pregnancy and breastfeeding compared to short-ARV prophylaxis to prevent mother-to-child transmission of HIV-1: the Kesho Bora randomized controlled clinical trial in five sites in Burkina Faso, Kenya and South Africa. Program and Abstracts of the 5th International AIDS Society Conference on HIV Pathogenesis, Treatment, and Prevention [abstract LBPE C01]. Capetown (South Africa), July 19–22, 2009.

24. Wade NA, Birkhead GS, French PT. Short courses of zidovudine and perinatal transmission of HIV [letter]. N Engl J Med 1999;340(13):1040–3.

25. Mirochnick M, Capparelli E, Connor J. Pharmacokinetics of zidovudine in infants: a population analysis across studies. Clin Pharmacol Ther 1999;66(1):16–24.

26. Caparelli E, Mirochnick M, Dankner WM, et al. Pharmacokinetics and tolerance of zidovudine in preterm infants. J Pediatr 2003;142(1):47–52.

27. Lorenzi P, Spicher VM, Laubereau B, et al. Antiretroviral therapies in pregnancy: maternal, fetal and neonatal effects. Swiss HIV Cohort Study, the Swiss Collaborative HIV and Pregnancy Study, and the Swiss Neonatal HIV Study. AIDS 1998;12:F241–7.

28. Sperling RS, Shapiro DE, McSherry GD, et al. Safety of the maternal infant zidovudine regimen utilized in the Pediatric ADIS Clinical Trial Group 076 Study. AIDS 1998;12:1805–13.

29. Le Chenadec J, Mayaux MJ, Guihenneuc-Jouyaux C, et al. Perinatal antiretroviral treatment and hematopoiesis in HIV-uninfected infants. AIDS 2003;17:2053–61.

30. Bellon Cano JM, Sanchez-Ramon S, Ciria L, et al. The effects on infants of potent antiretroviral therapy during pregnancy: a report from Spain. Med Sci Monit 2004; 10:CR179–84.

31. European Collaborative Study. Levels and patterns of neutrophil cell counts over the first 8 years of life in children of HIV-1-infected mothers. AIDS 2004;18:2009–17.
32. Bunders M, Thorne C, Newell ML. Maternal and infant factors and lymphocyte, CD4 and CD8 cell counts in uninfected children of HIV-1-infected mothers. AIDS 2005;19:1071–9.
33. Mussi-Pinhata MM, Rego MA, Freimanis L, et al. Maternal antiretrovirals and hepatic enzyme, hematologic abnormalities among human immunodeficiency virus type 1-uninfected infants: the NISDI Perinatal Study. Pediatr Infect Dis J 2007;26(11):1032–7.
34. Antiretroviral Pregnancy Registry Steering Committee. Antiretroviral pregnancy registry international interim report for 1 January 1989 through 31 July 2009. Available at: http://www.apregistry.com/forms/interim_report.pdf. Accessed June 21, 2010.
35. Patel D, Thorne C, Fiore S, et al. Does highly active antiretroviral therapy increase the risk of congenital abnormalities in HIV-infected women? J Acquir Immune Defic Syndr 2005;40:116–8.
36. Watts DH, Li D, Handelsman E, et al. Assessment of birth defects according to maternal therapy among infants in the Women and Infants Transmission Study. J Acquir Immune Defic Syndr 2007;44:299–305.
37. Townsend CL, Willey BA, Cortina-Borja M, et al. Antiretroviral therapy and congenital abnormalities in infants born to HIV-infected women in the UK and Ireland, 1990 to 2007. AIDS 2009;23:519–24.
38. Joao EC, Calvet GA, Krauss MR, et al. Maternal antiretroviral use during pregnancy and infant congenital anomalies: The NISDI Perinatal Study. J Acquir Immune Defic Syndr 2010;53(2):176–85.
39. European Collaborative Study. Swiss mother and Child HIV cohort study. Combination antiretroviral therapy and duration of pregnancy. AIDS 2000;14(18):2913–20.
40. Tuomala RE, Shapiro DE, Mofenson LM, et al. Antiretroviral therapy during pregnancy and the risk of an adverse outcome. N Engl J Med 2002;346(24):1863–70.
41. Thorne C, Patel D, Newell ML. Increased risk of adverse pregnancy outcomes in HIV-infected women treated with highly active antiretroviral therapy in Europe. AIDS 2004;18(17):2337–9.
42. Tuomala RE, Watts DH, Li D, et al. Improved obstetric outcomes and few maternal toxicities are associated with antiretroviral therapy, including highly active antiretroviral therapy during pregnancy. J Acquir Immune Defic Syndr 2005;38(4):449–73.
43. Szyld EG, Warley EM, Freimanis L, et al. Maternal antiretroviral drugs during pregnancy and infant low birth weight and preterm birth. AIDS 2006;20(18):2345–53.
44. Cotter AM, Garcia AG, Duthely ML, et al. Is antiretroviral therapy during pregnancy associated with an increased risk of preterm delivery, low birth weight, or stillbirth? J Infect Dis 2006;193(9):1195–201.
45. Kourtis AP, Schmid CH, Jamieson DJ, et al. Use of antiretroviral therapy in pregnancy HIV-infected women and the risk of premature delivery: a meta-analysis. AIDS 2007;21(5):607–15.
46. Townsend C, Cortina-Borja M, Peckham CS, et al. Antiretroviral therapy and premature delivery in diagnosed HIV-infected women in the United Kingdom and Ireland. AIDS 2007;21(8):1019–26.
47. Schulte J, Dominguez K, Sukalac T, et al. Declines in low birth weight and preterm birth among infants who were born to HIV-infected women during an era of

increased us of maternal antiretroviral drugs: Pediatric Spectrum of HIV Disease, 1989–2004. Pediatrics 2007;119(4):e900–6.

48. Ravizza M, Martinelli P, Bucceri A, et al. Treatment with protease inhibitors and coinfection with hepatitis C virus are independent predictors of preterm delivery in HIV-infected pregnant women. J Infect Dis 2007;195(6):913–4.

49. Grosch-Woerner I, Puch K, Maier RF, et al. Increased rate of prematurity associated with antenatal antiretroviral therapy in a German/Austrian cohort of HIV-1-infected women. HIV Med 2008;9(1):6–13.

50. Machado ES, Hofer CB, Costa TT, et al. Pregnancy outcome in women infected with HIV-1 receiving combination antiretroviral therapy before versus after conception. Sex Transm Infect 2009;85(2):82–7.

51. Patel K, Shapiro DE, Brogly SB, et al. Prenatal protease inhibitor use and risk of preterm birth among HIV-infected women initiating antiretroviral drugs during pregnancy. J Infect Dis 2010;201(7):1035–44.

52. Blanche S, Tardieu M, Rustin P, et al. Persistent mitochondrial dysfunction and perinatal exposure to antiretroviral nucleoside analogues. Lancet 1999; 354(9184):1084–9.

53. Barret B, Tardieu M, Rustin P, et al. Persistent mitochondrial dysfunction in HIV-1-exposed but uninfected infants: clinical screening in a large prospective cohort. AIDs 2003;17(12):1769–85.

54. The Perinatal Safety Review Working Group. Nucleoside exposure in the children of HIV-infected women receiving antiretroviral drugs: absence of clear evidence for mitochondrial disease in children who died before 5 years of age in five United States cohorts. J Acquir Immune Defic Syndr 2000;25(3):261–8.

55. Lipshultz SE, Easley KA, Orav EJ, et al. Absence of cardiac toxicity of zidovudine in infants. N Engl J Med 2000;353(11):759–66.

56. European Collaborative Study. Exposure to antiretroviral therapy in utero or early life: the health of uninfected children born to HIV-infected women. J Acquir Immune Defic Syndr 2003;32(4):380–7.

57. Alimenti A, Forbes JC, Oberlander TF, et al. A prospective controlled study of neurodevelopment in HIV-uninfected children exposed to combination antiretroviral drugs in pregnancy. Pediatrics 2006;118(40):e1139–45.

58. Brogly SB, Ylitalo N, Mofenson LM, et al. In utero nucleoside reverse transcriptase inhibitor exposure and signs of possible mitochondrial dysfunction in HIV-uninfected children. AIDS 2007;21(8):929–38.

59. Hankin C, Lyall H, Peckham C, et al. Monitoring death and cancer in children born to HIV-infected women in England and Wales: use of HIV surveillance and national routine data. AIDS 2007;21(7):867–9.

Prevention of Mother-to-Child Transmission of HIV: The Role of Cesarean Delivery

Jennifer K. Legardy-Williams, MPH[a],*,
Denise J. Jamieson, MD, MPH[a], Jennifer S. Read, MD, MS, MPH, DTM&H[b]

KEYWORDS

• Mother-to-child transmission • Cesarean delivery
• HIV • Prevention

An increasing proportion of deliveries in the United States are cesarean. In 2006, 31% of approximately 4.2 million live births in the United States were delivered via cesarean delivery.[1] Similar to overall trends, the proportion of HIV-infected women having a cesarean delivery has also increased,[2] presumably due, in part, to the role of cesarean delivery in the prevention mother-to-child transmission (MTCT) of HIV. Cesarean delivery before the onset of labor and before rupture of the amniotic membranes can decrease the risk of MTCT of HIV.[3,4]

In the context of HIV prevention, the term *elective cesarean delivery* (ECD) is used to denote cesarean deliveries performed prior to the onset of labor and prior to the rupture of membranes. The American College of Obstetricians and Gynecologists (ACOG) and the Department of Health and Human Services (DHHS) Panel on Treatment of HIV-Infected Pregnant Women and Prevention of Perinatal Transmission recommend ECD for HIV-infected women with plasma viral loads of more than 1,000 copies/mL.[5,6] This article discusses the rationale for the beneficial role of ECD in preventing

The authors have nothing to disclose.
The findings and conclusions in this report are those of the author(s) and do not necessarily represent the official position of the Centers for Disease Control and Prevention or the National Institutes of Health.
[a] Division of Reproductive Health, National Center for Chronic Disease Prevention and Health Promotion, Centers for Disease Control and Prevention, 4770 Buford Highway, MS-K-34, Atlanta, GA 30341, USA
[b] Pediatric, Adolescent, and Maternal AIDS Branch, Eunice Kennedy Shriver National Institute of Child Health and Human Development, National Institutes of Health, Executive Building, Room 4B11C, 6100 Executive Boulevard MSC 7510, Bethesda, MD 20892-7510, USA
* Corresponding author.
E-mail address: jlegardy@cdc.gov

Clin Perinatol 37 (2010) 777–785
doi:10.1016/j.clp.2010.08.013
0095-5108/10/$ – see front matter. Published by Elsevier Inc.

perinatology.theclinics.com

MTCT of HIV, the evidence for efficacy of ECD in preventing MTCT of HIV, recommendations for ECD as a prevention strategy in the United States, risk and morbidity of ECD in HIV-infected women and their infants, and unanswered questions.

RATIONALE FOR THE PREVENTIVE BENEFITS OF ECD

A large proportion of MTCT of HIV occurs intrapartum.[7–12] One potential mechanism of transmission is direct fetal exposure to infected maternal blood and cervicovaginal secretions in the maternal genital tract.[10,13–16] An early study of twins born to HIV-infected women found that the first-born twin was at higher risk for HIV transmission compared to the second twin.[13] This finding suggested that the first twin born vaginally may be at increased risk because of greater exposure to infected blood and secretions in the birth canal since the first twin is the first to pass through the birth canal and remains in the birth canal for a longer period of time. Although later findings from studies on twins did not confirm a higher risk in the first born,[17] this early study sparked debate about the potential protective role of cesarean delivery.

In addition, studies showed increased risk of MTCT of HIV with increased duration of ruptured membranes.[9,10,15,18] This suggested that transmission may be a result of ascending infection from the lower genital tract and that once the integrity of the amniotic membranes is breached, infants are at increased risk for HIV acquisition.[19] This provided further evidence to substantiate the hypothesis that performing a cesarean delivery may prevent MTCT of HIV.

Another potential mechanism for MTCT of HIV is microtransfusions of maternal blood during uterine contractions.[11,20,21] Placental microtransfusions occur when a small amount of maternal blood crosses the placenta to the fetus. Two studies assessing the levels of placental alkaline phosphatase, which is a marker of placental passage,[20,21] found that the lowest cord placental alkaline phosphatase level, thus volume of maternal–fetal transfusion, was among women undergoing ECD. This lent further support for performing ECD prior to the onset of uterine contractions.

EFFICACY OF ECD

In the late 1990s, groundbreaking results from a multicenter randomized clinical trial (RCT) and a large individual patient data meta-analysis showed the efficacy and effectiveness of ECD in reducing MTCT of HIV.[3,4] Researchers of the RCT, conducted in six European countries, investigated the risks and benefits of ECD and vaginal delivery among HIV-infected women. They found the risk of MTCT of HIV was 80% lower among women allocated to the ECD group. Analyses of the actual method of delivery showed that the risk of transmission was highest among women who delivered vaginally (10.2%), followed by those who had a cesarean delivery after onset of labor or ruptured membranes (8.8%), with the lowest risk among those who underwent ECD (2.4%).[4] An individual patient data meta-analysis from 15 prospective cohort studies found that, after controlling for advanced maternal age, receipt of antiretrovirals during pregnancy, and infant birth weight, ECD was associated with a lower risk of transmission of HIV (odds ratio, 0.43; 95% CI, 0.33–0.56) compared with other methods of delivery.[3]

Although these results clearly showed a benefit of ECD in reducing MTCT of HIV, these studies were primarily conducted before widespread use of combination antiretroviral regimens and viral load testing.

Current Recommendations

In the United States, the estimated number of women living with HIV was ~160,000 in 2007,[22] there were an estimated 8650–8900 births among HIV-infected women in 2006,[23] and 141 infants were diagnosed with HIV infection acquired through mother-to-child transmission in 2008.[22] This estimate is approximately 30% higher than estimates of births in 2002, thus, strategies for preventing MTCT are of utmost importance. Results from the individual-patient meta-analysis and the multisite, randomized controlled trial discussed earlier were the impetus for the ACOG and the DHHS Panel to issue recommendations regarding ECD.[24,25] Currently, ACOG and the DHHS Panel recommend that (1) HIV-infected women with plasma viral loads >1,000 copies/mL be counseled on the benefits of ECD to prevent MTCT; (2) ECD should be performed at 38 completed gestational weeks, based on the best clinical estimate, to minimize the odds of onset of labor and rupture of the membranes; (3) HIV-infected women should receive antiretrovirals during pregnancy and antiretrovirals should not be interrupted before the cesarean delivery; and (4) women receive intravenous zidovudine 3 hours before ECD.[5,6] Prior to the ACOG and DHHS Panel recommendations, 33% of infants born to HIV-infected women were delivered by ECD in the United States.[26] Since the release of these recommendations in the United States, 40% of infants born to HIV-infected women were delivered by ECD.[2,26] This shift in the proportion of infants delivered through ECD is believed to be attributed to the implementation of these policies and recommendations.

MORBIDITY AND RISKS OF ECD

Because cesarean deliveries are considered a major operative procedure, there are concerns about potential risks to the mothers and infants.

Maternal Morbidity

HIV-infected women have an increased risk of morbidity associated with cesarean delivery when compared with HIV-uninfected controls, and the risk of complications is correlated with the degree of immunosuppression.[27–31] In addition, cesarean delivery is associated with an increased risk of complications compared with vaginal delivery in women both infected and not infected with HIV. Women not infected with HIV have an increased risk of intra- and postoperative complications associated with cesarean deliveries, particularly in emergency cesarean deliveries, compared with vaginal deliveries.[32–37] Among HIV-infected women, there are several studies,[4,38–43] including one RCT, comparing postpartum morbidity according to the mode of delivery. These studies, which have been summarized in a Cochrane review,[44] also found that the risk of postpartum morbidity, primarily infectious (eg, urinary tract infection, pneumonia, wound infection, septicemia, and episiotomy infection), was highest with non-ECD, intermediate with ECD, and lowest with vaginal delivery. The DHHS Panel[6] concluded that the observed postpartum morbidity with ECD among HIV-infected women was not of sufficient frequency or severity to outweigh the benefit of decreased transmission of HIV to the infant. Due to the increased risk of infection associated with cesarean delivery, all women, regardless of HIV infection status, should receive prophylactic antibiotics perioperatively. Although ECD is beneficial, data suggest that HIV-infected women may be at an increased risk of postpartum morbidity and mortality as result of cesarean delivery in resource-limited countries.[45,46] Furthermore, countries that have high

HIV seroprevalence among pregnant women may not have adequate resources to perform cesarean deliveries for all HIV-infected women.

Neonatal Morbidity

Studies among women without HIV infection have shown that infants who are delivered before 39 of weeks gestation are at an increased risk for neonatal respiratory morbidity and other complications. Two recent prospective cohort studies describing birth outcomes among pregnant HIV-infected women found that the proportion of infants with respiratory morbidity, including respiratory distress syndrome, was higher among those delivered by ECD or other cesarean delivery compared with those delivered vaginally.[47,48] Kreitchmann and colleagues[47] found that 87 of 1086 HIV-exposed infants had some respiratory morbidity. Specifically, a significantly higher proportion experienced respiratory distress syndrome (RDS) when delivered via ECD and other cesarean delivery compared with vaginal delivery (4.4%, 5.2%, and 1.4%, respectively).[17,49] However, the consequences of this increased risk of respiratory distress syndrome and other respiratory morbidities (eg, requirement for mechanical ventilation, duration of intensive care unit stay, long-term sequelae) need to be more thoroughly evaluated. Currently, the benefits of cesarean delivery in preventing MTCT of HIV are believed to outweigh the small risk of respiratory morbidity among near-term infants.[48]

To strike a balance between minimizing the risks of iatrogenic prematurity and ensuring that the ECD is performed prior to the onset of labor, ACOG recommends that infants of HIV-infected women be delivered a week earlier (at 38 completed weeks of gestation) than is customary among uninfected women (39 completed weeks of gestation).[5] Although the ACOG recommends testing amniotic fluid if elective delivery is being considered before 39 weeks to determine fetal pulmonary maturity,[50] amniocentesis should not be routinely performed in HIV-infected women. Therefore, clinicians should generally depend on the best clinical estimate of gestational age to determine when to deliver.[51]

Another potential risk of cesarean delivery is inadvertent laceration of the infant at surgery, which could increase the risk of HIV acquisition. However, the risk of laceration at cesarean delivery is low.[52]

Unanswered Questions

Despite the tremendous advances in the field of prevention of MTCT of HIV, some unresolved questions remain, such as the need for an ECD in HIV-infected, pregnant women with low plasma viral loads (<1,000 copies/mL), whether ECD is beneficial in women who are using combination antiretroviral regimens, and in what timeframe is the benefit of ECD lost after the onset of labor or rupture of membranes.

Findings from several studies show low MTCT rates for HIV-infected women with low viral loads.[53–56] In one recent study, the MTCT rate among term births (including all modes of delivery) was 0.6% with maternal HIV-1 RNA levels at <400 copies/mL at delivery and 0.4% with levels <50 copies/mL.[52] Similarly, data regarding women receiving combination antiretroviral regimens indicate a very low risk of MTCT.[57] Recent European surveillance data showed a similarly low rate of transmission (0.8%) among women using combination antiretroviral regimens for at least the last 14 days of pregnancy, regardless of mode of delivery.[55] Given these very low transmission rates, a very large study would be needed to definitively evaluate the risk of MTCT of HIV according to mode of delivery among women with very low plasma viral loads or women who are using combination antiretroviral regimens. Those studies that have evaluated this issue are often underpowered and have yielded conflicting results.

Recent data from the European Collaborative Study[53] show an 80% reduction in transmission risk with ECD among women with viral loads of <400 copies/mL when adjusting for combination antiretroviral therapy and prematurity (adjusted odds ratio, 0.20; 95% CI 0.05–0.65). By contrast, other studies failed to show a significant protective effect of ECD, specifically among women who deliver at term with viral loads of <400 copies/mL[56] and among women on combination antiretroviral therapy when adjusting for viral load.[55] Another clinical question that arises but that has not been rigorously evaluated is whether there is a benefit of ECD for pregnant women presenting late in pregnancy who may not have a viral load measurement available prior to delivery. For those women who have not been taking antiretroviral therapy antenatally, it is unlikely that they will have maximal viral load suppression prior to delivery. Therefore, ECD is generally recommended for these women.[6]

Another unanswered question is the time after which there is no longer a benefit of cesarean delivery after the onset of labor or rupture of membranes. In the individual patient data meta-analysis regarding mode of delivery and MTCT of HIV,[3] women who underwent a cesarean delivery after onset of labor or after ruptured membranes were at increased risk of transmission compared with women who underwent delivery by ECD. Early studies showed an increased risk of MTCT of HIV when the rupture of membranes occurred 4 or more hours before delivery.[9,10,15,18,58] In a more recent individual patient meta-analysis of data from prospective studies regarding HIV-infected women with a duration of ruptured membranes of 24 hours or less, there was a statistically significant increased risk of MTCT of HIV of approximately 2% with each 1-hour increase in the duration of ruptured membranes.[58] It remains unclear how a pregnant woman with known HIV infection who presents in early labor or shortly after rupture of the membranes should be counseled about the optimal method of delivery.

SUMMARY

ECD has been shown to be efficacious and generally safe among HIV-infected women. The benefit of ECD for prevention of MTCT of HIV outweighs the potential risks of postpartum morbidity. Similarly, the risk to the infant (primarily related to iatrogenic prematurity) is outweighed by the benefit of ECD for prevention. Whether ECD is beneficial in HIV-infected pregnant women on highly active antiretroviral therapy with very low viral loads at the time of delivery, and whether it should still be performed in women who present after onset of labor or rupture of the membranes remain to be clarified.

REFERENCES

1. Martin JA, Hamilton BE, Sutton PD, et al. Births: final data for 2006. National vital statistics reports. Hyattsville (MD): National Center for Health Statistics; 2009;57(7).
2. Dominguez KL, Lindegren ML, D'Almada PJ, et al. Increasing trend of cesarean deliveries in HIV-infected women in the United States from 1994 to 2000. J Acquir Immune Defic Syndr 2003;33(2):232–8.
3. The International Perinatal HIV Group. The mode of delivery and the risk of vertical transmission of human immunodeficiency virus type 1—a meta-analysis of 15 prospective cohort studies. The International Perinatal HIV Group. N Engl J Med 1999;340(13):977–87.
4. The European Mode of Delivery Collaboration. Elective caesarean-section versus vaginal delivery in prevention of vertical HIV-1 transmission: a randomised clinical trial. The European Mode of Delivery Collaboration. Lancet 1999;353(9158): 1035–9.

5. ACOG Committee Opinion: Scheduled cesarean delivery and the prevention of vertical transmission of HIV infection. Number 234, May 2000 (replaces number 219, August 1999). Int J Gynaecol Obstet 2001;73(3):279–81.
6. Panel on treatment of HIV-infected pregnant women and prevention of perinatal transmission. Recommendations for use of antiretroviral drugs in pregnant HIV-1-infected women for maternal health and interventions to reduce perinatal HIV transmission in the United States. May 29, 2010. p. 1–117 NIH. Available at: http://aidsinfo.nih.gov/ContentFiles/PerinatalGL.pdf. Accessed May 26, 2010.
7. Kourtis AP, Bulterys M, Nesheim SR, et al. Understanding the timing of HIV transmission from mother to infant. JAMA 2001;285(6):709–12.
8. Kuhn L, Abrams EJ, Matheson PB, et al. Timing of maternal-infant HIV transmission: associations between intrapartum factors and early polymerase chain reaction results. New York City Perinatal HIV Transmission Collaborative Study Group. AIDS 1997;11(4):429–35.
9. Minkoff H, Burns DN, Landesman S, et al. The relationship of the duration of ruptured membranes to vertical transmission of human immunodeficiency virus. Am J Obstet Gynecol 1995;173(2):585–9.
10. Landesman SH, Kalish LA, Burns DN, et al. Obstetrical factors and the transmission of human immunodeficiency virus type 1 from mother to child. The Women and Infants Transmission Study. N Engl J Med 1996;334(25):1617–23.
11. Kalish LA, Pitt J, Lew J, et al. Defining the time of fetal or perinatal acquisition of human immunodeficiency virus type 1 infection on the basis of age at first positive culture. Women and Infants Transmission Study (WITS). J Infect Dis 1997;175(3):712–5.
12. De Cock KM, Fowler MG, Mercier E, et al. Prevention of mother-to-child HIV transmission in resource-poor countries: translating research into policy and practice. JAMA 2000;283(9):1175–82.
13. Goedert JJ, Duliege AM, Amos CI, et al. High risk of HIV-1 infection for first-born twins. The International Registry of HIV-exposed Twins. Lancet 1991;338(8781):1471–5.
14. Kwiek JJ, Mwapasa V, Milner DA Jr, et al. Maternal-fetal microtransfusions and HIV-1 mother-to-child transmission in Malawi. PLoS Med 2006;3(1):e10.
15. Mandelbrot L, Mayaux MJ, Bongain A, et al. Obstetric factors and mother-to-child transmission of human immunodeficiency virus type 1: The French Perinatal Cohorts. SEROGEST French Pediatric HIV Infection Study Group. Am J Obstet Gynecol 1996;175(3 Pt 1):661–7.
16. Scavalli CP, Mandelbrot L, Berrebi A, et al. Twin pregnancy as a risk factor for mother-to-child transmission of HIV-1: trends over 20 years. AIDS 2007;21(8):993–1002.
17. Biggar RJ, Cassol S, Kumwenda N, et al. The risk of human immunodeficiency virus-1 infection in twin pairs born to infected mothers in Africa. J Infect Dis 2003;188(6):850–5.
18. Mandelbrot L, Le CJ, Berrebi A, et al. Perinatal HIV-1 transmission: interaction between zidovudine prophylaxis and mode of delivery in the French Perinatal Cohort. JAMA 1998;280(1):55–60.
19. Nielsen K, Boyer P, Dillon M, et al. Presence of human immunodeficiency virus (HIV) type 1 and HIV-1-specific antibodies in cervicovaginal secretions of infected mothers and in the gastric aspirates of their infants. J Infect Dis 1996;173(4):1001–4.
20. Kaneda T, Shiraki K, Hirano K, et al. Detection of maternofetal transfusion by placental alkaline phosphatase levels. J Pediatr 1997;130(5):730–5.

21. Lin HH, Kao JH, Hsu HY, et al. Least microtransfusion from mother to fetus in elective cesarean delivery. Obstet Gynecol 1996;87(2):244–8.
22. Centers for Disease Control and Prevention. HIV Surveillance Report, 2008, vol. 20. Available at: http://www.cdc.gov/hiv/topics/surveillance/resources/reports/. Published June 2010. Accessed August 24, 2010.
23. Whitmore S, Zhang X, Taylor A. Estimated number of births to HIV+ women in the US, 2006 [abstract 924]. Program and abstracts of the 16th Conference on Retroviruses and Opportunistic Infections. Montreal (Canada), February 8–11, 2009.
24. ACOG Committee Opinion: scheduled cesarean delivery and the prevention of vertical transmission of HIV infection. Number 219, August 1999. Committee on Obstetric Practice. American College of Obstetricians and Gynecologists. Int J Gynaecol Obstet 1999;66(3):305–6.
25. Mofenson LM. U.S. Public health service task force recommendations for use of antiretroviral drugs in pregnant HIV-1-infected women for maternal health and interventions to reduce perinatal HIV-1 transmission in the United States. MMWR Recomm Rep 2002;51(RR–18):1–38.
26. Centers for Disease Control and Prevention. Enhanced perinatal surveillance-participating areas in the United States and dependent areas, 2000–2003. HIV/AIDS Surveillance Supplement Report, 2008. Available at: http://www.cdc.gov/hiv/topics/surveillance/resources/reports/2008supp_vol13no4/pdf/HIVAIDS_SSR_Vol13_No4.pdf. Accessed April 12, 2010.
27. Grubert TA, Reindell D, Kastner R, et al. Complications after caesarean section in HIV-1-infected women not taking antiretroviral treatment. Lancet 1999;354(9190):1612–3.
28. Maiques V, Garcia-Tejedor A, Perales A, et al. Intrapartum fetal invasive procedures and perinatal transmission of HIV. Eur J Obstet Gynecol Reprod Biol 1999;87(1):63–7.
29. Rodriguez EJ, Spann C, Jamieson D, et al. Postoperative morbidity associated with cesarean delivery among human immunodeficiency virus-seropositive women. Am J Obstet Gynecol 2001;184(6):1108–11.
30. Semprini AE, Castagna C, Ravizza M, et al. The incidence of complications after caesarean section in 156 HIV-positive women. AIDS 1995;9(8):913–7.
31. Coll O, Fiore S, Floridia M, et al. Pregnancy and HIV infection: a European consensus on management. AIDS 2002;16(Suppl 2):S1–18.
32. Miller JM Jr. Maternal and neonatal morbidity and mortality in cesarean section. Obstet Gynecol Clin North Am 1988;15(4):629–38.
33. Petitti DB. Maternal mortality and morbidity in cesarean section. Clin Obstet Gynecol 1985;28(4):763–9.
34. Nielsen TF, Hokegard KH. Cesarean section and intraoperative surgical complications. Acta Obstet Gynecol Scand 1984;63(2):103–8.
35. Hadar E, Melamed N, Tzadikevitch-Geffen K, et al. Timing and risk factors of maternal complications of cesarean section. Arch Gynecol Obstet 2010. [Epub ahead of print].
36. Chama CM, Morrupa JY. The safety of elective caesarean section for the prevention of mother-to-child transmission of HIV-1. J Obstet Gynaecol 2008;28(2):194–7.
37. Indications for cesarean section: final statement of the panel of the national consensus conference on aspects of cesarean birth. CMAJ 1986;134(12):1348–52.
38. Read JS, Tuomala R, Kpamegan E, et al. Mode of delivery and postpartum morbidity among HIV-infected women: the women and infants transmission study. J Acquir Immune Defic Syndr 2001;26(3):236–45.

39. Faucher P, Batallan A, Bastian H, et al. [Management of pregnant women infected with HIV at Bichat Hospital between 1990 and 1998: analysis of 202 pregnancies]. Gynecol Obstet Fertil 2001;29(3):211–25 [in French].

40. Fiore S, Newell ML, Thorne C. Higher rates of post-partum complications in HIV-infected than in uninfected women irrespective of mode of delivery. AIDS 2004; 18(6):933–8.

41. Marcollet A, Goffinet F, Firtion G, et al. Differences in postpartum morbidity in women who are infected with the human immunodeficiency virus after elective cesarean delivery, emergency cesarean delivery, or vaginal delivery. Am J Obstet Gynecol 2002;186(4):784–9.

42. Watts DH, Lambert JS, Stiehm ER, et al. Complications according to mode of delivery among human immunodeficiency virus-infected women with CD4 lymphocyte counts of < or = 500/microL. Am J Obstet Gynecol 2000;183(1): 100–7.

43. Duarte G, Read JS, Gonin R, et al. Mode of delivery and postpartum morbidity in Latin American and Caribbean countries among women who are infected with human immunodeficiency virus-1: the NICHD international site development initiative (NISDI) perinatal study. Am J Obstet Gynecol 2006;195(1): 215–29.

44. Read JS, Newell ML. Efficacy and safety of cesarean delivery for prevention of mother-to-child transmission of HIV-1. Cochrane Database Syst Rev 2005;4: CD005479.

45. Bjorklund K, Mutyaba T, Nabunya E, et al. Incidence of postcesarean infections in relation to HIV status in a setting with limited resources. Acta Obstet Gynecol Scand 2005;84(10):967–71.

46. Bulterys M, Chao A, Dushimimana A, et al. Fatal complications after cesarian section in HIV-infected women. AIDS 1996;10(8):923–4.

47. Kreitchmann R, Cohen R, Pinto J, et al. Mode of delivery and neonatal respiratory morbidity among HIV-exposed infants from Latin America and the Caribbean: the NISDI perinatal study [abstract 929]. 17th Conference on Retroviruses and Opportunistic Infections. Infant Outcome after Prenatal ART Exposure. San Francisco (CA), February 16–19, 2010.

48. Livingston E, Huo Y, Patel K, et al. Mode of delivery and infant respiratory morbidity among infants born to HIV-1-infected women. Obstet Gynecol 2010; 116(2 Pt 1):335–43.

49. Zanardo V, Simbi AK, Franzoi M, et al. Neonatal respiratory morbidity risk and mode of delivery at term: influence of timing of elective caesarean delivery. Acta Paediatr 2004;93(5):643–7.

50. Luo G, Norwitz ER. Revisiting amniocentesis for fetal lung maturity after 36 weeks' gestation. Rev Obstet Gynecol 2008;1(2):61–8.

51. Jamieson DJ, Read JS, Kourtis AP, et al. Cesarean delivery for HIV-infected women: recommendations and controversies. Am J Obstet Gynecol 2007;197 (Suppl 3):S96–100.

52. Moczygemba CK, Paramsothy P, Meikle S, et al. Route of delivery and neonatal birth trauma. Am J Obstet Gynecol 2010;202(4):361–6.

53. Boer K, England K, Godfried MH, et al. Mode of delivery in HIV-infected pregnant women and prevention of mother-to-child transmission: changing practices in western Europe. HIV Med 2010;11:368–78.

54. Ioannidis JP, Abrams EJ, Ammann A, et al. Perinatal transmission of human immunodeficiency virus type 1 by pregnant women with RNA virus loads <1000 copies/ml. J Infect Dis 2001;183(4):539–45.

55. Townsend CL, Cortina-Borja M, Peckham CS, et al. Low rates of mother-to-child transmission of HIV following effective pregnancy interventions in the United Kingdom and Ireland, 2000–2006. AIDS 2008;22(8):973–81.

56. Warszawski J, Tubiana R, Le CJ, et al. Mother-to-child HIV transmission despite antiretroviral therapy in the ANRS French Perinatal Cohort. AIDS 2008;22(2): 289–99.

57. European Collaborative Study. Mother-to-child transmission of HIV infection in the era of highly active antiretroviral therapy. Clin Infect Dis 2005;40(3):458–65.

58. The International Perinatal HIV Group. Duration of ruptured membranes and vertical transmission of HIV-1: a meta-analysis from 15 prospective cohort studies. AIDS 2001;15(3):357–68.

Immune-based Approaches to the Prevention of Mother-to-child Transmission of HIV-1: Active and Passive Immunization

Barb Lohman-Payne, PhD[a,b,c], Jennifer Slyker, PhD[b,c,d],
Sarah L. Rowland-Jones, MA (Cantab), BM BCh, DM (Oxon)[d,*]

KEYWORDS

• HIV-1 • Vaccine • Infant • Cofactor

Mother-to-child transmission (MTCT) of human immunodeficiency virus 1 (HIV-1) infection remains an important cause of new HIV-1 infections worldwide, despite the increasing implementation of prevention strategies using antiretroviral therapy (ART) across the developing world. In the year ending December 2008 an estimated 430,000 children less than the age of 15 years were newly infected with HIV-1 (UNAIDS Epidemic Update 2009), most of whom acquired the infection from their mothers in low- and middle-income countries. Despite clear evidence of significant progress, challenges remain for poor countries in providing comprehensive screening programs for pregnant women and implementing the full range of prevention services for those identified as HIV-1-infected.

For those children who acquire perinatal infection, disease progression seems to be unusually rapid compared with that of adults, particularly in developing countries,

[a] Department of Paediatrics and Child Health, University of Nairobi, Nairobi 00202, Kenya
[b] Department of Medicine, University of Washington, Seattle, WA 98104, USA
[c] Department of Global Health, University of Washington, Seattle, WA 98104, USA
[d] Nuffield Department of Medicine, University of Oxford, John Radcliffe Hospital, Oxford, OX3 9DS, UK
* Corresponding author.
E-mail address: sarah.rowland-jones@ndm.ox.ac.uk

Clin Perinatol 37 (2010) 787–805
doi:10.1016/j.clp.2010.08.005
0095-5108/10/$ – see front matter © 2010 Elsevier Inc. All rights reserved.

where mortality as high as 20% to 52% has been reported in the first 2 years of life.[1,2] A key factor contributing to the rapid disease progression observed in infants may be the persistently high levels of HIV-1 viremia observed throughout the first year of life, with the set-point viral load (VL) rarely decreasing more than 1 log less than the peak VL,[3,4] despite the early appearance of HIV-1-specific T-cell responses.[5] It is likely that coinfections acquired in babies in the developing world may play a role in rapid disease progression, such as human cytomegalovirus (CMV), which infects most West African children in the first year of life[6] and is associated with high VL in HIV-1-coinfected infants.[7] Coinfections, particularly malaria in pregnancy, may also contribute to the likelihood of transmission; therefore it is important to investigate and define the potential role of coinfections in MTCT so that these may be modified in preventive strategies.

MTCT OF HIV-1: AN IMMUNOLOGIC PERSPECTIVE

Vertical transmission of HIV-1 is not an inevitable consequence of exposure; in the absence of treatment 55% to 80% of infants exposed to HIV-1 remain uninfected by HIV-1. This finding is striking when the large volumes of maternal blood containing HIV-1-infected cells circulating through the placenta throughout gestation are considered; HIV-1 can be detected with relative ease in the placentas of both transmitting and nontransmitting mothers.[8] Moreover, infants breastfed by untreated HIV-1-uninfected mothers ingest hundreds of liters of HIV-1-contaminated milk but more than 80% of them remain uninfected.[9] It is generally assumed that there are no serious long-term consequences of exposure to HIV-1 in utero or in early life in children who escape infection. Nevertheless, uninfected babies born to HIV-1-infected mothers suffer from increased morbidity and mortality.[10,11] It has been difficult to distinguish the direct effect of HIV-1 exposure from the consequences of being born to a sick mother,[11] but there are some suggestions that exposed uninfected babies may present with severe infections that indicate clinical immunodeficiency.[12] With the widespread rollout of preventing MTCT (PMTCT) programs in resource-poor settings, this subject represents an important area for future investigation.

When transmission does occur, in utero (transplacental) transmission accounts for an estimated 5% to 10% of infections, and peripartum transmission (occurring during labor, delivery, and early breastfeeding) contributes 10% to 15% of infections, whereas breastfeeding transmission accounts for 5% to 20% of MTCT (reviewed in Ref.[13]). In the developed world, the successful deployment of intervention strategies has reduced the overall transmission rate to substantially less than 5%. Although antiretroviral regimens and risk-reduction counseling have been successfully used for pregnant women and their infants in many parts of the developing world, full implementation of these programs remains a challenge in many countries, especially where antenatal clinical attendance and HIV-1 screening are not widespread. In addition, the potential toxicities of and the development of drug resistance to ART in both mother and child are concerns. Therefore, the development of a safe effective immunoprophylaxis regimen begun at birth and continuing during breastfeeding, perhaps alongside neonatal chemoprophylaxis, remains an area of active research interest.

The major risk factors for MTCT include factors associated with maternal VL (duration and composition of antiretroviral regimen and VL at delivery) and infant exposure to infected fluids (duration of rupture of membranes, type of delivery, presence of other maternal sexually transmitted infections [STIs], and breastfeeding duration).[14,15] Breastfeeding considered alone is associated with a near doubling of the risk of MTCT of HIV.[16] Avoidance of breastfeeding and reduction of other maternal risk factors for

MTCT of HIV have led to remarkable declines in MTCT in settings with adequate resources. However, replacement feeding is advisable only when the AFASS criteria are met: namely, that formula feeding be culturally Acceptable, Feasible for the mother, Affordable, Sustainable and Safe (conditions rarely met in most areas of the world). Thus an ideal pediatric vaccine for PMTCT would combine the immediacy of passive immunization designed to protect the infant during the first vulnerable weeks of life with the durability of active immunization to protect against the repeated low-dose homologous virus exposure delivered multiple times a day via breastfeeding.

Why do such a large proportion of children exposed to HIV-1 and who remain uninfected resist infection? In utero transmission is believed to occur most commonly in the last trimester; it has been suggested that the placenta blocks the transmission of free HIV-1 virions[17] (by mechanisms as yet unidentified) and infection depends either on breaks in the placental barrier or the transcytosis of infected cells.[18] Some data suggest that uninfected infants exposed to HIV in utero, at delivery, or postnatally can develop HIV-1-specific T-cell responses,[19–22] which suggests that there has been sufficient exposure to replicating virus to prime such a response. Although the detection of an HIV-specific response in the absence of persistent infection does not necessarily imply that T-cell immunity contributes to protection, resistance to postnatal HIV-1 transmission was shown to correlate with the magnitude of the HIV-1-specific T-cell response in a prospective study in Nairobi, Kenya.[9] This finding provides some encouragement that enhancing the immune responses to HIV-1 through immunotherapeutic strategies in uninfected infants could confer protection against later infection.

VACCINE STRATEGIES TO PREVENT MTCT OF HIV-1
HIV-1 Vaccine Studies in Adults

Three large-scale human efficacy studies have been completed. In the first of these, Vaxgen used an envelope subunit protein construct with the aim of inducing a protective antibody response: however, a large phase III clinical trial showed no evidence of efficacy.[23] The field moved toward testing T-cell-inducing vaccines, and considerable hope was placed on a replication-defective adenovirus type 5 (Ad5)-based recombinant vaccine produced by Merck that appeared to be the most immunogenic available construct in human studies. This vaccine was tested in the phase 2b Step Trial (tested in high-risk volunteers), which was terminated prematurely because study subjects were neither protected from HIV-1 infection nor experienced reduced VL when infection occurred.[24,25] This failure led to a great deal of introspection in the HIV vaccine field, as it called into question whether or not a vaccine designed to elicit a cytotoxic T-lymphocyte (CTL) response could indeed protect against HIV-1 infection, as well as casting doubt on the nonhuman primate models of HIV infection that did not accurately predict the outcome of the human trial. However, progressive improvements in the constructs used to elicit T-cell responses have provided some encouragement in the macaque model: for example, a heterologous rAd26 prime/rAd5 boost vaccine regimen expressing simian immunodeficiency virus (SIV) Gag elicited broader and stronger cellular immune responses than had been seen with the homologous rAd5 regimen, which led to significantly lower set-point VLs as well as decreased AIDS-related mortality compared with control animals following challenge with a pathogenic SIV strain, SIVmac251.[26] More recently, a novel approach using rhesus CMV constructs induced effector memory T cells at mucosal sites that correlated with protection from infection in 4 of 12 macaques repeatedly challenged with the highly pathogenic SIVmac239 strain.[27] Further encouragement to the HIV vaccine field has come from the results of the rv144 phase III efficacy trial of a combination of canary-pox priming and HIV envelope protein boost tested in a low-risk population in Thailand.[28] Although the incidence of new infections was low in this study, meaning that significant efficacy was seen in only one of 3 analyses (the modified intention-to-treat analysis), the vaccine appeared to confer 31% protection against infection, the first indication of efficacy in any human study. The mechanisms of protection are not yet known, but are unlikely to include either neutralizing antibodies or CTLs, which are rarely induced by this vaccine approach.

Mucosal Vaccines

Mucosal immunization has been shown to induce mucosal responses, and because the first sites of SIV and recombinant simian-human immunodeficiency virus (SHIV) infection in neonatal rhesus macaques are mucosal surfaces, similar tissues are likely to be exposed in MTCT of HIV-1.[29,30] HIV-1-specific immunity present at these sites may be most relevant to preventing transmission. Many cellular and cytokine properties of the neonatal oral and intestinal tissues are known to differ from the adult; these could either represent protective or susceptibility factors and include the levels of $\gamma\delta$ T cells, natural killer (NK) cells, macrophages, dendritic cells (DC), IgG, IgA, and secretory IgA levels, and levels of cytokines such as tumor necrosis factor α and interferon γ (IFN-γ).[31]

Mucosal vaccines developed for PMTCT of HIV-1 could exploit the common mucosa-associated lymphoid tissue to explore oral or nasal delivery. Oral delivery, although attractive for neonates, has challenges such as induction of tolerance, limitations in the choice of safe effective adjuvants, requirement for large doses of antigen, and the need for antigen stability in the gut. This last concern has been addressed through the development of lipid vesicles or polymeric nanoparticles that act as immunostimulants and preserve immunogens from intestinal enzymes. So far only a limited number of orally administered vaccines against HIV have been tested in humans. An attenuated canarypox vector (vCP 205) and Salmonella vaccine vector (CKS257) vaccine platforms were both reportedly well tolerated in humans but with less than expected mucosal immunogenicity.[32,33] As opposed to oral vaccine delivery, the main advantage of nasally administered vaccine is the requirement for smaller doses of antigen. Several vaccine formulations have been tested in adults, including peptides, DNA, and live bacterial and viral vectors.[31] Mucosal vaccine development against HIV-1 seems to require the deployment of stronger adjuvants, the use of which may be associated with safety concerns in young children.

A pediatric vaccine to prevent HIV infection would rapidly induce both antibody and cellular responses detectable at mucosal surfaces that would remain at effective levels during the duration of breastfeeding. A greater understanding of the most important inductive and effector sites in the newborn would guide research to address such questions as to whether systemic immunization can induce sufficient mucosal immunity, if oral or nasal vaccines can be effective, and if appropriate adjuvants can be developed for an effective vaccine development strategy for use in HIV-1-exposed infants.

Neonatal Immunity

In conjunction with the challenges of designing an effective vaccine to prevent transmission across mucosal surfaces, pediatric vaccinologists have the additional difficulty of working with a neonatal immune system in a state of extreme change as the newborn adjusts to life outside its intrauterine environment.[34,35] Although neonates generally develop immune responses on immunization as well as cell-mediated responses to several acute viral infections, several deficiencies in the immunoregulatory pathways of T cells and antigen-presenting cells have been documented in human cord blood, with important implications for the development of immune-based therapies to prevent MTCT of HIV-1. Cord blood T cells have lower basal expression of CD3 and adhesion molecules, defects in cytokine production, and CD8+ T-cell activity,[36] whereas monocytes and DC express lower levels of costimulatory molecules, have altered differentiation pathways, and reduced cytokine/chemokine production.[37,38] Neonatal T cells have a bias against Th1-cell-polarizing cytokines that leaves the newborn susceptible to microbial infection and may contribute to the impairment of neonatal immune responses.[39,40] An exception is bacillus Calmette-Guérin (BCG) vaccination: newborns are capable of mounting a Th1-type response of similar magnitude to that given later in life.[41] Moreover, BCG itself can act as an adjuvant for other vaccines.[42] Pre- and postnatal exposure to environmental microbial products that activate innate immunity might accelerate this maturation, diminishing the Th2- and/or enhancing Th1-cell polarization, and this could be incorporated into adjuvant design. Both natural and inducible CD4+CD25+ regulatory T-cell (Treg) numbers are increased in infancy and are speculated to be required for maintaining peripheral T-cell tolerance through inhibition of Th1-cell immunity.[43-45] Exposure to foreign antigens, both alloantigens[46] and antigens from *Plasmodium falciparum* present in placental malaria,[47] promotes the development of regulatory T-cell populations at birth.

The B-cell compartment is also affected in newborns, with responses to vaccines characterized by lower antibody levels, restricted diversity of antibody repertoire and lower levels of IgG2 isotype compared with responses induced in adults.[48] The implications of these deficiencies in pediatric vaccine development may include a requirement for enhanced stimulation of antigen-presenting cells with increased avidity of CD3/TCR and costimulation molecule interactions to ensure immune activation.

Vaccine Strategies for PMTCT of HIV Infection

Animal models, especially the rhesus macaque-SIV/SHIV model, have been used to address areas of uncertainty in pediatric vaccine design, including the most appropriate vaccine, the timing of immunizations, and the duration of vaccine-elicited responses. The SIV models for vertical transmission of HIV-1 and for neonatal vaccine development were validated in the 1990s and many important proof of concepts have been shown, including protection of newborn macaques from oral SIV/SHIV challenge through maternal vaccination and through administration of passive hyperimmune serum (SIVIG/HIVIG) or neutralizing monoclonal antibodies at birth.[49-53] The mechanism of protection from infection could include antibody binding alone, classic viral neutralization, or NK-cell-mediated antibody-dependent cellular cytotoxicity. But does passive immunization to prevent MTCT of HIV-1 work? There are many challenges to this approach, particularly the composition of the antibody cocktail, which needs to be effective against more than one HIV-clade and circulating recombinant forms, and the scale-up delivery logistics are daunting. Alternatively, boosting of maternal antibody levels by vaccination represents an important strategy to augment passive immunity during the infant's early months of life, until the infant can be actively immunized: however, the role of maternal antibody in reducing the effectiveness of immune responses in the newborn, especially T-cell responses, is a concern. A phase III randomized clinical trial to compare the standard single-dose mother/infant nevirapine (NVP) regimen for PMTCT with the addition of HIV immune globulin (HIVIGLOB) or a second arm of extended infant NVP dosing compared with the standard single-dose NVP regimen alone without

HIVIGLOB was completed in Uganda in 2006 (http://www.mujhu.org/hiviglob2.html). The study enrolled 722 mothers with 204 in the HIVIGLOB arm. The data from the HIVIGLOB arm were pooled with other data from Johns Hopkins trials in Ethiopia and India, and results are not yet available.

Live attenuated vaccines have the advantage of prolonged antigen delivery and stimulation of both innate and adaptive immunity. Modified vaccinia virus Ankara (MVA) and canarypox viral vectors (ALVAC) have been tested in the rhesus macaque/SIV-SHIV models in advance of human trials. MVA expressing SIV gag, pol, and env or expressing SIVmac1A11was used to immunize infant macaques at birth and at 3 weeks of age.[54] The infants were challenged at 4 weeks of age with uncloned SIVmac251, using a multiple low-dose challenge model to deliver virus 3 times a day for 5 days to mimic breast milk exposure. The immunization regimen was unable to prevent infection; however, the immunized infants mounted antibody responses and had improved clinical outcome compared with controls. An attenuated recombinant canarypox vector expressing SIV gag, pol, and env (ALVAC-SIV) was used to immunize infant macaques at birth, 2, and 3 weeks of age, followed by repeated oral low-dose challenge.[55] In this experiment, significantly fewer immunized infants were infected (6 of 16) compared with the unimmunized controls (14 of 16), showing that neonatal immunization provided partial protection from infection. Lastly, a topical DNA vaccine containing HIV-1 gag and env (DermaVir) represents an immunization strategy that targets lymph node DC. Rhesus macaques immunized with DermaVir generated HIV-1-specific Th1 and Th2 cytokines and antigen-specific memory T cells, whereas serum antibody levels were boosted after p27/gp140 protein boosting. After mucosal challenge, none of the animals was protected from infection; however, 4 of 5 immunized monkeys had reduced peak and set-point viremia.[56]

Pediatric Clinical Trials of HIV Vaccines

The most recently reported clinical trials of live attenuated vaccine constructs tested as PACTG 326 part 1 and part 2 include the ALVAC constructs vCP205 and ALVAC-HIV vCP1452. Immunization of neonates was well tolerated and induced lymphoproliferative and/or cytotoxic T-cell responses in vaccinees: ~40% of infants immunized with ALVAC vCP205 and 75% of infants immunized with ALVAC vCP1452.[57,58] An MVA-vectored vaccine is also under evaluation in an open randomized phase I/II study evaluating safety and immunogenicity of a candidate HIV-1 vaccine, MVA-HIVA, administered to healthy infants born to HIV-1-infected mothers in Nairobi, Kenya. This active study is aiming to enroll 72 HIV-1-uninfected infants with 36 breastfeeding infants and 36 formula-feeding infants by the end of 2010, with infants in follow-up for 18 months. Within each feeding group, infants are randomized to receive MVA-HIVA or to remain unvaccinated. The design of the study allows for multiple secondary aims for comparison of immunogenicity in the different feeding groups and the response to other national immunization program vaccines in the MVA-HIVA-vaccinated or unvaccinated infants (Tomas Hanke, personal communication, 2010).

COINFECTIONS HAVE THE POTENTIAL TO ALTER VERTICAL HIV-1 TRANSMISSION AND VACCINE EFFICACY
Herpes Simplex Virus Type 2

Genital coinfections play an important role in both vertical and horizontal HIV-1 transmission. A study of HIV-1-discordant couples in Uganda showed that the presence of genital ulcers increased the probability of HIV-1 transmission per coital act 2.6-fold.[59] Herpes simplex type 2 (HSV-2) infection is the primary cause of genital ulcer disease in resource-poor settings. HSV-2 seroprevalence is high among HIV-1-infected populations globally, and is likely to have a significant population effect on HIV-1 transmission in endemic regions[60,61]; a recent meta-analysis of studies estimated HSV-2 infection confers a 3-fold increased risk of sexual HIV-1 acquisition.[62] Maternal HSV-2 seropositivity has also been associated with increased rates of peripartum HIV-1 transmission in some studies,[63,64] but not others.[65,66] Recurrent subclinical reactivation of HSV-2, characterized by HSV-2 shedding in the absence of ulcers, is common in HSV-2 infection.[67] The presence of genital ulcers, or genital shedding of HSV-2, proximal to delivery has been associated with an increased risk of vertical transmission of HIV.[14,66] Several mechanisms may explain this association. Ulcers may provide a physical breach in the mucosa that increases infant exposure to HIV-1 virions or infected cells beneath the epithelium. HSV-2 ulcers contain high levels of HIV-1 RNA,[68] and genital HIV-1 replication is a strong risk factor for transmission.[14] The concentration of HIV-1 in ulcers may result from the homing of activated CD4 T cells,[69,70] which are potential targets for HIV-1 infection. Even in the absence of ulcers, HSV-2 shedding is associated with increased HIV-1 shedding in the genital tract.[71,72] HSV-2 may also affect vertical transmission by more generalized effects on maternal systemic VL; plasma HIV-1 VL is increased during subclinical HSV-2 reactivation and declines with antiviral suppression of HSV-2 replication.[67,73] A randomized controlled trial (RCT) of valacyclovir versus placebo for 12 weeks showed a 0.53 $\log_{10}$ copies/mL decrease in HIV-1 plasma VL, and a 0.29 $\log_{10}$ decrease in HIV-1 RNA in the genital tract of HIV-1/HSV-2-coinfected women.[74] The effect of HSV-2 coinfection on systemic HIV-1 replication may result from increased immune activation or direct interactions between viruses (reviewed in Ref.[75]). In addition, acyclovir has been shown to have an inhibitory effect on HIV-1 replication in vitro.[76,77] Together, these data suggested that HSV-2 suppression may be an effective tool to prevent HIV-1 transmission. However, results from clinical trials of sexual transmission have been disappointing; HSV-2 suppression with acyclovir did not prevent either HIV-1 transmission or acquisition.[78–80] Acyclovir does not seem to affect egress of CD4 cells from lesion sites after healing, suggesting that HIV-1 target cells remain concentrated in the genital mucosa,[81] and this may explain in part the failure of acyclovir to prevent HIV-1 transmission despite reductions in VL. However, failure in the sexual transmission model may not exclude HSV-2 suppression as a strategy to reduce vertical transmission. A pharmacokinetic study showed acyclovir is actively transported to the amniotic fluid and breast milk[82]; if HSV-2 suppression reduces HIV-1 VL in these compartments, there is the potential for this approach to affect in utero or breast milk HIV-1 transmission. A randomized trial is under way in Kenya to address this question (NCT00530777).

Malaria

There is significant overlap between the malaria and HIV-1 epidemics (reviewed in Ref.[83]). Malaria coinfection is associated with a transient, but significant increase ($\sim 0.25 \log_{10}$) in plasma HIV-1 RNA VL,[84,85] but its role in transmission is unclear.[86] Ayouba and colleagues[87] reported higher rates of MTCT in Cameroon during the rainy season, and speculated that malaria may affect vertical HIV-1 transmission. A few studies have shown a trend for increased vertical transmission in women with blood parasitemia during pregnancy; however, this relationship disappears after adjusting for HIV-1 VL[88,89] and other studies have shown no association.[90,91] Placental malaria is more commonly detected in HIV-1-infected women,[88,89,92,93] and Malawian women with placental malaria were found to have a ~ 2.5-fold higher plasma HIV-1 RNA VL.[94] Some studies have shown an association between placental malaria and increased rates of vertical transmission independent of HIV-1 VL[89,92]; however, other studies have shown no association.[93] A study conducted in western Kenya found HIV-1 transmission risk to be increased when placenta parasitemia was high (>10,000 parasites/ mL) but reduced in cases of low parasitemia (<10,000 parasites/mL) compared with malaria-negative controls.[90] The potential protective effect of placental malaria was confirmed in a second study conducted in Mozambique.[91] These conflicting findings may be attributable to different methods of detecting placental parasitemia, different regional epidemics (seasonal, holoendemic), unrecorded self-treatment of malaria, and including breast-milk HIV-1 transmissions in the ascertainment of effect. Malaria may alter the risk of HIV-1 transmission in utero by causing inflammation in the placenta,[95] increasing CC-chemokine production,[96,97] shifting cytokine production from Th2- to Th1-type responses,[98] and increasing CCR5 expression on Hofbauer cells.[99] Together these data suggest malaria has the potential to alter the risk of vertical HIV-1 transmission, but further studies are needed to understand the interactions between immune responses to these 2 pathogens. Independent of HIV-1 infection, malaria during pregnancy is associated with obstetric problems and adverse birth outcomes, making malaria prevention, diagnosis, and treatment an important component of antenatal care for all women in malaria-endemic areas.

Bacterial Vaginosis and Other Vaginal Infections

In addition to HSV-2 as discussed earlier, other STIs are also associated with an increased risk of horizontal HIV-1 transmission and acquisition (reviewed in Ref.[100]). Ulcerative and nonulcerative STIs, as well as vaginitis and cervicitis of unknown causes, are associated with increased HIV-1 shedding in the female genital tract,[100–105] and treatment of genital infections is associated with declines in HIV-1 shedding.[104,106] Genital infections are likely to increase HIV-1 transmission via recruitment of activated HIV-1-infected cells to sites of inflammation. Disruption of healthy vaginal flora as a result of bacterial vaginosis (BV),[107–109] or vaginal washing has also been associated with an increased risk of HIV-1 acquisition.[110] A recent prospective study conducted in Kenya reported a 3-fold increased risk of in utero HIV-1 transmission from women diagnosed with BV at 32 weeks' gestation compared with women with normal vaginal flora.[111] However, a multisite RCT of metronidazole versus placebo in 3 African countries found no difference in rates of vertical transmission compared with placebo, despite a 16% reduction in BV.[112] Further studies are needed to determine whether restoration of normal vaginal flora can reduce vertical HIV-1 transmission.

Helminth Infection is Associated with Reduced Vaccine Responses

The greatest need for an HIV-1 vaccine is in Africa and Asia, where helminths may infect 25% to 76% of the healthy adults and children.[113–116] The first indication that helminths may compromise vaccine responses was the observation of reduced BCG efficacy in resource-poor countries.[117,118] Although helminths comprise a diverse group of organisms with heterogeneous routes and targets of infection, the most commonly encountered helminths (digenean flukes, cestodes, and nematodes) have similar effects on the host immune system; coinfection suppresses IFN-γ production and induces a Th2-type CD4 response in their hosts (reviewed in Ref.[119]). After BCG vaccination, newborns whose mothers had schistosomiasis or bancroftian filariasis infection had weaker IFN-γ responses to purified protein derivative (PPD) and increased production of interleukin 5 (IL-5).[120] This trend was also found at 14 months of age; PPD-specific CD4 responses in children exposed in utero to helminths had highly Th2-skewed responses, indicating that helminth exposure during priming of

CD4 responses in utero affected the profile of memory cells later in life.[120] Deworming before revaccination with BCG improves PPD-specific IFN-γ production and T-cell proliferation in adults.[121] Similarly, IFN-γ and IL-2 responses to cholera vaccination were improved by deworming of patients with Ascaris lumbricoides infection.[122]

Helminths may also affect HIV-1 disease progression and acquisition. Suppression of Th1-type responses may directly impair control viral replication, and helminth-induced systemic immune activation[123-125] may accelerate HIV-1 disease progression. The effect of helminths on the control over HIV-1 replication has been studied in vivo using primate models; after infection with SHIV-clade C, Schistosoma mansoni-infected rhesus macaques had higher SHIV VL compared with nonparasitized controls, and maintained higher IL-4 and IL-10 production.[126] Introduction of S mansoni into chronically SHIV-infected animals that were aviremic resulted in reactivation of SHIV replication and decline in CD4+CD29+ cells.[127] These experiments also showed that helminth infection may affect HIV-1 acquisition; S mansoni-coinfected animals became infected at lower SHIV doses compared with nonparasitized control animals, and had higher peak VLs and pro-VLs in central memory CD4 T cells.[128] One study in humans has found an increased risk of vertical HIV-1 transmission in the setting of maternal helminth infection.[88] Two RCTs have evaluated treatment of helminthic infections as a strategy to reduce HIV-1 disease progression. Treatment with albendazole improved CD4 counts in HIV-1-infected individuals with Ascaris lumbricoides infection, but no effect was found in patients infected with hookworm or Trichuris trichiura.[129] Similarly, Kallestrup and colleagues[130] found improved control over viral replication and increased CD4 counts in patients treated for schistosomiasis infection. In sub-Saharan Africa, periodic deworming is now a recommended component of comprehensive HIV-1 care of women and children.

Taking into consideration the local helminth burden of target populations enables the more strategic design and deployment of an HIV-1 vaccine. Deworming of vaccinees before or during immunization may improve the priming of a Th1-type response. In mouse models, elimination of S mansoni with praziquantel before immunization with an HIV-clade C DNA vaccine resulted in improved vaccine-specific IFN-γ responses.[131] In addition, infection with vaccinia virus expressing HIV-1 gp[160] resulted in stronger CTL responses and more rapid viral clearance in nonparasitized mice compared with S mansoni-infected mice.[132] Although deworming may improve immune responses to vaccination, reinfection rates are high, and this would be expected to reduce the benefit of deworming in vaccines requiring multiple doses or boosting. Continual reinfection with helminths may similarly impair the efficacy of a nonsterilizing therapeutic HIV-1 vaccine. An alternative approach is the design of vaccines targeted to overcome the Th2 bias induced by helminths, by the strategic use of adjuvants,[133,134] cytokines,[135] or Toll-like receptor signaling.[136,137]

Concerns Regarding Infant Vaccine Development

Many key questions regarding the development of a successful adult HIV-1 vaccine are equally valid for a neonatal immune-based intervention for PMTCT. However, pediatric vaccine development also faces a series of unique concerns. These concerns include, but are not limited to, regulatory/ethical issues applicable to vulnerable populations, physiologic constraints of blood volumes that may limit the degree of safety and immunogenicity testing, existing immunization schedules and potential vaccine interference, and simultaneous exposure to both vaccine and pathogen in the presence of maternal antibodies and the developing neonatal immune system.

There is general agreement that pediatric clinical trials are necessary for implementation of novel medical strategies for prevention or treatment of childhood illnesses. In the United States, several regulatory agencies have committed to ensure ethical conduct in research involving children and development of pharmaceutical formulations specific for children (http://www.fda.gov/cder/pediatric/). Although government programs and assurances provide a level of support to including infants in clinical trials of vaccines designed for PMTCT, in countries with historical imbalances in political and medical power, community-based opinion affects the support of local testing. Infants and children are also subject to cultural traditions; for example, within the family, who is empowered to grant consent? Who makes medical decisions? What is the relative value of family members? There is a need to include diverse populations in testing vaccines, and resources invested in community sensitization and education during all stages of the trial may help ensure continued involvement in subsequent trials.

A logistical concern for phase I/II studies in infants is the frequency and volume of blood collection, not only the physiologic limit of body size, but the psychological limit of the caregiver's tolerance to blood draws from healthy infants. Many assays and procedures have been optimized for minimal blood volumes, including Elispot assays for the detection of antigen-specific responses,[138] multicolor flow cytometry,[139] and detection of HIV-1 DNA in dried blood spots for monitoring infection status.[140] Continued development of assays that require minimal volumes of blood benefit pediatric clinical trials.

Currently infants are immunized worldwide against an array of infections delivered over the first 2 years of life, including BCG, polio, hepatitis B, diphtheria, pertussis, tetanus, pneumococcus and Hemophilus influenzae b (Hib). Investigations into the sequence of exposure to murine viruses have shown that the magnitude and specificity of the immune response elicited by the most recent infection are modified by the host's history of previous infections.[141] In newborn mice and humans Mycobacterium bovis BCG immunization induces a potent immune response and this response has been shown to alter immunity to unrelated vaccines.[42] Also, individual components of multivalent vaccines may induce responses that differ when given individually or in combination (reviewed in Ref.[142]). Therefore, the timing of introduction of new vaccines into the existing Expanded Program on Immunization (EPI) has the potential to modify responses to both previous and subsequent vaccines.

Maternal antibodies have been clearly shown to interfere with the effectiveness of measles virus vaccination, although not affecting the immunogenicity of other vaccines administered in the presence of maternal antibodies.[143] Passively transferred maternal antibodies may form antigen-antibody complexes with vaccine antigens, thereby limiting vaccine exposure before the development of an infant-specific immune response, although there is evidence for many vaccines of B-cell priming with development of protective antibody titers after boosting.[144] Antigen-antibody complexes are efficiently taken up via Fc-mediated mechanism by professional antigen-presenting cells, which may facilitate the development of antigen-specific T- and B-cell responses. However in the setting of PMTCT of HIV, potential exists for cocirculation not only of maternal antibody and vaccine constructs aimed at priming immunity in the infant but also maternal antibody and cell-free HIV-1 acquired from breast milk. Thus, Fc-mediated uptake of antigen-antibody complexes by antigen-presenting cells could potentially lead to enhancement of HIV infection (reviewed in Ref.[145]).

Vaccine constructs and adjuvants may also react differently in infants, although thus far, recombinant HIV-1 gp120 delivered either in alum or MF59, and recombinant canarypox vectored vaccines for HIV have proved safe in pediatric populations (PACTG 230, 326, and HPTN 027), whereas the testing of adjuvant CRM_{197} for use in multivalent pediatric vaccines has shown improve immunogenicity of certain vaccines.[146] Live attenuated SIV vaccines tested in neonatal macaques have also proved safe, with the rare exception of a multiply deleted SIVmac239 that when administered to neonates showed unexpected pathogenicity not initially observed in adults. Pathogenesis in adults was later documented in ~25% of vaccinated adults after a median of ~3 years of infection.[147]

These concerns can be addressed readily through investment in the use of animal models, of continued testing in adults, and of basic research into underlying mechanisms of neonatal immune regulation, maternal antibody interference, and vaccine interference.

SUMMARY AND FUTURE DIRECTIONS

Although HIV vaccines still have some way to go before an effective vaccine to prevent infection becomes available, the special issues of MTCT and infant immunization deserve further study. We have highlighted the approaches tested to date and the potentially modifiable infectious cofactors that can facilitate transmission of HIV-1 from mother to child in the developing world. Some of the issues that need to be considered in the development of a pediatric HIV vaccine have been discussed. Even if deployment of strategies to prevent vertical transmission of HIV-1 becomes universal, a scenario that currently seems some distance away in resource-poor settings, it is likely that a prophylactic HIV vaccine needs to be given as part of the EPI. Therefore a better understanding of infant immune responses to candidate vaccine antigens and adjuvants is an important area for future investigation.

REFERENCES

1. Obimbo EM, Mbori-Ngacha DA, Ochieng JO, et al. Predictors of early mortality in a cohort of human immunodeficiency virus type 1-infected African children. Pediatr Infect Dis J 2004;23(6):536–43.
2. Newell ML, Coovadia H, Cortina-Borja M, et al. Mortality of infected and uninfected infants born to HIV-infected mothers in Africa: a pooled analysis. Lancet 2004;364(9441):1236–43.
3. Richardson BA, Mbori-Ngacha D, Lavreys L, et al. Comparison of human immunodeficiency virus type 1 viral loads in Kenyan women, men, and infants during primary and early infection. J Virol 2003;77(12):7120–3.
4. Mphatswe W, Blanckenberg N, Tudor-Williams G, et al. High frequency of rapid immunological progression in African infants infected in the era of perinatal HIV prophylaxis. AIDS 2007;21(10):1253–61.
5. Lohman BL, Slyker JA, Richardson BA, et al. Longitudinal assessment of human immunodeficiency virus type 1 (HIV-1)-specific gamma interferon responses during the first year of life in HIV-1-infected infants. J Virol 2005;79(13):8121–30.
6. Miles DJ, van der Sande M, Jeffries D, et al. Cytomegalovirus infection in Gambian infants leads to profound CD8 T-cell differentiation. J Virol 2007;81(11):5766–76.
7. Slyker JA, Lohman-Payne BL, John-Stewart GC, et al. Acute cytomegalovirus infection in Kenyan HIV-infected infants. AIDS 2009;23(16):2173–81.
8. Maury W, Potts BJ, Rabson AB. HIV-1 infection of first-trimester and term human placental tissue: a possible mode of maternal-fetal transmission. J Infect Dis 1989;160(4):583–8.
9. John-Stewart GC, Mbori-Ngacha D, Payne BL, et al. HIV-1-Specific cytotoxic T lymphocytes and breast milk HIV-1 transmission. J Infect Dis 2009;199(6):889–98.

10. Mussi-Pinhata MM, Freimanis L, Yamamoto AY, et al. Infectious disease morbidity among young HIV-1-exposed but uninfected infants in Latin American and Caribbean countries: the National Institute of Child Health and Human Development International Site Development Initiative Perinatal Study. Pediatrics 2007;119(3):e694–704.

11. Kuhn L, Kasonde P, Sinkala M, et al. Does severity of HIV disease in HIV-infected mothers affect mortality and morbidity among their uninfected infants? Clin Infect Dis 2005;41(11):1654–61.

12. Slogrove AL, Cotton MF, Esser MM. Severe infections in HIV-exposed uninfected infants: clinical evidence of immunodeficiency. J Trop Pediatr 2010;56(2):75–81.

13. Lehman DA, Farquhar C. Biological mechanisms of vertical human immunodeficiency virus (HIV-1) transmission. Rev Med Virol 2007;17(6):381–403.

14. John GC, Nduati RW, Mbori-Ngacha DA, et al. Correlates of mother-to-child human immunodeficiency virus type 1 (HIV-1) transmission: association with maternal plasma HIV-1 RNA load, genital HIV-1 DNA shedding, and breast infections. J Infect Dis 2001;183(2):206–12.

15. Becquet R, Bland R, Leroy V, et al. Duration, pattern of breastfeeding and post-natal transmission of HIV: pooled analysis of individual data from West and South African cohorts. PLoS One 2009;4:e3797.

16. John-Stewart G, Mbori-Ngacha D, Ekpini R, et al. Breast-feeding and transmission of HIV-1. J Acquir Immune Defic Syndr 2004;35(2):196–202.

17. Dolcini G, Derrien M, Chaouat G, et al. Cell-free HIV type 1 infection is restricted in the human trophoblast choriocarcinoma BeWo cell line, even with expression of CD4, CXCR4 and CCR5. AIDS Res Hum Retroviruses 2003;19(10):857–64.

18. Lagaye S, Derrien M, Menu E, et al. Cell-to-cell contact results in a selective translocation of maternal human immunodeficiency virus type 1 quasispecies across a trophoblastic barrier by both transcytosis and infection. J Virol 2001; 75(10):4780–91.

19. Cheynier R, Langlade-Demoyen P, Marescot MR, et al. Cytotoxic T lymphocyte responses in the peripheral blood of children born to HIV-1-infected mothers. Eur J Immunol 1992;22:2211–7.

20. Rowland-Jones SL, Nixon DF, Aldhous MC, et al. HIV-specific CTL activity in an HIV-exposed but uninfected infant. Lancet 1993;341:860–1.

21. Aldhous MC, Watret KC, Mok JY, et al. Cytotoxic T lymphocyte activity and CD8 subpopulations in children at risk of HIV infection. Clin Exp Immunol 1994;97(1): 61–7.

22. Kuhn L, Coutsoudis A, Moodley D, et al. T-helper cell responses to HIV envelope peptides in cord blood: protection against intrapartum and breast-feeding transmission. AIDS 2001;15(1):1–9.

23. Pitisuttithum P, Gilbert P, Gurwith M, et al. Randomized, double-blind, placebo-controlled efficacy trial of a bivalent recombinant glycoprotein 120 HIV-1 vaccine among injection drug users in Bangkok, Thailand. J Infect Dis 2006; 194(12):1661–71.

24. Buchbinder SP, Mehrotra DV, Duerr A, et al. Efficacy assessment of a cell-mediated immunity HIV-1 vaccine (the Step Study): a double-blind, randomised, placebo-controlled, test-of-concept trial. Lancet 2008;372(9653):1881–93.

25. McElrath MJ, De Rosa SC, Moodie Z, et al. HIV-1 vaccine-induced immunity in the test-of-concept Step Study: a case-cohort analysis. Lancet 2008;372(9653): 1894–905.

26. Liu J, O'Brien KL, Lynch DM, et al. Immune control of an SIV challenge by a T-cell-based vaccine in rhesus monkeys. Nature 2009;457(7225):87–91.

27. Hansen SG, Vieville C, Whizin N, et al. Effector memory T cell responses are associated with protection of rhesus monkeys from mucosal simian immunodeficiency virus challenge. Nat Med 2009;15(3):293–9.

28. Rerks-Ngarm S, Pitisuttithum P, Nitayaphan S, et al. Vaccination with ALVAC and AIDSVAX to prevent HIV-1 infection in Thailand. N Engl J Med 2009;361(23): 2209–20.

29. Abel K, Pahar B, Van Rompay KK, et al. Rapid virus dissemination in infant macaques after oral simian immunodeficiency virus exposure in the presence of local innate immune responses. J Virol 2006;80:6357–67.

30. Kumar RB, Maher DM, Herzberg MC, et al. Expression of HIV receptors, alternate receptors and co-receptors on tonsillar epithelium: implications for HIV binding and primary oral infection. J Virol 2006;3:25–38.

31. Azizi A, Ghunaim H, Diaz-Mitoma F, et al. Mucosal HIV vaccines: a holy grail or a dud? Vaccine 2010;28:4015–26.

32. Wright PF, Mestecky J, McElrath MJ, et al. Comparison of systemic and mucosal delivery of 2 canarypox virus vaccines expressing either HIV-1 genes or the gene for rabies virus G protein. J Infect Dis 2004;189:1221–31.

33. Kotton CN, Lankowski AJ, Scott N, et al. Safety and immunogenicity of attenuated *Salmonella enterica* serovar *Typhimurium* delivering an HIV-1 gag antigen via the *Salmonella* Type III secretion system. Vaccine 2006;24: 6216–24.

34. Jaspan HB, Lawn SD, Safrit JT, et al. The maturing immune system: implications for development and testing HIV-1 vaccines for children and adolescents. AIDS 2006;20:483–94.

35. Marchant A, Newport M. Prevention of infectious diseases by neonatal and early infantile immunization: prospects for the new millennium. Curr Opin Infect Dis 2000;13:241–6.

36. Adkins B, Leclerc C, Marshall-Clarke S. Neonatal adaptive immunity comes of age. Nature Rev 2004;4:553–64.

37. Levy O. Innate immunity of HTE newborn: basic mechanisms and clinical correlates. Nat Rev Immunol 2007;7:379–89.

38. Velilla PA, Rugeles MT, Chougnet CA. Defective antigen-resenting cell function in human neonates. Clin Immunol 2006;121:251–9.

39. Chheda S, Palkowetz KH, Garofalo R, et al. Decreased interleukin-10 production by neonatal monocytes and T cells: relationship to decreased production and expression of tumor necrosis factor - [alpha] and its receptors. Pediatr Res 1996;40:475–83.

40. Lilic D, Cant AJ, Abinun M, et al. Cytokine production differs in children and adults. Pediatr Res 1997;42:237–40.

41. Marchant A, Goetghebuer T, Ota MO, et al. Newborns develop a Th1-type immune response to *Mycobacterium bovis* bacillus Calmette-Guerin vaccination. J Immunol 1999;163:2249–55.

42. Ota MO, Vekemans J, Schlegel-Haueter SE, et al. Influence of *Mycobacterium bovis* bacillus Calmette-Guerin on antibody and cytokine responses to human neonatal vaccination. J Immunol 2002;168(2):919–25.

43. Godfrey WR, Spoden DJ, Ge YG, et al. Cord blood CD4+CD25+-derived T regulatory cell lines express FoxP3 protein and manifest potent suppressor function. Blood 2005;105:750–8.

44. Legrand FA, Nixon DF, Loo CP, et al. Strong HIV-1-specific T cell responses in HIV-1-exposed uninfected infants and neonates revealed after regulatory T cell removal. PLoS One 2006;1:e102.

45. Hartigan-O'Connor DJ, Abel K, McCune JM. Suppression of SIV-specific CD4+ T cells by infant but not adult macaque regulatory T cells: implications for SIV disease progression. J Exp Med 2007;204:2679–92.

46. Mold JE, Michaelsson J, Burt TD, et al. Maternal alloantigens promote the development of tolerogenic fetal regulatory T cells in utero. Science 2008;322(5907):1562–5.

47. Flanagan KL, Halliday A, Burl S, et al. The effect of placental malaria infection on cord blood and maternal immunoregulatory responses at birth. Eur J Immunol 2010;40(4):1062–72.

48. Gans H, Yasukawa L, Rinki M, et al. Immune responses to measles and mumps vaccination of infants at 6, 9, and 12 months. J Infect Dis 2001;184:817–26.

49. Van Rompay KKA, Otsyula MG, Tarara RP, et al. Vaccination of pregnant macaques protects newborns against mucosal simian immunodeficiency virus infection. J Infect Dis 1996;173:1327–35.

50. Van Rompay KK, Berardi CJ, Dillard-Telm S, et al. Passive immunization of newborn rhesus macaques prevents oral simian immunodeficiency virus infection. J Infect Dis 1998;177:1247–59.

51. Hofmann-Lehmann R, Vlasak J, Rasmussen RA, et al. Postnatal passive immunization of neonatal macaques with a triple combination of human monoclonal antibodies against oral simian-human immunodeficiency virus challenge. J Virol 2001;75:7470–80.

52. Ferrantelli F, Rasmussen RA, Buckley KA, et al. Complete protection of neonatal rhesus macaques against oral exposure to pathogenic simian-human immunodeficiency virus by human anti-HIV monoclonal antibodies. J Infect Dis 2004; 189:2149–53.

53. Ferrantelli F, Buckley KA, Rasmussen RA, et al. Time dependence of protective post-exposure prophylaxis with human monoclonal antibodies against pathogenic SHIV challenge in newborn macaques. Virology 2007;358:69–78.

54. Van Rompay KK, Greenier JL, Cole KS, et al. Immunization of newborn rhesus macaques with simian immunodeficiency virus (SIV) vaccines prolongs survival after oral challenge with virulent SIVmac251. J Virol 2003;77:179–90.

55. Van Rompay KK, Abel K, Lawson JR, et al. Attenuated poxvirus-based simian immunodeficiency virus (SIV) vaccines given in infancy partially protect infant and juvenile macaques against repeated oral challenge with virulent SIV. J Acquir Immune Defic Syndr 2005;38:124–34.

56. Cristillo AD, Lisziewicz J, He L, et al. HIV-1 prophylactic vaccine comprised of topical DermaVir prime and protein boost elicits cellular immune responses and controls pathogenic R5 SHIV162P3. Virology 2007;366:197–211.

57. McFarland EJ, Johnson DC, Muresan P, et al. HIV-1 vaccine induced immune responses in newborns of HIV-1 infected mothers. AIDS 2006;20(11):1481–9.

58. Johnson DC, McFarland EJ, Muresan P, et al. Safety and immunogenicity of an HIV-1 recombinant canarypox vaccine in newborns and infants of HIV-1-infected women. J Infect Dis 2005;192:2129–33.

59. Gray RH, Wawer MJ, Brookmeyer R, et al. Probability of HIV-1 transmission per coital act in monogamous, heterosexual, HIV-1-discordant couples in Rakai, Uganda. Lancet 2001;357(9263):1149–53.

60. Corey L, Wald A, Celum CL, et al. The effects of herpes simplex virus-2 on HIV-1 acquisition and transmission: a review of two overlapping epidemics. J Acquir Immune Defic Syndr 2004;35(5):435–45.

61. Hitti J, Watts DH, Burchett SK, et al. Herpes simplex virus seropositivity and reactivation at delivery among pregnant women infected with human immunodeficiency virus-1. Am J Obstet Gynecol 1997;177(2):450–4.

62. Freeman EE, Weiss HA, Glynn JR, et al. Herpes simplex virus 2 infection increases HIV acquisition in men and women: systematic review and meta-analysis of longitudinal studies. AIDS 2006;20(1):73–83.

63. Cowan FM, Humphrey JH, Ntozini R, et al. Maternal herpes simplex virus type 2 infection, syphilis and risk of intra-partum transmission of HIV-1: results of a case control study. AIDS 2008;22(2):193–201.

64. Bollen LJ, Whitehead SJ, Mock PA, et al. Maternal herpes simplex virus type 2 coinfection increases the risk of perinatal HIV transmission: possibility to further decrease transmission? AIDS 2008;22(10):1169–76.

65. Chen KT, Tuomala RE, Chu C, et al. No association between antepartum serologic and genital tract evidence of herpes simplex virus-2 coinfection and perinatal HIV-1 transmission. Am J Obstet Gynecol 2008;198(4):399, e1-395.

66. Drake AL, John-Stewart GC, Wald A, et al. Herpes simplex virus type 2 and risk of intrapartum human immunodeficiency virus transmission. Obstet Gynecol 2007;109(2 Pt 1):403–9.

67. Schacker T, Zeh J, Hu H, et al. Changes in plasma human immunodeficiency virus type 1 RNA associated with herpes simplex virus reactivation and suppression. J Infect Dis 2002;186(12):1718–25.

68. Schacker T, Ryncarz AJ, Goddard J, et al. Frequent recovery of HIV-1 from genital herpes simplex virus lesions in HIV-1-infected men. JAMA 1998;280(1):61–6.

69. Cunningham AL, Turner RR, Miller AC, et al. Evolution of recurrent herpes simplex lesions. An immunohistologic study. J Clin Invest 1985;75(1):226–33.

70. Koelle DM, Abbo H, Peck A, et al. Direct recovery of herpes simplex virus (HSV)-specific T lymphocyte clones from recurrent genital HSV-2 lesions. J Infect Dis 1994;169(5):956–61.

71. Mbopi-Keou FX, Gresenguet G, Mayaud P, et al. Interactions between herpes simplex virus type 2 and human immunodeficiency virus type 1 infection in African women: opportunities for intervention. J Infect Dis 2000;182(4):1090–6.

72. McClelland RS, Wang CC, Overbaugh J, et al. Association between cervical shedding of herpes simplex virus and HIV-1. AIDS 2002;16(18):2425–30.

73. Mole L, Ripich S, Margolis D, et al. The impact of active herpes simplex virus infection on human immunodeficiency virus load. J Infect Dis 1997;176(3):766–70.

74. Nagot N, Ouedraogo A, Foulongne V, et al. Reduction of HIV-1 RNA levels with therapy to suppress herpes simplex virus. N Engl J Med 2007;356(8):790–9.

75. Van de Perre P, Segondy M, Foulongne V, et al. Herpes simplex virus and HIV-1: deciphering viral synergy. Lancet Infect Dis 2008;8(8):490–7.

76. McMahon MA, Siliciano JD, Lai J, et al. The antiherpetic drug acyclovir inhibits HIV replication and selects the V75I reverse transcriptase multidrug resistance mutation. J Biol Chem 2008;283(46):31289–93.

77. Lisco A, Vanpouille C, Tchesnokov EP, et al. Acyclovir is activated into a HIV-1 reverse transcriptase inhibitor in herpesvirus-infected human tissues. Cell Host Microbe 2008;4(3):260–70.

78. Celum C, Wald A, Hughes J, et al. Effect of aciclovir on HIV-1 acquisition in herpes simplex virus 2 seropositive women and men who have sex with men: a randomised, double-blind, placebo-controlled trial. Lancet 2008;371(9630): 2109–19.

79. Celum C, Wald A, Lingappa JR, et al. Acyclovir and transmission of HIV-1 from persons infected with HIV-1 and HSV-2. N Engl J Med 2010;362(5):427–39.

80. Watson-Jones D, Weiss HA, Rusizoka M, et al. Effect of herpes simplex suppression on incidence of HIV among women in Tanzania. N Engl J Med 2008;358(15):1560–71.

81. Zhu J, Hladik F, Woodward A, et al. Persistence of HIV-1 receptor-positive cells after HSV-2 reactivation is a potential mechanism for increased HIV-1 acquisition. Nat Med 2009;15(8):886–92.
82. Kimberlin DF, Weller S, Whitley RJ, et al. Pharmacokinetics of oral valacyclovir and acyclovir in late pregnancy. Am J Obstet Gynecol 1998;179(4):846–51.
83. Rowland-Jones SL, Lohman B. Interactions between malaria and HIV infection-an emerging public health problem? Microbes Infect 2002;4(12):1265–70.
84. Kublin JG, Patnaik P, Jere CS, et al. Effect of Plasmodium falciparum malaria on concentration of HIV-1-RNA in the blood of adults in rural Malawi: a prospective cohort study. Lancet 2005;365(9455):233–40.
85. Hoffman IF, Jere CS, Taylor TE, et al. The effect of Plasmodium falciparum malaria on HIV-1 RNA blood plasma concentration. AIDS 1999;13(4):487–94.
86. Whitworth JA, Hewitt KA. Effect of malaria on HIV-1 progression and transmission. Lancet 2005;365(9455):196–7.
87. Ayouba A, Nerrienet E, Menu E, et al. Mother-to-child transmission of human immunodeficiency virus type 1 in relation to the season in Yaounde, Cameroon. Am J Trop Med Hyg 2003;69(4):447–9.
88. Gallagher M, Malhotra I, Mungai PL, et al. The effects of maternal helminth and malaria infections on mother-to-child HIV transmission. AIDS 2005;19(16): 1849–55.
89. Brahmbhatt H, Sullivan D, Kigozi G, et al. Association of HIV and malaria with mother-to-child transmission, birth outcomes, and child mortality. J Acquir Immune Defic Syndr 2008;47(4):472–6.
90. Ayisi JG, van Eijk AM, Newman RD, et al. Maternal malaria and perinatal HIV transmission, western Kenya. Emerg Infect Dis 2004;10(4):643–52.
91. Naniche D, Lahuerta M, Bardaji A, et al. Mother-to-child transmission of HIV-1: association with malaria prevention, anaemia and placental malaria. HIV Med 2008;9(9):757–64.
92. Brahmbhatt H, Kigozi G, Wabwire-Mangen F, et al. The effects of placental malaria on mother-to-child HIV transmission in Rakai, Uganda. AIDS 2003;17(17):2539–41.
93. Inion I, Mwanyumba F, Gaillard P, et al. Placental malaria and perinatal transmission of human immunodeficiency virus type 1. J Infect Dis 2003;188(11):1675–8.
94. Mwapasa V, Rogerson SJ, Molyneux ME, et al. The effect of Plasmodium falciparum malaria on peripheral and placental HIV-1 RNA concentrations in pregnant Malawian women. AIDS 2004;18(7):1051–9.
95. Moormann AM, Sullivan AD, Rochford RA, et al. Malaria and pregnancy: placental cytokine expression and its relationship to intrauterine growth retardation. J Infect Dis 1999;180(6):1987–93.
96. Abrams ET, Brown H, Chensue SW, et al. Host response to malaria during pregnancy: placental monocyte recruitment is associated with elevated beta chemokine expression. J Immunol 2003;170(5):2759–64.
97. Chaisavaneeyakorn S, Moore JM, Mirel L, et al. Levels of macrophage inflammatory protein 1 alpha (MIP-1 alpha) and MIP-1 beta in intervillous blood plasma samples from women with placental malaria and human immunodeficiency virus infection. Clin Diagn Lab Immunol 2003;10(4):631–6.
98. Fried M, Muga RO, Misore AO, et al. Malaria elicits type 1 cytokines in the human placenta: IFN-gamma and TNF-alpha associated with pregnancy outcomes. J Immunol 1998;160(5):2523–30.
99. Tkachuk AN, Moormann AM, Poore JA, et al. Malaria enhances expression of CC chemokine receptor 5 on placental macrophages. J Infect Dis 2001; 183(6):967–72.

100. Fleming DT, Wasserheit JN. From epidemiological synergy to public health policy and practice: the contribution of other sexually transmitted diseases to sexual transmission of HIV infection. Sex Transm Infect 1999;75(1):3–17.
101. Wolday D, Gebremariam Z, Mohammed Z, et al. The impact of syndromic treatment of sexually transmitted diseases on genital shedding of HIV-1. AIDS 2004; 18(5):781–5.
102. Kreiss J, Willerford DM, Hensel M, et al. Association between cervical inflammation and cervical shedding of human immunodeficiency virus DNA. J Infect Dis 1994;170(6):1597–601.
103. John GC, Nduati RW, Mbori-Ngacha D, et al. Genital shedding of human immunodeficiency virus type 1 DNA during pregnancy: association with immunosuppression, abnormal cervical or vaginal discharge, and severe vitamin A deficiency. J Infect Dis 1997;175(1):57–62.
104. Ghys PD, Fransen K, Diallo MO, et al. The associations between cervicovaginal HIV shedding, sexually transmitted diseases and immunosuppression in female sex workers in Abidjan, Cote d'Ivoire. AIDS 1997;11(12): F85–93.
105. Mostad SB, Overbaugh J, DeVange DM, et al. Hormonal contraception, vitamin A deficiency, and other risk factors for shedding of HIV-1 infected cells from the cervix and vagina. Lancet 1997;350(9082):922–7.
106. McClelland RS, Wang CC, Mandaliya K, et al. Treatment of cervicitis is associated with decreased cervical shedding of HIV-1. AIDS 2001;15(1):105–10.
107. Atashili J, Poole C, Ndumbe PM, et al. Bacterial vaginosis and HIV acquisition: a meta-analysis of published studies. AIDS 2008;22(12):1493–501.
108. Taha TE, Hoover DR, Dallabetta GA, et al. Bacterial vaginosis and disturbances of vaginal flora: association with increased acquisition of HIV. AIDS 1998;12(13): 1699–706.
109. van de Wijgert JH, Morrison CS, Cornelisse PG, et al. Bacterial vaginosis and vaginal yeast, but not vaginal cleansing, increase HIV-1 acquisition in African women. J Acquir Immune Defic Syndr 2008;48(2):203–10.
110. McClelland RS, Lavreys L, Hassan WM, et al. Vaginal washing and increased risk of HIV-1 acquisition among African women: a 10-year prospective study. AIDS 2006;20(2):269–73.
111. Farquhar C, Mbori-Ngacha D, Overbaugh J, et al. Illness during pregnancy and bacterial vaginosis are associated with in-utero HIV-1 transmission. AIDS 2010; 24(1):153–5.
112. Taha TE, Brown ER, Hoffman IF, et al. A phase III clinical trial of antibiotics to reduce chorioamnionitis-related perinatal HIV-1 transmission. AIDS 2006; 20(9):1313–21.
113. Belyhun Y, Medhin G, Amberbir A, et al. Prevalence and risk factors for soil-transmitted helminth infection in mothers and their infants in Butajira, Ethiopia: a population based study. BMC Public Health 2010;10:21.
114. Naish S, McCarthy J, Williams GM. Prevalence, intensity and risk factors for soil-transmitted helminth infection in a South Indian fishing village. Acta Trop 2004; 91(2):177–87.
115. Yatich NJ, Yi J, Agbenyega T, et al. Malaria and intestinal helminth co-infection among pregnant women in Ghana: prevalence and risk factors. Am J Trop Med Hyg 2009;80(6):896–901.
116. Nguyen PH, Nguyen KC, Nguyen TD, et al. Intestinal helminth infections among reproductive age women in Vietnam: prevalence, co-infection and risk factors. Southeast Asian J Trop Med Public Health 2006;37(5):865–74.

117. Ponnighaus JM, Fine PE, Sterne JA, et al. Efficacy of BCG vaccine against leprosy and tuberculosis in northern Malawi. Lancet 1992;339(8794):636–9.

118. Fine PE. Variation in protection by BCG: implications of and for heterologous immunity. Lancet 1995;346(8986):1339–45.

119. van Riet E, Hartgers FC, Yazdanbakhsh M. Chronic helminth infections induce immunomodulation: consequences and mechanisms. Immunobiology 2007; 212(6):475–90.

120. Malhotra I, Mungai P, Wamachi A, et al. Helminth- and Bacillus Calmette-Guerin-induced immunity in children sensitized in utero to filariasis and schistosomiasis. J Immunol 1999;162(11):6843–8.

121. Elias D, Wolday D, Akuffo H, et al. Effect of deworming on human T cell responses to mycobacterial antigens in helminth-exposed individuals before and after bacille Calmette-Guerin (BCG) vaccination. Clin Exp Immunol 2001; 123(2):219–25.

122. Cooper PJ, Chico M, Sandoval C, et al. Human infection with Ascaris lumbricoides is associated with suppression of the interleukin-2 response to recombinant cholera toxin B subunit following vaccination with the live oral cholera vaccine CVD 103-HgR. Infect Immun 2001;69(3):1574–80.

123. Weisman Z, Kalinkovich A, Borkow G, et al. Infection by different HIV-1 subtypes (B and C) results in a similar immune activation profile despite distinct immune backgrounds. J Acquir Immune Defic Syndr 1999;21(2):157–63.

124. Bentwich Z, Weisman Z, Moroz C, et al. Immune dysregulation in Ethiopian immigrants in Israel: relevance to helminth infections? Clin Exp Immunol 1996; 103(2):239–43.

125. Kalinkovich A, Weisman Z, Greenberg Z, et al. Decreased CD4 and increased CD8 counts with T cell activation is associated with chronic helminth infection. Clin Exp Immunol 1998;114(3):414–21.

126. Chenine AL, Buckley KA, Li PL, et al. Schistosoma mansoni infection promotes SHIV clade C replication in rhesus macaques. AIDS 2005;19(16):1793–7.

127. Ayash-Rashkovsky M, Chenine AL, Steele LN, et al. Coinfection with Schistosoma mansoni reactivates viremia in rhesus macaques with chronic simian-human immunodeficiency virus clade C infection. Infect Immun 2007; 75(4):1751–6.

128. Chenine AL, Shai-Kobiler E, Steele LN, et al. Acute Schistosoma mansoni infection increases susceptibility to systemic SHIV clade C infection in rhesus macaques after mucosal virus exposure. PLoS Negl Trop Dis 2008;2(7):e265.

129. Walson JL, Otieno PA, Mbuchi M, et al. Albendazole treatment of HIV-1 and helminth co-infection: a randomized, double-blind, placebo-controlled trial. AIDS 2008;22(13):1601–9.

130. Kallestrup P, Zinyama R, Gomo E, et al. Schistosomiasis and HIV-1 infection in rural Zimbabwe: effect of treatment of schistosomiasis on CD4 cell count and plasma HIV-1 RNA load. J Infect Dis 2005;192(11):1956–61.

131. Da'dara AA, Harn DA. Elimination of helminth infection restores HIV-1C vaccine-specific T cell responses independent of helminth-induced IL-10. Vaccine 2010; 28(5):1310–7.

132. Actor JK, Shirai M, Kullberg MC, et al. Helminth infection results in decreased virus-specific CD8+ cytotoxic T-cell and Th1 cytokine responses as well as delayed virus clearance. Proc Natl Acad Sci U S A 1993;90(3):948–52.

133. Ayash-Rashkovsky M, Weisman Z, Diveley J, et al. Generation of Th1 immune responses to inactivated, gp120-depleted HIV-1 in mice with a dominant Th2 biased immune profile via immunostimulatory [correction of imunostimulatory]

oligonucleotides–relevance to AIDS vaccines in developing countries. Vaccine 2002;20(21-22):2684–92.

134. Ayash-Rashkovsky M, Weisman Z, Zlotnikov S, et al. Induction of antigen-specific Th1-biased immune responses by plasmid DNA in schistosoma-infected mice with a preexistent dominant Th2 immune profile. Biochem Biophys Res Commun 2001;282(5):1169–76.

135. Kusakabe K, Xin KQ, Katoh H, et al. The timing of GM-CSF expression plasmid administration influences the Th1/Th2 response induced by an HIV-1-specific DNA vaccine. J Immunol 2000;164(6):3102–11.

136. Wille-Reece U, Flynn BJ, Lore K, et al. HIV Gag protein conjugated to a Toll-like receptor 7/8 agonist improves the magnitude and quality of Th1 and CD8+ T cell responses in nonhuman primates. Proc Natl Acad Sci U S A 2005; 102(42):15190–4.

137. Sieling PA, Chung W, Duong BT, et al. Toll-like receptor 2 ligands as adjuvants for human Th1 responses. J Immunol 2003;170(1):194–200.

138. Lalvani A, Brookes R, Wilkinson RJ, et al. Human cytolytic and interferon gamma-secreting CD8+ T lymphocytes specific for *Mycobacterium tuberculosis*. Proc Natl Acad Sci U S A 1998;95(1):270–5.

139. Maino VC, Maecker HT. Cytokine flow cytometry: a multiparametric approach for assessing cellular immune responses to viral antigens. Clin Immunol 2003;110: 222–31.

140. DeVange Panteleeff D, John GC, Nduati R, et al. Rapid method for screening dried blood samples on filter paper for human immunodeficiency virus type 1 DNA. J Clin Microbiol 1999;37:350–3.

141. Selin LK, Lin M-L, Kraemer KA, et al. Attrition of T cell memory: selective loss of LCMV epitope-specific memory CD8 T cells following infections with heterologous viruses. Immunity 1999;11:733–42.

142. Vidor E. The nature and consequences of intra- and inter-vaccine interference. J Comp Pathol 2007;137(Suppl 1):S62–6.

143. Gans HA, Arvin AM, Galinus J, et al. Deficiency of the humoral immune response to measles vaccine in infants immunized at 6 months of age. JAMA 1998;280:527–32.

144. Siegrist CA, Cordova M, Brandt C, et al. Determinants of infant responses to vaccines in presence of maternal antibodies. Vaccine 1998;16:1409–14.

145. Stoiber H. Complement, Fc receptors and antibodies: a Trojan horse in HIV infection? Curr Opin HIV AIDS 2009;4:394–9.

146. Shinefield HR. Overview of the development and current use of CRM197 conjugate vaccines for pediatric use. Vaccine 2010;28:4335–9.

147. Baba TW, Liska V, Khimani AH, et al. Live attenuated, multiply deleted simian immunodeficiency virus causes AIDS in infant and adult macaques. Nat Med 1999;5:194–203.

HIV-1 and Breastfeeding: Biology of Transmission and Advances in Prevention

Marc Bulterys, MD, PhD[a,b], Sascha Ellington, MSPH[c],
Athena P. Kourtis, MD, PhD, MPH[c],*

KEYWORDS

- Breastfeeding • HIV-1 • Mother-to-child HIV transmission
- Antiretroviral prophylactic treatment

In 2008 there were an estimated 430,000 new infections of human immunodeficiency virus type 1 (HIV-1) in children younger than 15 years of age, and there were 2.1 million children living with HIV-1.[1] The same year there were 280,000 AIDS-related deaths among children.[1] Most new cases of HIV-1 infection in children are acquired through mother-to-child transmission (MTCT) in utero, intrapartum, or postpartum through breastfeeding[1]; pre-mastication of food by HIV-1–infected care providers has also caused postnatal infant HIV-1 infections in some settings.[2] Among children with known timing of infection, as much as 42% of MTCT of HIV-1 is attributable to breastfeeding.[3,4]

The benefits of breastfeeding are well recognized and include providing the infant with optimal nutrition during the first months of life, reducing infant morbidity and mortality owing to diarrheal and lower respiratory infections, protecting against common childhood infections, and promoting child spacing, which is associated with higher child survival.[5,6] These benefits are particularly important in areas where the water supply is unsafe and infant mortality high.

---

[a] Division of HIV/AIDS, Center for Global Health, Centers for Disease Control and Prevention (CDC), Atlanta, GA 30333, USA
[b] CDC Global AIDS Program, China, Suite #403, Dongwai Diplomatic Office, 23 Dongzhimenwai Dajie, Beijing, China
[c] Division of Reproductive Health, National Center for Chronic Disease Preventation and Health Promotion, Centers for Disease Control and Prevention 4770 Buford Highway, NE, MS-K34, Atlanta, GA 30341, USA
* Corresponding author. WHFB/DRH/NCCDPHP/CDC, MS-K34, 4770 Buford Highway, NE, Atlanta, GA 30341.
E-mail address: apk3@cdc.gov

Clin Perinatol 37 (2010) 807–824
doi:10.1016/j.clp.2010.08.001
0095-5108/10/$ – see front matter. Published by Elsevier Inc.

Since 1985, the US Centers for Disease Control and Prevention (CDC) has recommended that HIV-1–infected women in the United States avoid breastfeeding.[7] Because replacement feeding is safe, affordable, and culturally acceptable for women in the United States and other resource-rich settings, postnatal MTCT of HIV-1 is nearly zero in such settings. For most HIV-1–infected mothers in resource-limited settings, however, breastfeeding remains the only feasible option for infant feeding, given the unsafe water and poor hygiene, cultural norms that stigmatize mothers who do not breastfeed, and the prohibitive costs and lack of availability of infant formula. That is why the World Health Organization (WHO) recommends that in resource-limited settings HIV-1–infected women breastfeed their infants if safe formula feeding is not possible.[8]

BIOLOGY OF TRANSMISSION OF HIV-1 TO THE INFANT THROUGH BREASTFEEDING
Virology

HIV-1 in breast milk of infected mothers can originate either from blood cell–free virus released into breast milk or can be produced by local replication in macrophages and in ductal and alveolar mammary epithelial cells.[9,10] HIV-1 is detected both in the cellular compartment of breast milk and in cell-free milk with varying frequencies in different studies (39%–89%).[11,12] Detection is associated with lower maternal CD4+ T-cell count and vitamin A deficiency,[9] as well as with clinical and subclinical mastitis.[13,14] HIV-1 load in breast milk seems to be highest just after birth.[12] Intermittent shedding and differences in viral load between the 2 breasts have been noted in several studies.[14,15] The concentration of HIV-1 in cell-free breast milk is generally lower than in plasma by about 2 logs.[11,16] Highly active antiretroviral therapy (HAART) started during pregnancy or postpartum suppresses HIV-1 RNA but may not suppress DNA in breast milk.[17,18]

Immunology

Breast milk contains many antimicrobial and immunomodulatory factors with diverse effects on HIV-1: some have in vitro anti-HIV-1 activity (including secretory leukocyte protease inhibitor [SLPI], lactoferrin, RANTES, interferon-γ, and α- and β-defensins), whereas others have proinflammatory activity that might promote local HIV-1 replication (including interleukin [IL]-6, IL-8, IL-7, IL-1β, and tumor necrosis factor [TNF]-α).[9,19–21] Some studies have also reported protective effects of long-chain polyunsaturated fatty acids in breast milk.[22] HIV-1–specific antibodies are detected in breast milk, predominantly of the IgG isotype.[23] The specificity of IgG and IgA anti-HIV-1 antibodies in breast milk can differ from that of the antibodies in the serum of the same woman.[23] Lower likelihood of postnatal transmission of HIV-1 to the infant has been associated with the presence of HIV-1–specific secretory IgA and IgM in the breast milk in some[20,24] but not all studies.[25–27] The role that HIV-1 neutralizing antibodies in breast milk play in postnatal transmission of HIV-1 to the infant has not been evaluated so far.

Breast milk also contains many immune cell types such as lymphocytes and macrophages. Breast milk lymphocytes have an activated phenotype and express chemokine receptors and mucosal homing markers.[28] The macrophages in the breast milk express, when stimulated with IL-4, DC-SIGN, a dendritic cell receptor for HIV-1,[29] which may play a role in HIV-1 transmission through mucosal membranes.[30,31] There is some evidence that infant HIV-1–specific cytotoxic T-lymphocyte responses may be associated with protection from breastfeeding transmission of HIV-1.[32] Particular human leukocyte antigen (HLA) alleles have been associated with protection against

MTCT of HIV-1; in particular, HLA B18 may protect the infant against breastfeeding transmission.[33] There is also some evidence that maternal HLA homozygosity and mother-child HLA concordance may increase the risk of transmission of HIV-1 via breastfeeding.[34]

Role of Mucosal Factors

Several studies have shown that the type of infant feeding has a substantial effect on postnatal transmission of HIV-1. Exclusive breastfeeding is associated with a lower risk of transmission than mixed feeding.[35-37] This may be attributable to damage to the gut mucosa induced from early introduction of non–breast milk foods, leading to delayed closure of the enterocyte junctions in the intestinal mucosal barrier, or, alternatively, from intestinal immune activation resulting from early introduction of foreign antigens or pathogens. Both of these mechanisms can increase the risk of HIV-1 transmission to the infant.[38] In addition, infrequent breast emptying, which might occur with nonexclusive breastfeeding, may increase the risk of ductal inflammation in the breast, with production of cytokines and other inflammatory mediators, leading to subclinical mastitis and increases in mammary epithelial permeability. Elevations in breast milk sodium in the absence of clinical symptoms (subclinical mastitis) and symptomatic breast inflammation (mastitis) have been associated with higher levels of HIV-1 in breast milk and increased risk of postnatal transmission.[21] However, a recent study indicated that laboratory markers of mastitis, such as increased sodium level and cell count, are poor predictors of HIV-1 RNA levels in breast milk.[39]

FACTORS AFFECTING BREASTFEEDING TRANSMISSION OF HIV-1
Duration of Breastfeeding

Longer duration of breastfeeding leads to a higher risk of transmission.[4,9,20,40,41] Data from Malawi found a risk of postnatal transmission of HIV-1 of 0.6% to 0.7% per month in the first year from months 1 to 12, and 0.3% per month in the second year of lactation.[41,42] Some studies suggest that the highest risk of breast milk transmission of HIV-1 is in the immediate neonatal period.[4,11,12,41,43] A meta-analysis suggested a more constant risk of postnatal transmission of HIV-1 of 0.9% per month after the first month of life[44]; the risk persists with prolonged breastfeeding.[45] It is difficult to differentiate between early breast milk transmission and intrapartum transmission. Two studies estimated postnatal HIV-1 transmission based on differences in transmission between mothers who breastfed and those who used formula from birth.[4,43] Both found a very high risk of transmission for the breastfed compared with the formula-fed infants in the early weeks of life: a 6.3% difference in the Nairobi trial from birth to 6 weeks (or 1%/week) and a 5.6% difference in the SAINT trial in South Africa over 8 weeks (or 0.7% per week).[4,43]

HIV-1 Load in Breast Milk

HIV-1 level in breast milk is one of the most important determinants of breast milk transmission risk. Cell-associated virus is a stronger predictor for HIV-1 transmission to the infant than cell-free virus.[16,46] A 2-fold increase in MTCT risk for every 10-fold increase in cell-free HIV-1 RNA and a 3-fold increase in MTCT risk for every 10-fold increase in infected cells harboring HIV-1 DNA has been estimated.[12,16,44,46,47] It should be noted that abrupt weaning may increase concentrations of HIV-1 RNA in breast milk.[48] Local breast inflammation resulting from mastitis (clinical or subclinical) or breast abscess can also increase breast milk virus levels and MTCT risk.[49]

Type of Breastfeeding

As mentioned, several studies have shown that postnatal HIV-1 transmission is lower with exclusive breastfeeding compared with mixed feeding.[36,37,50] In the ZVITAMBO trial in Zimbabwe, the rate of postnatal transmission of HIV-1 was 5.1, 6.7, and 10.5 infections per 100 child-years of breastfeeding for infants who were exclusively breastfed, predominantly breast-fed (feeding breast milk and other nonmilk fluids), and mixed fed, respectively.[36] Many infant feeding policies encouraged HIV-1–infected women to wean abruptly to avoid mixed feeding. Abrupt weaning, however, was associated with maternal illness (fever, mastitis) and elevations in breast milk sodium in a study in Zambia.[48] In addition, large increases in breast milk HIV-1 RNA were also observed, as previously mentioned, indicating that abrupt weaning may expose the infants to a higher risk of HIV-1 acquisition. Weaning infants at 4 to 6 months of age was also shown to be associated with increased diarrheal morbidity and mortality in several studies.[51–53] These results have led WHO to revise its recommendations about duration of breastfeeding, as is described later in this article.[8]

Maternal and Infant Conditions

Advanced maternal disease, higher plasma viral load, lower CD4+ T-cell counts, and poor maternal nutritional status increase the risk of breast milk transmission of HIV-1 to the infant.[50,54,55] It has been postulated that malnutrition and poor maternal health, other concurrent, subacute infections, and nonexclusive breastfeeding may be contributing factors to breast milk stasis and subclinical mastitis.[56–59] Cracked nipples and infant conditions such as thrush and oral ulcers may also increase the risk for HIV-1 transmission via breastfeeding (reviewed in Kourtis and colleagues[38]).

ANTIRETROVIRAL DRUGS DURING BREASTFEEDING

The effect of maternal HAART on the HIV-1 load in breast milk has been reported in recent studies from Africa. In Mozambique, HAART in breastfeeding women decreased cell-free HIV-1 RNA load in breast milk.[17] A study in Botswana among women with CD4+ T-cell counts lower than 200 cells/mm^3 showed that HAART decreased HIV-1 RNA but had no apparent effect on HIV-1 DNA load in breast milk.[18] A third study from Kenya similarly showed the suppression of cell-free HIV-1 RNA in breast milk without suppression of HIV-1 DNA.[60] **Box 1** summarizes the factors affecting MTCT of HIV-1 via breastfeeding.

Box 1
Risk factors for HIV-1 transmission from mother to infant through breastfeeding

Higher HIV-1 load in maternal plasma and breast milk

Lower maternal CD4+ T-cell count

Advanced maternal disease

Maternal malnutrition

Prolonged duration of breastfeeding

Nonexclusive breastfeeding

Clinical and subclinical mastitis, breast abscess, cracked nipples

Elevated breast milk Na/K ratio

Infant thrush, oral ulcers

Antiretroviral Approaches for Prevention of Mother-to-Child Transmission of HIV-1 through Breastfeeding

For more than a decade, antiretroviral (ARV) regimens administered to the mother during pregnancy and delivery and to the infant postnatally have proven very effective in reducing in utero and intrapartum transmission of HIV-1; this has included simplified short-course regimens in resource-limited settings.[61–66] Development of effective strategies to reduce postnatal transmission in breastfeeding populations has comparatively lagged behind. Recently, however, several studies have shown that ARV prophylaxis given either to the infant or the mother during breastfeeding is highly effective in reducing breastfeeding transmission of HIV-1 to infants.[67–74]

Infant Antiretroviral Prophylaxis

Results from an observational and several open-label randomized clinical trials that evaluated the use of extended ARV prophylaxis among infants of breastfeeding HIV-1–infected mothers are now available.[67,69,74,75] The Mitra study was an observational study in which daily lamivudine given to the breastfeeding infant for up to 6 months resulted in a low cumulative HIV-1 infection rate of 4.9% at 6 months, with an HIV-1 infection risk of 1.2% between 6 weeks and 6 months.[75] The Six-Week Extended-Dose Nevirapine (SWEN) trials, which evaluated the effectiveness of 6 weeks of extended nevirapine (NVP) given to breastfeeding infants, found a significant reduction in HIV-1 transmission at 6 weeks, compared with the control arm, from 5.3% to 2.5%.[67] However, there was no statistically significant difference of HIV-1 transmission at 6 months between the 2 arms, suggesting that a longer duration of prophylaxis would be required to protect the infant from ongoing breastfeeding transmission.[67] The PEPI (Post Exposure Prophylaxis of Infants) trial in Malawi found that extended prophylaxis with either NVP or NVP plus zidovudine through 14 weeks of infant age significantly reduced postnatal HIV-1 transmission compared with the control arm of single-dose NVP and 1 week of zidovudine.[69] There were no significant differences in the effectiveness of the extended prophylaxis arms in PEPI; however, the NVP plus zidovudine regimen was associated with significantly more adverse events, primarily neutropenia.[69] Last, the recently completed Breastfeeding, Antiretrovirals, and Nutrition (BAN) Study, also in Malawi, evaluated 6 months of extended NVP infant prophylaxis; the estimated risk of HIV-1 transmission through breastfeeding at 28 weeks was 1.7%, compared with 5.7% for infants in the control arm of single-dose NVP and 7 days of zidovudine and lamivudine.[74]

The results from the SWEN, PEPI, and BAN trials showed infant NVP prophylaxis to be a safe and effective strategy in reducing breastfeeding transmission of HIV-1; however, infants who continued to breastfeed after prophylaxis ended were at continued risk of becoming HIV-1-infected in both the SWEN and PEPI studies. Combined, these results suggest greater protection with longer duration of NVP prophylaxis; infants may benefit from daily NVP throughout the entire duration of breastfeeding. Extended infant NVP prophylaxis is a low-cost, single daily regimen associated with little toxicity and is feasible for many resource-limited settings.[76] There is, however, concern that failure of such prophylaxis will result in an increased rate of NVP resistance in the HIV-1–infected infant, thereby reducing future treatment options for the infant.[77] Indeed, 92% of infants who became HIV-1 infected during the first 6 weeks of life (period of NVP prophylaxis) in the SWEN study had NVP resistance; the risk, however, was much lower (15%) for infants who became infected after prophylaxis had stopped.[67,78]

An additional infant prophylaxis study, PROMISE-PEP (Peri-Exposure Prophylaxis), began enrollment in December 2009. The PROMISE-PEP study is a multisite, double-blinded, randomized clinical trial comparing twice-daily lopinavir-ritonavir to twice-daily lamivudine. Both regimens will be administered to the infant from day 7 through 4 weeks after cessation of breastfeeding with a maximum duration of 50 weeks of prophylaxis.[79]

Maternal ARV Prophylaxis

WHO currently recommends that all pregnant, HIV-1–infected women with CD4 counts of 350 cells/mm^3 or less initiate ARV therapy for their own health. But even for mothers with higher CD4+ T-cell counts, ARV prophylaxis may be an approach to prevent postnatal transmission of HIV-1 to the infant. From 2007 to 2009, results from observational studies had suggested that maternal ARVs did indeed reduce the risk of transmitting HIV-1 to the infant through breast milk.[68,70,71] Results are now available from several randomized clinical trials, proving that maternal ARVs are an effective prophylactic strategy to reduce postnatal HIV-1 transmission.[72–74] Furthermore, both observational and randomized studies have shown that when ARV prophylaxis is started during the antenatal period, very low rates of postnatal HIV-1 transmission are achievable at 6 months.[68,70,72,73,80] For example, in the Mitra Plus study, an observational study in which most women started HAART at 34 weeks of gestation, the risk of infant HIV-1 infection between 6 weeks and 6 months was just 1.0%; between 6 weeks and 18 months it was 2.1%.[68] Of all PMTCT studies conducted in breastfeeding populations, the Mma Bana trial, which initiated ARVs between 26 and 34 weeks of gestation in women with CD4+ T-cell counts higher than 200 cells/mm^3, had the lowest rate of infant HIV-1 infection at 6 months, with a cumulative infant transmission rate of just 1%.[72] In contrast, in the BAN study, which enrolled women with CD4+ T-cell counts higher than 250 cells/mm^3, maternal prophylaxis was not initiated until labor/delivery; the HIV-1 transmission rate to the infant in the maternal-ARV arm was 2.9% between 2 and 28 weeks, which was significantly lower than the transmission rate in the control arm (5.7%).[74] Taken together, these results suggest that maternal prophylaxis may need to start antenatally to achieve maximal reduction of postnatal HIV-1 transmission to the infant.

Although maternal ARV prophylaxis is effective in reducing postnatal HIV-1 transmission, this benefit needs to be considered along with any harm or discomfort the regimen may pose to the mother. Maternal toxicities, HAART interruption at the end of breastfeeding, and poor adherence may increase the mother's risk of developing resistance and limit her future treatment options.[81,82] Also, failure of such prophylaxis has the potential for transmission of a resistant virus, limiting the infant's future treatment options as well-indeed 67% of infants infected postnatally in the KiBS trial had drug-resistant virus.[71,81] Some ARV agents enter breast milk—zidovudine appears to be present at levels similar or slightly lower than those in maternal plasma, NVP levels are about 70% those in maternal plasma, and 3TC appears to concentrate in breast milk at levels 3 to 5 times those of maternal plasma, whereas protease inhibitors seem to have very limited penetration.[83] Breastfed infants may thus be ingesting subtherapeutic levels of ARV present in breast milk, leading to the potential for development of resistance. Other prophylactic ARV regimens in the nursing HIV-1–infected mothers, including tenofovir, tenofovir/emtricitabine, efavirenz, and lopinavir/ritonavir combinations, will be evaluated for their safety and efficacy in a number of ongoing and planned trials (**Table 1**).[73,84,85]

The Mitra and Mitra-Plus observational studies of infant prophylaxis and maternal prophylaxis, respectively, had similar rates of postnatal transmission at 6 months.[68,75]

However, the studies were observational and were conducted sequentially at the same site. The BAN study is the only randomized controlled trial to date to have both a maternal and an infant prophylaxis arm, each of which was compared with the control arm. Although the study was not powered to directly compare the 2 interventions, there was a suggestion that HIV-1–free survival at 28 weeks may be greater with infant, compared with maternal prophylaxis ($P = .07$).[74] A more direct comparison of the 2 approaches is planned[84] (see **Table 1**). Although effective maternal and infant ARV prophylactic strategies are now available to reduce postnatal HIV-1 transmission through breastfeeding, more research is needed to determine the optimal method that balances benefits and risks for mothers and infants and is feasible for a particular resource-limited setting.

Immune-Based Approaches

An effective neonatal vaccine could prevent transmission of HIV-1 via breast milk and protect the infant long term; however, the lack of efficacy of gp120 vaccine in adults has tempered enthusiasm for this approach in infants.[86] Replication-defective recombinant viral vaccines have been evaluated: a canarypox vector (ALVAC vCP205) was shown to have limited immunogenicity in infants in the PACTG 326 study.[87] The HIV Prevention Trials Network (HPTN) recently completed a phase I randomized trial evaluating the safety and immunogenicity of an HIV-1 vaccine candidate using a canarypox vector (ALVAC-HIV vCP1521), in infants born to HIV-1–infected mothers in Uganda. Sixty breastfed infants were randomly assigned to receive 4 injections of vaccine or placebo during the first 3 months of life. The results of the trial are not yet available.[88] A phase I/II trial evaluating the safety and immunogenicity of a Modified-Vaccinia Ankara (vaccine vector) (MVA)-HIV-1 vaccine in 20-week-old breastfed and formula-fed infants of HIV-1–infected mothers is planned in Kenya.[89] A trial in Uganda evaluated a different approach, that of passive immunization: HIV-1 immune globulin (HIVIGLOB) was given as an infusion to mothers at 36 to 37 weeks of gestation and to the newborn, and was found safe and well-tolerated.[90] This was compared with daily infant NVP for 6 weeks in a recently completed phase II/III trial; results have not yet become available.[91]

Inactivation of HIV-1 in Breast Milk

In resource-limited settings, inactivation of HIV-1 in breast milk may provide for a nutritionally adequate and safe alternative to traditional breastfeeding for HIV-1–infected mothers. Several methods to inactivate the virus have been proposed, including chemical and heat treatment processes. A preliminary study of treating breast milk with sodium dodecyl sulfate has shown promise.[92] Although the antimalarial agent chloroquine and its hydroxyl analog have in vitro activity against HIV-1 replication, studies have not shown a significant effect of chloroquine on breast milk viral loads of HIV-1–infected women.[93–95] A number of studies have been successful in inactivating HIV-1 in breast milk with heat treatments. Placing breast milk in glass jars in boiling water for 12 to 15 minutes, a method called Pretoria pasteurization, was shown to be effective in reducing bacterial contamination and inactivating HIV-1 in breast milk.[96–99] Another study demonstrated that flash-heating inactivates cell-free HIV-1 in naturally infected breast milk from HIV-1–infected women and could be implemented over an outdoor fire or in a kitchen.[100] Heat-treated milk appears to have a similar nutritional and immune composition to untreated milk; however, this needs further assessment.[101] WHO endorses the need for continued research to find safe, feasible, and effective methods to heat-treat expressed breast milk.[8]

Table 1
Summary of ongoing and planned clinical trials for prevention of mother-to-child transmission of HIV-1 through breastfeeding

Trial (Location, Status)	Study Arm	Antepartum	Intrapartum	Postpartum (Mother)	Postnatal (Infant) Regimen
BAN (N = 2369) Phase III randomized clinical trial in Lilongwe, Malawi, study completed January 2010	Arm 1 (Maternal Prophylaxis)	No drug	sdNVP	ZDV/3TC/LPV/rv × 6 mo	sdNVP plus ZDV/3TC × 1 wk EBF × 6 mo with rapid weaning over 4 wk
	Arm 2 (Infant Prophylaxis)	No drug	sdNVP	ZDV/3TC × 1wk	ZDV/3TC × 1 wk plus NVP daily × 6 mo EBF × 6mo with rapid weaning over 4 wk
	Arm 3 (control)	No drug	sdNVP	ZDV/3TC × 1wk	sdNVP plus ZDV/3TC × 1 wk EBF × 6 mo with rapid weaning over 4 wk
Kesho Bora (N = 805) Phase III, multisite, randomized clinical trial in Burkina Faso, Kenya and South Africa, follow-up ongoing, study completed June 2010	Arm 1 (Maternal Prophylaxis)	ZDV/3TC/LPV/rv from 28–36 wk	ZDV/3TC/LPV/rv	ZDV/3TC/LPV/rv × 6 mo	sdNVP plus ZDV × 1 wk EBF × 5.5 mo with rapid weaning over 2 wk
	Arm 2 (Control)	ZDV from 28–36 wks	ZDV/3TC/sdNVP	ZDV/3TC × 1 wk	sdNVP plus ZDV × 1 wk EBF × 5.5 mo with rapid weaning over 2 wk
Mma Bana (N = 560) Phase III randomized clinical trial in Botswana, follow-up ongoing, study completed May 2009	Arm 1 (Maternal Prophylaxis)	ZDV/3TC/Abacavir from 26–34 wk	ZDV/3TC/Abacavir	ZDV/3TC/Abacavir × 6 mo or for duration of BF (if <6 mo)	sdNVP plus ZDV × 1 mo EBF × 6 mo then weaned
	Arm 2 (Maternal Prophylaxis)	ZDV/3TC/LPV/rv (Trizivir) from 26–34 wks	ZDV/3TC/LPV/rv	ZDV/3TC/LPV/rv × 6mo	sdNVP plus ZDV × 1 mo EBF × 6 mo then weaned
HPTN 046 (ongoing, N = 1670) Phase III, multisite, double blind clinical trial in South Africa, Tanzania, Uganda, and Zimbabwe, closed to accrual, study completion expected March 2011	Arm 1	Local ARV standard of care for PMTCT	Local ARV standard of care for PMTCT	No drug	Open-label NVP × 6 wk then daily NVP through 6 mo or for the duration of BF (if < 6 mo) EBF × 6 mo and encouraged to wean
	Arm 2 (control)	Local ARV standard of care for PMTCT	Local ARV standard of care for PMTCT	No drug	Open-Label NVP × 6 wk then placebo through 6 mo or for the duration of BF (if <6mo) EBF × 6 mo and encouraged to wean

PROMISE-PEP (Planned N = 1500) Phase III, multisite, randomized, double-blind clinical trial in Burkina Faso, Uganda, Zambia, and South Africa, ongoing	Arm 1 (3TC)	Any perinatal ARV prophylaxis, per local standard	Any perinatal ARV prophylaxis, per local standard	No drug	sdNVP plus ZDV × 1 wk then *3TC from day 7 until 4 wk after BF cessation for a maximum of 50 wk* EBF recommended for 6 mo-weaning over 8 wk
	Arm 2 (LPV/rv)	Any perinatal ARV prophylaxis, per local standard	Any perinatal ARV prophylaxis, per local standard	No drug	sdNVP plus ZDV × 1 wk then *LPV/rv from day 7 until 4 wk after BF cessation for a maximum of 50 wk* EBF recommended for 6 mo-weaning over 8 wk
IMPAACT PROMISE 1077 (Postpartum Component - Planned N = 12,536 for all components) Phase III, multisite, randomized clinical trial, sites and start date to be determined	Arm 1 (Maternal Prophylaxis)	Triple ARV regimen starting at 28 wk (dependent on randomization in antepartum portion)	Triple ARV regimen (dependent on randomization in antepartum portion)	*Truvada plus LPV/rv for the duration of BF or 18 mo (whichever occurs first)*	*NVP × 6 wk*
	Arm 2 (Infant Prophylaxis)	Triple ARV regimen starting at 28 wk (dependent on randomization in antepartum portion)	Triple ARV regimen (dependent on randomization in antepartum portion)	*No drug*	*Daily NVP for the duration of BF or 18 mo (whichever occurs first)*
UMA (Planned N = 960) Phase III, multisite, randomized clinical trial in Côte D'Ivoire and Zambia	Arm 1 (Maternal Prophylaxis)	*EFV/TDF/FTC* (formulated as Atripla) from 20 wk	*EFV/TDF/FTC*	*EFV/TDF/FTC for the duration of BF with advice to cease at 6 mo*	Daily ZDV syrup from birth through 1 wk or updated with a prophylaxis regimen recommended by WHO Advise BF cessation at 6 mo
	Arm 2 (Maternal Prophylaxis)	*ZDV/3TC/LPV/rv* from 20 wk	*ZDV/3TC/LPV/rv*	*ZDV/3TC/LPV/rv for the duration of BF with advice to cease at 6 mo*	Daily ZDV syrup from birth through 1 wk or updated with a prophylaxis regimen recommended by WHO Advise BF cessation at 6 mo

(continued on next page)

Table 1
(continued)

Trial (Location, Status)	Study Arm	Antepartum	Intrapartum	Postpartum (Mother)	Postnatal (Infant) Regimen
HIVIGLOB (2 of the 3 study arms included in SWEN) phase II/III, single-site, randomized clinical trial in Uganda (study completed in 2008, results not yet published, N = 722)	Arm 1	*HIV hyperimmune globulin at 36–37 wk*	sdNVP	No drug	*NVP × 6 wk* This arm was included in SWEN trials (extended prophylaxis)
	Arm 2	*HIV hyperimmune globulin at 36–37 wk*	sdNVP	No drug	*sdNVP plus HIV hyperimmune globulin within 18 hr of birth* sdNVP
	Arm 3 (control)	*HIV hyperimmune globulin at 36–37 wk*	sdNVP	No drug	This arm was included in SWEN trials (control)
ALVAC-HIV vCP1521 trial (Uganda, completed, N = 60) Phase I, double-blind, randomized clinical trial, completed	Arm 1	Standard of care	Standard of care	Standard of care	Standard of care plus vaccine *(birth, wk 4, wk 8, wk 12)*
	Arm 2 (control)	Standard of care	Standard of care	Standard of care	Standard of care
PedVac002 Study (Planned, N = 72) Phase I/II, single-site, randomized clinical trial in Kenya, planned to start in 2010	Arm 1	Standard of care	Standard of care	Standard of care	*Candidate MVA HIV-1 Vaccine given at 20 wk plus standard of care*
	Arm 2 (Control)	Standard of care	Standard of care	Standard of care	Standard of care

Abbreviations: ARV, antiretroviral drugs; BF, breastfeeding; EBF, exclusive breastfeeding; EFV, efavirenz; FTC, emtricitabine; LPV/rv, lopinavir/ritonavir; MTCT, mother-to-child transmission; MVA, Modified-Vaccinia Ankara (vaccine vector)NVP, nevirapine; sd, single dose; TDF, tenofovir; Trizivir, zidovudine/lamivudine/abacavir; Truvada, tenofovir/emtricitabine; ZDV, zidovudine; 3TC, lamivudine.
For further information on some of these clinical trials, please see http://www.clinicaltrials.gov.

WHO RECOMMENDATIONS FOR BREASTFEEDING AMONG HIV-1–INFECTED MOTHERS IN RESOURCE-LIMITED SETTINGS

WHO recommendations have undergone many revisions over the years, as scientific knowledge has evolved and clinical trial results have increasingly become available in this rapidly changing field. In November 2009, WHO revised the breastfeeding guidelines for HIV-1–infected mothers in resource-limited settings once again, based on the most recent evidence.[8] The new rapid advice recommends that women who received a 3-drug ARV regimen during pregnancy should continue this regimen through breastfeeding and until 1 week after all exposure of the infant to breast milk has ended. If a woman received only zidovudine during pregnancy, daily NVP is recommended for her child from birth until 1 week after the end of breastfeeding.

WHO further recommended that national health authorities should decide whether they will counsel HIV-1–infected mothers to either avoid all breastfeeding or to breastfeed and receive either maternal or infant prophylaxis.[8] If breastfeeding is recommended, then the HIV-1–infected mothers should exclusively breastfeed their infants for the first 6 months of life, introducing appropriate complementary foods thereafter, and continue breastfeeding for the first 12 months. Breastfeeding should be stopped only once a nutritionally adequate and safe diet without breast milk can be provided. Enabling breastfeeding in the presence of ARV interventions to continue to 12 months avoids many of the complexities associated with stopping breastfeeding and with providing a safe and adequate diet without breast milk to the infant between 6 and 12 months of age. HIV-1–infected mothers who decide to stop breastfeeding at any time should stop gradually within 1 month.

A systematic review examined the effect of prolonged breastfeeding on the health of HIV-1–infected mothers.[102] This review indicated that there was no clear evidence of harm to the mother if she continued breastfeeding. One study that did report increased mortality in breastfeeding mothers[103] was in conflict with several others, including the meta-analysis that did not confirm this outcome.[102]

In infants and young children known to be HIV-1 infected, mothers are strongly encouraged to exclusively breastfeed for the first 6 months of life and continue breastfeeding as per the recommendations for the general population, that is up to 2 years.

In a randomized controlled trial in Zambia in which infants of HIV-1–infected breastfeeding mothers either stopped all breastfeeding at 4 months of age or continued to breastfeed, mortality at 24 months was 55% among those infants who were already HIV-1 infected and were randomized to continued breastfeeding, compared with 74% among those who were HIV-1 infected who stopped breastfeeding early.[104] In a study in Botswana that randomized HIV-1–exposed infants to either breast milk or infant formula, among infants who were already HIV-1 infected, mortality at 6 months of age was 7.5% in those who breastfed, compared with 33% in those randomized to receive infant formula.[105]

Considerations for the Future

As the most recent advice from WHO highlights, ARV drugs in the mother or infant should be used throughout breastfeeding to reduce postnatal transmission of HIV-1 to the infant in resource-limited settings; breastfeeding should be completely avoided in resource-rich settings where safe infant feeding alternatives exist. In the current WHO guidelines, 12 months is advised as the breastfeeding duration for resource-limited settings; however, there is a compelling need to determine the minimum period for which infants born to HIV-1–infected mothers should be breastfed to provide adequate nutrition and immunologic benefits while minimizing exposure to the virus and to ARV drugs. There is also a need to evaluate the optimal weaning practices to minimize exposure to supplemental foods that may have infectious risks. The safety for mother and infants and the efficacy of other, newer ARV drugs or drugs of newer ARV classes during breastfeeding need to be tested, as well as immunologic approaches of active or passive immunization. The safety of stopping ARV prophylaxis for the mothers after cessation of breastfeeding and whether maternal, versus infant, prophylaxis is preferable for different settings need further assessment.[106] Exclusive breastfeeding needs to be vigorously supported. Finally, whether breastfeeding with ARV prophylaxis is an acceptable strategy in middle-income or resource-rich settings for the HIV-1–infected women who strongly wish to breastfeed their infants has not been evaluated; a formal assessment of its risk/benefit ratio may deserve more study. Linking HIV-1 prevention, care, and treatment services with family planning, antenatal and child health services, and building the health infrastructure required to implement MTCT prevention programs remains a critical need for resource-limited settings.

NOTE

The findings and conclusions in this report are those of the authors and do not necessarily represent the official position of the Centers for Disease Control and Prevention.

REFERENCES

1. UNAIDS. AIDS Epidemic update: November 2009. Available at: http://data.unaids.org/pub/Report/2009/jc1700_epi_update_2009_en.pdf. Geneva (Switzerland). Accessed May 14, 2010
2. Gaur AH, Dominguez KL, Kalish ML, et al. Practice of feeding premasticated food to infants: a potential risk factor for HIV transmission. Pediatrics 2009; 124:658–66.
3. Horvath T, Madi BC, Iuppa IM, et al. Interventions for preventing late postnatal mother-to-child transmission of HIV. Cochrane Database Syst Rev 2009;1: CD006734.
4. Nduati R, John G, Mbori-Ngacha D, et al. Effect of breastfeeding and formula feeding on transmission of HIV-1: a randomized clinical trial. JAMA 2000;283: 1167–74.
5. World Health Organization. HIV transmission through breastfeeding: a review of available evidence. 2010. Available at: http://www.unfpa.org/upload/lib_pub_file/276_filename_HIV_PREV_BF_GUIDE_ENG.pdf. Accessed April 20, 2010.
6. World Health Organization. Report of a WHO technical consultation on birth spacing. 2005. Available at: http://www.who.int/making_pregnancy_safer/documents/birth_spacing.pdf. Accessed April 20, 2010.
7. Achievements in public health. Reduction in perinatal transmission of HIV infection—United States, 1985-2005. MMWR Morb Mortal Wkly Rep 2006;55:592-7.
8. World Health Organization. Rapid advice: revised WHO principles and recomendations on infant feeding in the context of HIV — November 2009. Available at: http://www.searo.who.int/LinkFiles/HIV-AIDS_Rapid_Advice_Infant_feeding (web).pdf. 2009. Geneva (Switzerland). Accessed April 20, 2010.
9. Kourtis AP, Butera S, Ibegbu C, et al. Breast milk and HIV-1: vector of transmission or vehicle of protection? Lancet Infect Dis 2003;3:786–93.
10. Toniolo A, Serra C, Conaldi PG, et al. Productive HIV-1 infection of normal human mammary epithelial cells. AIDS 1995;9:859–66.
11. Lewis P, Nduati R, Kreiss JK, et al. Cell-free human immunodeficiency virus type 1 in breast milk. J Infect Dis 1998;177:34–9.

12. Rousseau CM, Nduati RW, Richardson BA, et al. Longitudinal analysis of human immunodeficiency virus type 1 RNA in breast milk and of its relationship to infant infection and maternal disease. J Infect Dis 2003;187:741–7.
13. Lunney KM, Iliff P, Mutasa K, et al. Associations between breast milk viral load, mastitis, exclusive breast-feeding, and postnatal transmission of HIV. Clin Infect Dis 2010;50:762–9.
14. Willumsen JF, Filteau SM, Coutsoudis A, et al. Breastmilk RNA viral load in HIV-infected South African women: effects of subclinical mastitis and infant feeding. AIDS 2003;17:407–14.
15. Hartmann SU, Berlin CM, Howett MK. Alternative modified infant-feeding practices to prevent postnatal transmission of human immunodeficiency virus type 1 through breast milk: past, present, and future. J Hum Lact 2006;22:75–88.
16. Rousseau CM, Nduati RW, Richardson BA, et al. Association of levels of HIV-1-infected breast milk cells and risk of mother-to-child transmission. J Infect Dis 2004;190:1880–8.
17. Giuliano M, Guidotti G, Andreotti M, et al. Triple antiretroviral prophylaxis administered during pregnancy and after delivery significantly reduces breast milk viral load: a study within the Drug Resource Enhancement Against AIDS and Malnutrition Program. J Acquir Immune Defic Syndr 2007;44:286–91.
18. Shapiro RL, Ndung'u T, Lockman S, et al. Highly active antiretroviral therapy started during pregnancy or postpartum suppresses HIV-1 RNA, but not DNA, in breast milk. J Infect Dis 2005;192:713–9.
19. Farquhar C, VanCott TC, Mbori-Ngacha DA, et al. Salivary secretory leukocyte protease inhibitor is associated with reduced transmission of human immunodeficiency virus type 1 through breast milk. J Infect Dis 2002;186:1173–6.
20. Van de Perre P, Simonon A, Hitimana DG, et al. Infective and anti-infective properties of breastmilk from HIV-1-infected women. Lancet 1993;341:914–8.
21. Walter J, Kuhn L, Aldrovandi GM. Advances in basic science understanding of mother-to-child HIV-1 transmission. Curr Opin HIV AIDS 2008;3:146–50.
22. Villamor E, Koulinska IN, Furtado J, et al. Long-chain n-6 polyunsaturated fatty acids in breast milk decrease the risk of HIV transmission through breastfeeding. Am J Clin Nutr 2007;86:682–9.
23. Becquart P, Hocini H, Garin B, et al. Compartmentalization of the IgG immune response to HIV-1 in breast milk. AIDS 1999;13:1323–31.
24. Van de Perre P, Simonon A, Msellati P, et al. Postnatal transmission of human immunodeficiency virus type 1 from mother to infant. A prospective cohort study in Kigali. Rwanda. N Engl J Med 1991;325:593–8.
25. Becquart P, Hocini H, Levy M, et al. Secretory anti-human immunodeficiency virus (HIV) antibodies in colostrum and breast milk are not a major determinant of the protection of early postnatal transmission of HIV. J Infect Dis 2000;181:532–9.
26. Duprat C, Mohammed Z, Datta P, et al. Human immunodeficiency virus type 1 IgA antibody in breast milk and serum. Pediatr Infect Dis J 1994;13:603–8.
27. Kuhn L, Trabattoni D, Kankasa C, et al. HIV-specific secretory IgA in breast milk of HIV-positive mothers is not associated with protection against HIV transmission among breast-fed infants. J Pediatr 2006;149:611–6.
28. Kourtis AP, Ibegbu CC, Theiler R, et al. Breast milk CD4+ T cells express high levels of C chemokine receptor 5 and CXC chemokine receptor 4 and are preserved in HIV-infected mothers receiving highly active antiretroviral therapy. J Infect Dis 2007;195:965–72.
29. Ichikawa M, Sugita M, Takahashi M, et al. Breast milk macrophages spontaneously produce granulocyte-macrophage colony-stimulating factor and differentiate into

dendritic cells in the presence of exogenous interleukin-4 alone. Immunology 2003;108:189–95.

30. Naarding MA, Dirac AM, Ludwig IS, et al. Bile salt-stimulated lipase from human milk binds DC-SIGN and inhibits human immunodeficiency virus type 1 transfer to CD4+ T cells. Antimicrob Agents Chemother 2006;50:3367–74.

31. Requena M, Bouhlal H, Nasreddine N, et al. Inhibition of HIV-1 transmission in trans from dendritic cells to CD4+ T lymphocytes by natural antibodies to the CRD domain of DC-SIGN purified from breast milk and intravenous immuno-globulins. Immunology 2008;123:508–18.

32. John-Stewart GC, Mbori-Ngacha D, Payne BL, et al. HIV-1-specific cytotoxic T lymphocytes and breast milk HIV-1 transmission. J Infect Dis 2009;199:889–98.

33. Farquhar C, Rowland-Jones S, Mbori-Ngacha D, et al. Human leukocyte antigen (HLA) B*18 and protection against mother-to-child HIV type 1 transmission. AIDS Res Hum Retroviruses 2004;20:692–7.

34. Mackelprang RD, John-Stewart G, Carrington M, et al. Maternal HLA homozy-gosity and mother-child HLA concordance increase the risk of vertical transmis-sion of HIV-1. J Infect Dis 2008;197:1156–61.

35. Coutsoudis A, Pillay K, Spooner E, et al. Influence of infant-feeding patterns on early mother-to-child transmission of HIV-1 in Durban, South Africa: a prospec-tive cohort study. South African Vitamin A Study Group. Lancet 1999;354: 471–6.

36. Iliff PJ, Piwoz EG, Tavengwa NV, et al. Early exclusive breastfeeding reduces the risk of postnatal HIV-1 transmission and increases HIV-free survival. AIDS 2005; 19:699–708.

37. Kuhn L, Sinkala M, Kankasa C, et al. High uptake of exclusive breastfeeding and reduced early post-natal HIV transmission. PLoS One 2007;2:e1363.

38. Kourtis AP, Jamieson DJ, de Vincenzi I, et al. Prevention of human immunodefi-ciency virus-1 transmission to the infant through breastfeeding: new develop-ments. Am J Obstet Gynecol 2007;197:S113–22.

39. Gantt S, Shetty AK, Seidel KD, et al. Laboratory indicators of mastitis are not associated with elevated HIV-1 DNA loads or predictive of HIV-1 RNA loads in breast milk. J Infect Dis 2007;196:570–6.

40. Dunn DT, Newell ML, Ades AE, et al. Risk of human immunodeficiency virus type 1 transmission through breastfeeding. Lancet 1992;340:585–8.

41. Miotti PG, Taha TE, Kumwenda NI, et al. HIV transmission through breastfeed-ing: a study in Malawi. JAMA 1999;282:744–9.

42. Embree JE, Njenga S, Datta P, et al. Risk factors for postnatal mother-child transmission of HIV-1. AIDS 2000;14:2535–41.

43. Moodley D, Moodley J, Coovadia H, et al. A multicenter randomized controlled trial of nevirapine versus a combination of zidovudine and lamivudine to reduce intrapartum and early postpartum mother-to-child transmission of human immu-nodeficiency virus type 1. J Infect Dis 2003;187:725–35.

44. Coutsoudis A, Dabis F, Fawzi W, et al. Late postnatal transmission of HIV-1 in breast-fed children: an individual patient data meta-analysis. J Infect Dis 2004;189:2154–66.

45. Bulterys M, Chao A, Dushimimana A, et al. HIV-1 seroconversion after 20 months of age in a cohort of breastfed children born to HIV-1-infected women in Rwanda. AIDS 1995;9:93–4.

46. Koulinska IN, Villamor E, Msamanga G, et al. Risk of HIV-1 transmission by breastfeeding among mothers infected with recombinant and non-recombinant HIV-1 genotypes. Virus Res. 2006;120:191–8.

47. Gantt S, Katzenstein D, Shetty A, et al. Associations between breast milk cellularity, microbial pathogens, and viral shedding in HIV-1-infected women. 13th Annual Conference on Retroviruses and Opportunistic Infections. Available at: http://www.retroconference.org/2006/Abstracts/26205.HTM. Accessed May 2, 2006.

48. Thea DM, Aldrovandi G, Kankasa C, et al. Post-weaning breast milk HIV-1 viral load, blood prolactin levels and breast milk volume. AIDS 2006;20:1539–47.

49. John GC, Nduati RW, Mbori-Ngacha DA, et al. Correlates of mother-to-child human immunodeficiency virus type 1 (HIV-1) transmission: association with maternal plasma HIV-1 RNA load, genital HIV-1 DNA shedding, and breast infections. J Infect Dis 2001;183:206–12.

50. Coovadia HM, Rollins NC, Bland RM, et al. Mother-to-child transmission of HIV-1 infection during exclusive breastfeeding in the first 6 months of life: an intervention cohort study. Lancet 2007;369:1107–16.

51. Kafulafula G, Hoover DR, Taha TE, et al. Frequency of gastroenteritis and gastroenteritis-associated mortality with early weaning in HIV-1-uninfected children born to HIV-infected women in Malawi. J Acquir Immune Defic Syndr 2010; 53:6–13.

52. Kuhn L, Sinkala M, Semrau K, et al. Elevations in mortality associated with weaning persist into the second year of life among uninfected children born to HIV-infected mothers. Clin Infect Dis 2010;50:437–44.

53. Onyango-Makumbi C, Bagenda D, Mwatha A, et al. Early weaning of HIV-exposed uninfected infants and risk of serious gastroenteritis: findings from two perinatal HIV prevention trials in Kampala, Uganda. Marc J Acquir Immune Defic Syndr 2010;53:20–7.

54. Leroy V, Karon JM, Alioum A, et al. Postnatal transmission of HIV-1 after a maternal short-course zidovudine peripartum regimen in West Africa. AIDS 2003;17:1493–501.

55. Mmiro FA, Aizire J, Mwatha AK, et al. Predictors of early and late mother-to-child transmission of HIV in a breastfeeding population: HIV Network for Prevention Trials 012 experience, Kampala, Uganda. J Acquir Immune Defic Syndr 2009; 52:32–9.

56. Fultz PN. HIV-1 superinfections: omens for vaccine efficacy? AIDS 2004;18: 115–9.

57. Kumwenda N, Miotti PG, Taha TE, et al. Antenatal vitamin A supplementation increases birth weight and decreases anemia among infants born to human immunodeficiency virus-infected women in Malawi. Clin Infect Dis 2002;35:618–24.

58. Phiri W, Kasonka L, Collin S, et al. Factors influencing breast milk HIV RNA viral load among Zambian women. AIDS Res Hum Retroviruses 2006;22:607–14.

59. Semba RD, Kumwenda N, Taha TE, et al. Mastitis and immunological factors in breast milk of lactating women in Malawi. Clin Diagn Lab Immunol 1999;6:671–4.

60. Lehman DA, Chung MH, John-Stewart GC, et al. HIV-1 persists in breast milk cells despite antiretroviral treatment to prevent mother-to-child transmission. AIDS 2008;22:1475–85.

61. Dabis F, Msellati P, Meda N, et al. 6-month efficacy, tolerance, and acceptability of a short regimen of oral zidovudine to reduce vertical transmission of HIV in breastfed children in Cote d'Ivoire and Burkina Faso: a double-blind placebo-controlled multicentre trial. DITRAME study group. Diminution de la transmission mèrè-enfant. Lancet 1999;353:786–92.

62. Guay LA, Musoke P, Fleming T, et al. Intrapartum and neonatal single-dose nevirapine compared with zidovudine for prevention of mother-to-child

transmission of HIV-1 in Kampala, Uganda: HIVNET 012 randomised trial. Lancet 1999;354:795–802.

63. Connor EM, Sperling RS, Gelber R, et al. Reduction of maternal-infant transmission of human immunodeficiency virus type 1 with zidovudine treatment. Pediatric AIDS Clinical Trials Group Protocol 076 Study Group. N Engl J Med 1994;331:1173–80.

64. Cooper ER, Charurat M, Mofenson L, et al. Combination antiretroviral strategies for the treatment of pregnant HIV-1-infected women and prevention of perinatal HIV-1 transmission. J Acquir Immune Defic Syndr 2002;29:484–94.

65. Shaffer N, Chuachoowong R, Mock PA, et al. Short-course zidovudine for perinatal HIV-1 transmission in Bangkok, Thailand: a randomised controlled trial. Bangkok collaborative perinatal HIV transmission study group. Lancet 1999; 353:773–80.

66. Wiktor SZ, Ekpini E, Karon JM, et al. Short-course oral zidovudine for prevention of mother-to-child transmission of HIV-1 in Abidjan, Cote d'Ivoire: a randomised trial. Lancet 1999;353:781–5.

67. Bedri A, Gudetta B, Isehak A, et al. Extended-dose nevirapine to 6 weeks of age for infants to prevent HIV transmission via breastfeeding in Ethiopia, India, and Uganda: an analysis of three randomised controlled trials. Lancet 2008;372: 300–13.

68. Kilewo C, Karlsson K, Ngarina M, et al. Prevention of mother-to-child transmission of HIV-1 through breastfeeding by treating mothers with triple antiretroviral therapy in Dar es Salaam, Tanzania: the Mitra plus study. J Acquir Immune Defic Syndr 2009;52:406–16.

69. Kumwenda NI, Hoover DR, Mofenson LM, et al. Extended antiretroviral prophylaxis to reduce breast-milk HIV-1 transmission. N Engl J Med 2008;359:119–29.

70. Palombi L, Marazzi MC, Voetberg A, et al. Treatment acceleration program and the experience of the DREAM program in prevention of mother-to-child transmission of HIV. AIDS 2007;21(Suppl 4):S65–71.

71. Thomas R, Masaba R, Ndivo R, et al. Kisumu breastfeeding study team. prevention of mother-to-child transmission of HIV-1 among breastfeeding mothers using haart: the kisumu breastfeeding study, kisumu, kenya, 2003–2007. 15th Conference on Retroviruses and Opportunistic Infections. 2008. Available at: http://www.retroconference.org/2008/Abstracts/33397.htm. Accessed May 4, 2010.

72. Shapiro RL, Hughes M, Ogwu A, et al. Antiretroviral regimens in pregnancy and breast-feeding in Botswana. N Engl J Med 2010;362:2282–94.

73. de Vincenzi, I, Kesho Bora Study Group. Triple-antiretroviral (ARV) prophylaxis during pregnancy and breastfeeding compared to short-ARV prophylaxis to prevent mother-to-child transmission of HIV-1 (MTCT): the Kesho Bora randomized controlled clinical trial in five sites in Burkina Faso, Kenya. Proceedings of the 5th International AIDS Society Conference on HIV Pathogenesis, Treatment and Prevention. 2009. Accessed July 19, 2009.

74. Chasela C, Hudgens M, Jamieson D, et al. Maternal or infant antiretroviral drugs to reduce HIV-1 transmission. N Engl J Med 2010;362:2271–81.

75. Kilewo C, Karlsson K, Massawe A, et al. Prevention of mother-to-child transmission of HIV-1 through breast-feeding by treating infants prophylactically with lamivudine in Dar es Salaam, Tanzania: the Mitra study. J Acquir Immune Defic Syndr 2008;48:315–23.

76. Bulterys M, Fowler MG, Van Rompay KK, et al. Prevention of mother-to-child transmission of HIV-1 through breast-feeding: past, present, and future. J Infect Dis 2004;189:2149–53.

77. Mofenson LM. Prevention of breast milk transmission of HIV: the time is now. J Acquir Immune Defic Syndr 2009;52:305–8.
78. Moorthy A, Gupta A, Bhosale R, et al. Nevirapine resistance and breast-milk HIV transmission: effects of single and extended-dose nevirapine prophylaxis in subtype C HIV-infected infants. PLoS One 2009;4:e4096.
79. ClinicalTrials.gov. Comparison of efficacy and safety of infant peri-exposure prophylaxis with lopinavir/ritonavir versus lamivudine to prevent HIV-1 transmission by breastfeeding. Available at: http://clinicaltrials.gov/ct2/show/NCT00640263. updated April 8, 2010. Accessed April 30, 2010.
80. Peltier CA, Ndayisaba GF, Lepage P, et al. Breastfeeding with maternal antiretroviral therapy or formula feeding to prevent HIV postnatal mother-to-child transmission in Rwanda. AIDS 2009;23:2415–23.
81. Zeh C, Weidle P, Nafisa L, et al. Emergence of HIV-1 drug resistance among breastfeeding infants born to hiv-infected mothers taking antiretrovirals for prevention of mother-to-child transmission of hiv: the kisumu breastfeeding study, kenya. 15th Conference on Retroviruses and Opportunistic Infections. 2008. Available at: www.retroconference.org/AbstractSearch/Default.aspx?Conf=19. Accessed April 20, 2010.
82. Darwich L, Esteve A, Ruiz L, et al. Variability in the plasma concentration of efavirenz and nevirapine is associated with genotypic resistance after treatment interruption. Antivir Ther 2008;13:945–51.
83. Mirochnick M, Thomas T, Capparelli E, et al. Antiretroviral concentrations in breast-feeding infants of mothers receiving highly active antiretroviral therapy. Antimicrob Agents Chemother 2009;53:1170–6.
84. ClinicalTrials.gov. Evaluating strategies to reduce mother-to-child transmission of HIV infection in resource-limited countries (PROMISE). Available at: http://clinicaltrials.gov/ct2/show/NCT01061151. updated April 14, 2010. Accessed April 30, 2010.
85. ClinicalTrials. gov: Universal Use of EFV-TDF-FTC and AZT-3TC-LPV/r Combinations for HIV-1 PMTCT in Pregnant and breastfeeding women: a Phase 3 Trial (UMA). Available at: http://clinicaltrials.gov/ct2/show/NCT00936195?term=UMA&rank=1. updated August 6, 2009. Accessed April 30, 2010.
86. Luzuriaga K, Newell ML, Dabis F, et al. Vaccines to prevent transmission of HIV-1 via breastmilk: scientific and logistical priorities. Lancet 2006;368:511–21.
87. Cunningham CK, McFarland E. Vaccines for prevention of mother-to-child transmission of HIV. Curr Opin HIV AIDS 2008;3:151–4.
88. HIV Prevention Trials Network: HPTN 027. A Phase I Study to Evaluate the Safety and Immunogenicity of ALVAC-HIV vCP1521 in Infants Born to HIV-1 Infected Women in Uganda. 2010. Available at: http://www.hptn.org/research_studies/hptn027.asp. Accessed April 20, 2010.
89. ClinicalTrials.gov. Safety and immunogenicity study of candidate HIV-1 vaccine given to healthy infants born to hiv-1-infected mothers (PedVacc002). Available at: http://clinicaltrials.gov/ct2/show/NCT00981695. updated October 10, 2009. Accessed April 20, 2010.
90. Guay LA, Musoke P, Hom DL, et al. Phase I/II trial of HIV-1 hyperimmune globulin for the prevention of HIV-1 vertical transmission in Uganda. AIDS 2002;16:1391–400.
91. ClinicalTrials.gov. Nevirapine Study for the Prevention of Maternal-Infant HIV Transmission in Uganda. Available at: http://clinicaltrials.gov/ct2/show/NCT00639938. updated April 1, 2008. Accessed April 20, 2010.

92. Hartmann SU, Wigdahl B, Neely EB, et al. Biochemical analysis of human milk treated with sodium dodecyl sulfate, an alkyl sulfate microbicide that inactivates human immunodeficiency virus type 1. J Hum Lact 2006;22: 61–74.

93. Boelaert JR, Yaro S, Augustijns P, et al. Chloroquine accumulates in breast-milk cells: potential impact in the prophylaxis of postnatal mother-to-child transmission of HIV-1. AIDS 2001;15:2205–7.

94. Savarino A, Gennero L, Chen HC, et al. Anti-HIV effects of chloroquine: mechanisms of inhibition and spectrum of activity. AIDS 2001;15:2221–9.

95. Luchters SM, Veldhuijzen J, Nsanzabera D. A phase I/II randomized, placebo controlled study to evaluate chloroquine administration to reduce HIV-1 RNA in breast milk in an HIV-1 infected breastfeeding population: the CHARGE Study. Proceedings of the 15th International AIDS Conference. 2004. Accessed November 7, 2004.

96. Jeffery BS, Mercer KG. Pretoria pasteurisation: a potential method for the reduction of postnatal mother to child transmission of the human immunodeficiency virus. J Trop Pediatr 2000;46:219–23.

97. Jeffery BS, Webber L, Mokhondo KR, et al. Determination of the effectiveness of inactivation of human immunodeficiency virus by Pretoria pasteurization. J Trop Pediatr 2001;47:345–9.

98. Jeffery BS, Soma-Pillay P, Makin J, et al. The effect of Pretoria Pasteurization on bacterial contamination of hand-expressed human breastmilk. J Trop Pediatr 2003;49:240–4.

99. Orloff SL, Wallingford JC, McDougal JS. Inactivation of human immunodeficiency virus type I in human milk: effects of intrinsic factors in human milk and of pasteurization. J Hum Lact 1993;9:13–7.

100. Israel-Ballard K, Donovan R, Chantry C, et al. Flash-heat inactivation of HIV-1 in human milk: a potential method to reduce postnatal transmission in developing countries. J Acquir Immune Defic Syndr 2007;45:318–23.

101. Chantry CJ, Israel-Ballard K, Moldoveanu Z, et al. Effect of flash-heat treatment on immunoglobulins in breast milk. J Acquir Immune Defic Syndr 2009;51: 264–7.

102. Breastfeeding and HIV International Transmission Study Group. Mortality among HIV-1-infected women according to children's feeding modality: an individual patient data meta-analysis. J Acquir Immune Defic Syndr 2005;39:430–8.

103. Nduati R, Richardson BA, John G, et al. Effect of breastfeeding on mortality among HIV-1 infected women: a randomised trial. Lancet 2001;357:1651–5.

104. Kuhn L, Aldrovandi GM, Sinkala M, et al. Effects of early, abrupt weaning on HIV-free survival of children in Zambia. N Engl J Med 2008;359:130–41.

105. Thior I, Lockman S, Smeaton LM, et al. Breastfeeding plus infant zidovudine prophylaxis for 6 months vs formula feeding plus infant zidovudine for 1 month to reduce mother-to-child HIV transmission in Botswana: a randomized trial: the Mashi study. JAMA 2006;296:794–805.

106. Bulterys M, Wilfert CM. HAART during pregnancy and during breastfeeding among HIV-infected women in the developing world: has the time come? [editorial]. AIDS 2009;23:2473–7.

HIV Drug Resistance and Mother-to-Child Transmission of HIV

Paul J. Weidle, PharmD, MPH*, Steven Nesheim, MD

KEYWORDS

- HIV • Antiretroviral resistance
- Mother-to-child transmission • Infant

BASIC PRINCIPLES OF HIV DRUG RESISTANCE

Emergence of resistance to antiretroviral drugs can be quite virologically complex, yet has principles that can be simple to understand as a clinician.[1] HIV characteristically has a high rate of viral replication, which, coupled with continuous mutation and recombination events, enables it to develop resistance to any and all of the more than 20 antiretroviral drugs licensed for use.[1,2] Drugs that target the reverse-transcriptase enzyme include those characterized as nucleoside/nucleotide analogs because they are structurally related to endogenous nucleosides. Non-nucleoside reverse-transcriptase inhibitors are a broad group of drugs that also target reverse-transcriptase, but are structurally dissimilar to endogenous nucleosides and to each other. Protease inhibitors target the protease enzyme to interrupt assembly of the mature virion. Integrase inhibitors target the integrase enzyme to block integration of HIV into cellular DNA. Two drug classes target entry of HIV into the cell: fusion inhibitors and those that block the CCR5 receptor.

Retroviruses, such as HIV, do not have proofreading mechanisms when synthesizing new nucleic acid strands that results in frequent incorporation of unintended nucleotides during chain elongation.[1] This random substitution of nucleotides, coupled with the high turnover of HIV in vivo, enables virtually any and all genotypic mutations to occur. Some of these changes in genetic structure are associated with decreased susceptibility to antiretroviral drugs, with some single-point mutations conferring a high degree of resistance to certain drugs (eg, lamivudine, nevirapine, efavirenz); whereas, multiple mutations are needed to develop resistance to other drugs.

Conflict of interest: Neither of the authors report conflicts of interest.
Disclaimer: The opinions and conclusions in this report are those of the authors and do not necessarily represent the views of the US Centers for Disease Control and Prevention.
Epidemiology Branch, Division of HIV/AIDS Prevention, National Center for HIV, Viral Hepatitis, STD, and TB Prevention, Centers for Disease Control and Prevention, 1600 Clifton Road, MS E-45, Atlanta, GA 30333, USA
* Corresponding author.
E-mail address: pweidle@cdc.gov

Clin Perinatol 37 (2010) 825–842
doi:10.1016/j.clp.2010.08.009
0095-5108/10/$ – see front matter. Published by Elsevier Inc.

perinatology.theclinics.com

There are two types of commercial HIV resistance tests available: genotypic tests and phenotypic tests. Both tests typically require a plasma HIV viral load greater than 1000 to 2000 copies/mL, and will only detect resistance that is present in greater than 10% to 20% of the circulating HIV in plasma. The phenotypic test is more expensive than the genotypic test. Genotypic resistance testing is the most common test performed and involves sequencing the nucleic acids that make up all 99 codons of the protease gene, the first approximately 335 codons of the reverse-transcriptase gene, and targeted portions of the integrase gene and envelope gene.[3] The sequence derived from the plasma of patients is compared with a consensus HIV-1, group M, subtype B virus (the most common strain in North America). Mutations are described by the letter indicating the consensus B wild-type amino acid followed by the amino acid number, followed by a letter indicating the amino acid mutant.[3] For example, T215Y (a common mutation associated with resistance to zidovudine) denotes a change at position 215 of the reverse-transcriptase gene from threonine (the consensus wild-type amino acid at that position) to tyrosine (the mutant amino acid). If there is a mixture of more than one amino acid detected at a position, each amino acid detected is denoted after the number. For example, T215T/Y indicates a detection of both the wild-type amino acid and the mutant. The phenotypic test measures the ability of HIV to replicate in the presence of a drug and reports results as a fold change in the inhibitory concentration compared with a sensitive strain of HIV. Phenotypic fold change may be reported in 2 manners: (1) as the fold change at which there is a reduction in antiviral activity and (2) the fold change above which there is essentially no drug activity.

Some drugs have a low genetic barrier to resistance because a single-point nucleic acid mutation can engender resistance.[3] For instance, a change of one nucleic acid in the reverse-transcriptase gene at amino acid 184 results in a change from methionine to valine (M184V), which confers high-level resistance to lamivudine and emtricitabine. For non-nucleoside reverse-transcriptase inhibitors, a single-point mutation at several positions of the reverse-transcriptase gene, most commonly 103 from lysine to asparagine (K103N) or 181 from tyrosine to cysteine (Y181C), are associated with high-level resistance to the first generation of non-nucleoside reverse-transcriptase inhibitors, nevirapine and efavirenz. The second generation, non-nucleoside reverse-transcriptase inhibitor, etravirine, maintains virologic activity in the presence of the K103N mutation; however, resistance to etravirine can be present if the Y181C mutation is also accompanied by additional mutations.

Resistance to protease inhibitors is complex with resistance-associated mutations documented at approximately 25% of the 99 amino acid positions.[1–3] Major mutations in the protease gene are those selected first in the presence of the drug (these may vary considerably by drug) and are typically the primary contact amino acid for that drug or are mutations that substantially reduce susceptibility to that drug. Minor mutations generally emerge over time and may improve the replicative capacity of viruses containing a major mutation. These mutations are sometimes referred to as compensatory mutations because they tend not to occur naturally in subtype B. However, some minor mutations in subtype B are also common polymorphisms in non-B subtypes. Protease inhibitors are typically coadministered with ritonavir to take advantage of its unique property to decrease the hepatic metabolism of many other drugs, including most protease inhibitors, resulting in what is commonly referred to as boosted protease inhibitors. Often, numerous mutations in the protease gene are necessary to impact virologic response to ritonavir-boosted regimens, and most boosted protease inhibitor-based regimens are said to have a high genetic barrier to resistance.[3]

Antiretroviral Therapy for Pregnant Women and Infants for Prevention of Mother-to-Child Transmission of HIV

Transmission of HIV from mother to child mainly occurs in utero during the third trimester of pregnancy, or in the short interval during which the placenta detaches, labor occurs, and the infant passes through the birth canal. Overall, rates of transmission are 15% to 40% without preventive interventions.[4] Maternal HIV viral load correlates with the risk of HIV transmission to the infant; low HIV viral load (typically <50 copies/mL) is associated with an extremely low, but not absent, chance of transmission.[5–7] Antiretroviral drugs reduce transmission of HIV through reduction in plasma and genital tract viral load and through an independent effect in addition to viral suppression. Transplacental passage of antiretroviral drugs is one mechanism of protection against transmission of HIV. Antiretroviral drugs are detectable in infant plasma immediately after birth following chronic maternal dosing during pregnancy and labor.[8–10] With all of these considerations, antiretroviral drug use during pregnancy for prevention of mother-to-child transmission (PMTCT) of HIV should be discussed with and provided to all women regardless of viral load.[4]

Since 2002, guidelines have recommended that HIV-infected pregnant women be tested before the initiation of treatment for the presence of mutations indicative of antiretroviral resistance in their HIV strains.[4] Whether or not the clinician need wait for documentation of antiretroviral resistance in an HIV-infected pregnant woman will depend on the gestational age of the pregnancy. In some cases, antiretroviral therapy will need to begin before the results of genotyping are available; for instance, if a woman is first diagnosed with HIV late in the pregnancy, the clinician may need to start treatment while awaiting the results of the resistance test. If a woman begins antiretroviral therapy for the first time, or changes to a new regimen, it is vital to document a response. Viral load testing should be performed at least monthly until it is suppressed (typically <50 copies/mL) and, regardless of that result, performed at 34 to 36 gestational weeks to plan for mode of delivery. If a woman is infected with HIV that is resistant to zidovudine, it is still recommended to administer intravenous zidovudine during labor, and oral zidovudine to the infant for 6 weeks; some experts recommend an additional antiretroviral for such an infant.[4]

Existing data regarding antiretroviral resistance and PMTCT of HIV are predominantly based on genotypic testing. It has been suggested that phenotypic resistance data add little to the data that are provided by genotypic testing for evaluating prevalence of resistance in pregnant women or neonates.[11] Genotypic testing of HIV is usually performed on plasma specimens, although data from peripheral blood mononuclear cells are considered comparable.[12] Few data are available about the degree to which genotypic testing for antiretroviral resistance has been implemented for HIV-infected pregnant women. In the United Kingdom, with data available on 60% of HIV-infected women in the national database during 2006 to 2009, approximately 60% were tested for antiretroviral resistance (Pat Tookey, personal communication, 2010).

Several scenarios and options for antiretroviral treatment are provided below. More detailed and specific discussions are continuously updated at http://aidsinfo.nih.gov. Furthermore, in most situations, in management of pregnant HIV-infected women, consultation with an infectious diseases consultant is advisable. Expert clinical advice on HIV/AIDS management for health care providers is also available at the National Clinicians Consultation Center (http://www.nccc.ucsf.edu/).

HIV-infected pregnant women on therapy for their own health

For women who require antiretroviral therapy for their own health, for instance a CD4+ cell count less than 350 cells/µL, symptomatic HIV disease, or history of an

AIDS-defining illness, the treatment approach is similar to that of nonpregnant adults with the goal of viral load suppression below the level of detection of the available assay (typically <50 copies/mL).[4] However, for pregnant women the regimen should include zidovudine because it has been studied and used the most extensively for PMTCT of HIV, unless there is severe toxicity or documented resistance to zidovudine.[4] Genotypic resistance testing is recommended for all HIV-infected pregnant women with detectable viremia.[4] Generally, the result of the antiretroviral resistance test should be available to aid the choice of drugs, but antiretroviral therapy should not be delayed while awaiting the results, especially in the third trimester.

If the pregnant woman is already taking antiretroviral therapy, viral load should be checked and, if the viral load is detectable, a genotypic resistance test should be performed. Combining the results of the genotypic test with knowledge of prior antiretroviral history and prior HIV resistance test results, the clinician can make an informed decision for selecting antiretroviral drugs with the best possibility of suppressing viral load. In women with a complicated antiretroviral history and prior resistance test results, the obstetrician may want to consult with an infectious disease specialist knowledgeable about the intricacy of these results, preferably the specialist that constructed prior regimens for that woman.

HIV-infected pregnant women not on therapy

If a woman is diagnosed with HIV infection during pregnancy, the physician needs to assess whether she meets current criteria for antiretroviral treatment or whether antiretroviral drugs will be used during the pregnancy only for PMTCT. In both cases, triple combination antiretroviral therapy is preferred,[4] but, when given solely for PMTCT, there are a couple of options. Initiation of combination antiretroviral therapy can be delayed until after the first trimester. Although controversial, zidovudine alone may be considered for women whose viral load is less than 1000 copies/mL.[4]

An HIV-infected woman who has received no antiretroviral therapy before labor may be treated with zidovudine as a continuous infusion during labor.[4] The likelihood of resistance to zidovudine emerging in the woman in such cases is extremely low. In addition to zidovudine as a continuous infusion, 2010 guidelines include an option to add a single dose of nevirapine and lamivudine during labor.[4] Nevirapine can be detected in maternal plasma 2 to 3 weeks after a single dose, resulting effectively in monotherapy against HIV with an agent that has a low barrier to resistance.[13] Maternal zidovudine/lamivudine for 7 days postpartum is suggested if single-dose nevirapine is used, to limit the emergence of resistance to nevirapine.[4]

Infants

Infants may acquire a drug-resistant strain of HIV without having been treated for HIV. This infection can occur if the mother harbors a resistant virus while pregnant or if the woman's antiretroviral therapy does not result in complete suppression of viral load and allows resistance to emerge while pregnant. The infant can acquire a drug-resistant strain of HIV directly from the mother if the dominant HIV strain in the mother becomes the dominant HIV strain in the infant or if the infant acquires a minor resistant strain of HIV that is selected in the child during perinatal antiretroviral prophylaxis (**Fig. 1**).[14,15] In the United States, all HIV-exposed infants should receive a 6-week course of zidovudine.[4] In the case where the mother was not on antiretroviral therapy before labor but was given a single dose of nevirapine along with continuous infusion zidovudine during labor, the infant should also receive a single dose of nevirapine within the first 2 to 3 days postpartum along with 6 weeks of zidovudine. In this case, 1 week of lamivudine therapy to the infant may be considered to decrease the

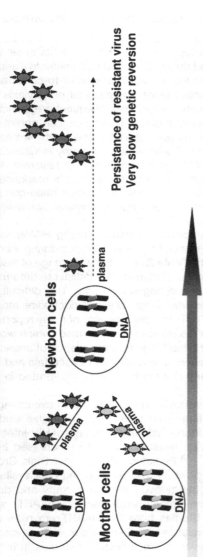

Fig. 1. Mechanisms of antiretroviral resistance acquisition in HIV-1 infected newborns. Wild-type viruses are shown in green and resistance viruses in red. The length of the yellow-to-red arrow indicates the duration of perinatal prophylaxis and thus the risk of resistance selection (*A, B*). PTME, Prévention de la transmission de la mère à l'enfant (Prevention of mother-to-child transmission of HIV, PMTCT). (*Reprinted from* Delaugerre C, Chaix ML, Blanche S, Warszawski J, Cornet D, Dollfus C, et al. Perinatal acquisition of drug-resistant HIV-1 infection: mechanisms and long-term outcome. Retrovirology 2009;685; with permission.)

emergence of resistance mutations to nevirapine, in the event the child was HIV-infected at birth.[4] The newborn could acquire a wild-type sensitive strain of HIV in utero or during the peripartum period, but have resistance emerge while on antiretroviral prophylaxis during the first weeks of life.

Antiretroviral Resistance Among HIV-infected Pregnant Women and HIV-infected Infants in Industrialized Countries

Antiretroviral resistance can affect HIV-infected women and their infants in several ways. If antiretroviral resistance is undetected during pregnancy, an ineffective antiretroviral regimen may be prescribed, leading to the possibility of mother-to-child transmission. If resistance develops while a woman takes antiretroviral prophylaxis for PMTCT, there is potential for affecting preventive efforts in subsequent pregnancies. In addition, antiretroviral resistance that develops during pregnancy can potentially reduce the effectiveness of antiretroviral therapy used at a later time for the woman's treatment. Whether resistance is discovered in a woman when therapy is initiated or while she takes antiretroviral drugs for PMTCT, infant acquisition of resistant virus will affect the selection of antiretroviral drugs and, in turn, the infant's response to therapy. Even if antiretroviral therapy is initiated in the infant early, replication-competent HIV strains, including antiretroviral-resistant strains, may become archived within the infant's T cells and remain detectable for years.[14,16]

Several reports have documented antiretroviral resistance among HIV-infected pregnant women (**Table 1**). Antiretroviral resistance has also developed during administration of antiretroviral prophylaxis to infants (**Table 2**). With the wide range of results found in both women and infants in cross-sectional studies, it is difficult to determine whether the resistance rate in either group has changed over time. This difficulty is increased by the fact that most of the studies were from the era of zidovudine monotherapy or dual antiretroviral therapy for PMTCT. The denominator of many reports is based on the number of women who had a resistance test performed, which would have excluded women with undetectable viral load. The true prevalence of antiretroviral drug resistance among pregnant women in care is difficult to ascertain and the percentages of women with resistance in any one study must be interpreted in the context of the constraints of that study.

Few studies have addressed whether antiretroviral resistance rates have changed among pregnant women or HIV-infected infants over time. Two successive studies performed by the New York State laboratory found that the percentage of HIV-infected pregnant women with any major antiretroviral resistance mutation increased from 12.1% (1997–1998) to 19.1% (2001–2002).[17,18] Pediatric AIDS Clinical Trials Group 316 was a study of single-dose nevirapine given to women receiving best available therapy or prophylaxis, which overlapped the zidovudine monotherapy and dual-therapy era and the era of highly active antiretroviral therapy (HAART) with triple-combination antiretroviral therapy.[19] Studies from the HAART era have not demonstrated a clear trend in increasing prevalence of antiretroviral resistance among pregnant women over time.[16,19,20–24] However, 2 cross-sectional studies from the HAART era have documented a high prevalence of antiretroviral resistance mutations in the late 1990s and early 2000s.[22,23]

In the Women and Infants Transmission Study (WITS) during the 1991 to 2001 time frame, 18.3% of pregnant women tested for antiretroviral resistance had resistance mutations; in addition, the overall rate of major mutations in therapy-experienced patients increased to 34%, and in therapy-naïve patients to 18%, by the final 3 years of the study.[24] Furthermore, for therapy-experienced patients, between 1997 to 1998 and 1999 to 2001, non-nucleoside reverse-transcriptase inhibitor resistance increased from 5.9% to 21.9%, and protease inhibitor resistance increased from 9.8% to 15.6%, respectively. In therapy-naïve patients, major resistance mutations to non-nucleoside reverse-transcriptase inhibitors or protease inhibitors did not occur until 1999 to 2001, reflecting the fact that resistance to a class of drugs was not detected among pregnant women until after the use of that class of drugs became prevalent in the community. For antiretroviral-naïve women, the resistance rate was 7.1% for non-nucleoside reverse-transcriptase inhibitors and protease inhibitors in that period.[24] Also from WITS, during a later time frame (1998–2005), 43.0% of women had major mutations to at least 1 drug class, 6.1% to 2 drug classes, but 0% to 3 drug classes.[21]

Clinical factors that have been associated with the development of antiretroviral resistance include low maternal CD4+ cell count,[11,25–28] elevated maternal HIV viral load,[11,26,28] and prior therapy with antiretroviral drugs.[11,22,25–28] Fewer antiretroviral resistance mutations were noted in antiretroviral-naïve women in the AIDS Clinical Trials Group 076 study.[25] In a study from the early HAART era, there were no major mutations in therapy-naïve women and no major antiretroviral resistance mutations were found among those whose only previous antiretroviral exposure had been for PMTCT.[23] Although this finding is in contrast to what others have found, most studies do not distinguish effects of treatment from those of prophylaxis for PMTCT. Overall, in the longitudinal WITS, major mutations were detected more often in therapy-experienced than in therapy-naïve women (25.6% versus 8.6%, respectively).[24]

Emergence of antiretroviral resistance has occurred while on antiretroviral drugs for PMTCT; this occurrence is particularly common with lamivudine and nevirapine. The mutation M184V, which results in high-level resistance to lamivudine, has occurred when dual prophylaxis (lamivudine combined with zidovudine) is administered.[26,29,30] After administration of intrapartum nevirapine, 15% of women in the ACTG 315 study developed nevirapine resistance.[19] While receiving pregnancy-limited antiretroviral therapy, resistance emerged in recipients of dual-therapy prophylaxis more frequently than with triple-therapy prophylaxis (65.0% versus 28.7%, respectively).[21] On the other hand, postponing prophylaxis until later in pregnancy to limit the time on antiretrovirals and to reduce the chance of developing resistance might delay the initiation of antiretroviral therapy until too late, perhaps increasing the risk of mother-to-child transmission of HIV.[31]

An association between antiretroviral resistance and mother-to-child transmission has been addressed in only a few studies. A positive association was found in 2 studies, both from the WITS early in the antiretroviral era, one using genotypic testing[28] and the other using phenotypic testing.[11] In addition, 2 studies failed to find a statistical association between antiretroviral resistance and mother-to-child transmission;[26,27] whereas, many studies make no attempt to relate the two. Failure to find an effect of HIV resistance leading to increased transmission of HIV in earlier studies might be attributable to small sample size and the small number of transmissions.[11] The failure of later studies to show that effect might be the result of accommodations made as a result of the detected resistance, that is, selection of an effective regimen because of more genotypic-driven prophylaxis. Such a possibility is supported by the high prevalence of antiretroviral resistance mutations, which itself indicates the need for alternative antiretroviral drugs.

Antiretroviral Resistance among HIV-infected Pregnant Women and HIV-infected Infants in Resource-limited Settings

Worldwide, less than one-third of HIV-exposed infants receive perinatal HIV prophylaxis.[32] One of the most important developments of the past decade regarding

Table 1
Prevalence of HIV resistance associated with antiretroviral prophylaxis against maternal-to-child transmission of HIV among women

Author	Study, Location	N	Years	Resistance was Associated with Transmission	Maternal Regimen	Resistance Documented to:		
						Nucleoside Reverse-transcriptase Inhibitors	Non-nucleoside Reverse-transcriptase Inhibitors	Protease Inhibitors
Eastman[25]	PACTG 076, United States	96	1991–1993	No	Zidovudine	Zidovudine 4.3% at delivery	N/A	N/A
Welles[28]	WITS, United States	142	1989–1994	Yes	Zidovudine	Zidovudine 24% at delivery	N/A	N/A
Bauer[11]	WITS, United States	74	1989–1994	Yes	Zidovudine	Zidovudine 39% at delivery (by phenotypic resistance testing)	N/A	N/A
Frenkel[15]	United States	16	Pre-1995	—	Zidovudine (35% treatment-naïve)	Zidovudine 25% at delivery	N/A	N/A
Palumbo[27]	PACTS, United States	220	1991–1997	No	Zidovudine (6 lamivudine, 6 didanosine, 3 protease inhibitor, 2 delavirdine)	Zidovudine 17.3% Lamivudine 2.7%	2.3%	Major mutation <1%
Kully[58]	Swiss HIV and Pregnancy Study, Switzerland	62	1995	—	Zidovudine (n = 51)	Zidovudine 9.6% (only tested for T215Y mutation)	N/A	N/A
Mandelbrot[26]	ANRS 075, France	445	1997–1998	No	Zidovudine/lamivudine	Zidovudine 6.8% Lamivudine 39% six weeks after delivery	N/A	N/A

Author	Country	n	Years		Regimen			
Clarke[30]	United Kingdom	19	1995	No	Zidovudine (n = 14; 10 tested for resistance) Zidovudine/ lamivudine (n = 5)	Zidovudine 20% Lamivudine 80% women tested before or at delivery	N/A	N/A
Cunningham[19]	PACTG 316, United States & France	217	1997–2000	No	Zidovudine (n = 65) Combination without protease inhibitor (n = 79) Combination with protease inhibitor (n = 73) plus single intrapartum dose of nevirapine (n = 95)	Zidovudine 16% Lamivudine 44% at 6 weeks post partum	New NNRTI mutations 15% at 6 weeks post partum	Major mutation 9% Minor mutation 2% at 6 weeks post partum
Jeuthner[59]	St Louis, Missouri, United States	18	2000–2001	No	ART-naive	0%	17%	0%
Shah[22]	New York City, New York, United States	45	2000–2002	—	Various	27%	24%	Major mutation 2%

(continued on next page)

Table 1
(continued)

Author	Study, Location	N	Years	Resistance was Associated with Transmission	Maternal Regimen	Resistance Documented to:		
						Nucleoside Reverse-transcriptase Inhibitors	Non-nucleoside Reverse-transcriptase Inhibitors	Protease Inhibitors
Paredes, 2007[20]	WITS, United States	134 women 64 women had resistance data	1998–2004	—	Zidovudine/lamivudine with or without nelfinavir or nevirapine	Lamivudine 9.4% within 14 days of starting therapy	2% within 14 days of starting therapy	Major mutation 6.3% within 14 days of starting therapy
Paredes 2010[21]	WITS, United States	114	1998–2004	—	Zidovudine/lamivudine (n = 114) with or without nelfinavir (n = 111) or nevirapine (n = 8) for >28 days during pregnancy and stopped post partum	Zidovudine 25% on dual therapy 5% on 3 drugs Lamivudine 65% on dual therapy 29% on 3 drugs 2-month or 6-month postpartum visit	38% (3 of 8 women on nevirapine) 2-month or 6-month postpartum visit	1% (1 of 87 women on nelfinavir) 2-month or 6-month postpartum visit

The denominator of many reports is based on the number of women who had a resistance test performed, which often excluded women with undetectable viral load or for whom a resistance test was not successful. The true prevalence of antiretroviral drug resistance among pregnant women in care is difficult to ascertain and the percentages of women with resistance in any one study must be interpreted in the context of the constraints of that study.

Abbreviations: ANRS, Agence Nationale de Recherches sur le SIDA; ART, antiretroviral therapy; N/A, not applicable; PACTG, Pediatric AIDS Clinical Trials Group; PACTS, Pediatric AIDS Collaborative Transmission Study; WITS, Women and Infants Transmission Study; PACTS, Pediatric AIDS Collaborative Transmission Study; ANRS, Agence Nationale de Recherches sur le SIDA.

antiretroviral drug resistance in resource-limited settings has been the administration of a single intrapartum dose of nevirapine to women at the onset of labor, with or without short-term antepartum administration of 1 or 2 nucleoside reverse-transcriptase inhibitors. For the mothers, mutations that confer resistance to nevirapine (and other non-nucleoside reverse-transcriptase inhibitors) emerge in plasma HIV-RNA within the first 6 weeks post partum in a high proportion of single-dose nevirapine-exposed women, appear to decline by 1 year, but can be detected with ultrasensitive resistance testing for an extended period of time in some populations.[33–37] Virologic response is diminished if a nevirapine-based regimen is started within 6 to 12 months of exposure to single-dose nevirapine.[33,38–40] However, if nevirapine-based therapy is started more than 12 months after single-dose nevirapine, virologic response is similar to women who have not been exposed to single-dose nevirapine.

One strategy to limit the emergence of resistance in the mother after single-dose nevirapine administration is to treat the mothers with a 1- to 2-week course of dual nucleoside reverse-transcriptase inhibitors or a single-dose of tenofovir/emtricitabine (both drugs have long half-lives in plasma) often referred to as an *antiretroviral tail*.[41,42] Many resource-limited settings are moving toward universal treatment with a 3-drug antiretroviral therapy regimen for all pregnant women or at least for those with a CD4+ cell count less than 350 cells/μL.[43] This strategy provides suppressive combination therapy to women during the time of greatest risk of perinatal HIV transmission.

Single-dose nevirapine to the newborn infant within the first 72 hours of life protects the infant from HIV infection during the early postpartum period, but results in emergence of mutations that confer resistance to nevirapine (and efavirenz) in a high proportion of infants who are HIV-infected in utero, during the intrapartum period, or infected within the first few weeks after delivery from early breastfeeding.[34,44,45] Extended infant nevirapine prophylaxis during breastfeeding reduces transmission of HIV to infants, but there is a high risk of developing resistance to nevirapine among those infants who become HIV infected.[46–48]

Breastfeeding presents a problem that is unique to resource-limited settings, especially sub-Saharan Africa, because substituting formula for breast milk results in higher mortality caused by pneumonia and diarrhea among both HIV-infected and HIV-uninfected infants born to HIV-infected mothers.[49] Exclusive breastfeeding, in contrast to mixtures of breast milk and other foods, reduces early transmission of HIV[50] and is recommended by the World Health Organization. Nevirapine resistance can be detected in HIV RNA in the breast milk of lactating women even after a single dose of intrapartum nevirapine, raising the possibility of transmitting resistant HIV to infants during breastfeeding.[51] Treating HIV-infected nursing women or their children with combination antiretrovirals to prevent breast-milk transmission reduces, but does not eliminate, HIV transmission during the breastfeeding period.[52] Several studies in humans have demonstrated that antiretroviral drugs (including zidovudine, lamivudine, nevirapine, efavirenz, and nelfinavir) administered to lactating women are present in breast milk.[9,53,54] Some antiretroviral drugs, but perhaps not all, are transferred via breastfeeding; the magnitude of infant drug concentrations from exposure to maternally administered drug differs for each drug as well as with the time post partum. Because of the frequency of feeding even low concentrations of antiretrovirals in breast milk may result in biologically significant antiretroviral concentrations in the nursing infant.[55] Ingestion of antiretroviral drugs in breastmilk has led to resistance emerging in HIV-infected children whose mothers take antiretroviral drugs whether the child was infected in utero, during the peripartum period, or via breastfeeding.[56]

Table 2
Prevalence of HIV resistance associated with antiretroviral prophylaxis against mother-to-child transmission of HIV among infants

Author	Study, Location	N	Years	Infant ART Exposure		Resistance Documented to (%)		
				Maternal Regimen	Infant Regimen	Nucleoside Reverse-transcriptase Inhibitors	Non-nucleoside Reverse-transcriptase Inhibitors	Protease Inhibitor
Masquelier[60]	French Perinatal Cohort, France	34	1994–1996	Zidovudine alone 55% Combination therapy 32% No therapy 13%	Zidovudine	Zidovudine 20%	N/A	N/A
Palumbo[27]	PACTS, United States	22	1991–1997	Zidovudine	Zidovudine	Zidovudine 9%	N/A	N/A
Fiscus[61]	North Carolina, United States	59	1993–1997	Antepartum and intrapartum zidovudine 4% in 1993 to 78% in 1997	Zidovudine 4% in 1993 to 78% in 1997	Zidovudine 9%	N/A	0%
Mandelbrot[26]	ANRS 075, France	5	1997–1998	Zidovudine/lamivudine	Zidovudine/lamivudine	Zidovudine 40% Lamivudine 40%	—	—
Parker[18]	New York State, United States	91	1998–1999	Combination therapy 44% No therapy 56%	—	Zidovudine 7.7% Lamivudine 3.3 (3/91)	Nevirapine 3.3% Zidovudine 3.3% Lamivudine 3.3%	3.3%

Reference	Location	N	Years					
Karchava[17]	New York State, United States	42	2001–2002	Zidovudine-containing regimens 67%	Zidovudine 93%	Lamivudine 7%	Nevirapine 12%	2%
Delaugerre[62]	French Perinatal Cohort, France	60	1997–2004	Zidovudine dual or triple combination therapy (% not specified)	Zidovudine, lamivudine (% not specified)	Zidovudine 13% Lamivudine 5%	Nevirapine 3%	2%
Persaud[16]	PACTG 1030, United States and Brazil	21	2002–2005	Zidovudine 59% Zidovudine, nevirapine 5% Zidovudine, lamivudine, nevirapine 5% Zidovudine, lamivudine 5% None 23%	Zidovudine 59% Zidovudine, nevirapine 14% Zidovudine, lamivudine, nevirapine 5% None 23%	Zidovudine 5% Lamivudine 14%	Nevirapine 18%	N/A

The denominator of many reports is based on the number of infants who had a resistance test performed. The true prevalence of antiretroviral drug resistance among infants in care is difficult to ascertain and the percentages of infants with resistance in any one study must be interpreted in the context of the constraints of that study.

Abbreviations: ANRS, Agence Nationale de Recherches sur le SIDA; ART, antiretroviral therapy; N/A, not applicable; PACTG, Pediatric AIDS Clinical Trials Group; PACTS, Pediatric AIDS Collaborative Transmission Study.

Resistance to nevirapine among HIV-infected newborn infants is associated with poorer virologic response when the infant is taking nevirapine-based therapy.[57] The lack of readily available real-time resistance testing to determine if an infant is infected with a resistant strain of HIV can be addressed by using protease-inhibitor–based antiretroviral therapy for infants if the mother or infant received nevirapine prophylaxis. However, infant-friendly formulations of protease inhibitors may not be available in all resource-limited settings, leaving some programs with no options other than nevirapine-based therapy.

SUMMARY

Pregnant women who are HIV-infected may harbor resistant HIV from acquisition of a resistant strain or emergence of a resistant strain while taking antiretroviral drugs. Clinicians can address HIV drug resistance by ordering an HIV resistance test for pregnant women with no prior antiretroviral therapy, with prior antiretroviral therapy that has been interrupted, and with current antiretroviral therapy that has not fully suppressed viral load. An antiretroviral regimen should be chosen with the results of the antiretroviral resistance test considered, as well as current and past history of antiretroviral therapy and prior resistance tests. In complicated cases, it may be prudent to consult with a clinician who is an expert in managing antiretroviral therapy. In the infant, antiretroviral-resistant HIV can be transferred from mother to child in utero, during the perinatal period, or can emerge in the infant from antiretroviral prophylaxis. In settings where breastfeeding remains recommended for HIV-infected pregnant women, antiretroviral-resistant HIV may be transmitted via breast milk or it may emerge in HIV-infected infants via passive ingestion of antiretroviral drugs from breast milk if the mother is taking antiretroviral therapy. The extent that antiretroviral resistance directly influences the infrequent, but continuing, transmission of HIV from mother to child in the United States cannot be fully ascertained.

ACKNOWLEDGMENTS

Susie Danner, BA, Centers for Disease Control and Prevention, for assistance with research and manuscript preparation.

REFERENCES

1. Clavel F, Hance AJ. HIV drug resistance. N Engl J Med 2004;350(10):1023–35.
2. Hirsch MS, Gunthard HF, Schapiro JM, et al. Antiretroviral drug resistance testing in adult HIV-1 infection: 2008 recommendations of an International AIDS Society-USA panel. Clin Infect Dis 2008;47(2):266–85.
3. Johnson VA, Brun-Vezinet F, Clotet B, et al. Update of the drug resistance mutations in HIV-1: December 2009. Top HIV Med 2009;17(5):138–45.
4. Panel on Treatment of HIV-Infected Pregnant Women and Prevention of Perinatal Transmission. Recommendations for use of antiretroviral drugs in pregnant HIV-1-infected women for maternal health and interventions to reduce perinatal HIV transmission in the United States. May 24, 2010. Available at: http://aidsinfo.nih.gov/ContentFiles/PerinatalGL.pdf. Accessed May 24, 2010.
5. Cooper ER, Charurat M, Mofenson L, et al. Combination antiretroviral strategies for the treatment of pregnant HIV-1-infected women and prevention of perinatal HIV-1 transmission. J Acquir Immune Defic Syndr 2002;29(5):484–94.
6. Mofenson LM, Lambert JS, Stiehm ER, et al. Risk factors for perinatal transmission of human immunodeficiency virus type 1 in women treated with zidovudine.

pediatric AIDS clinical trials group study 185 team. N Engl J Med 1999;341(6): 385–93.

7. Warszawski J, Tubiana R, Le CJ, et al. Mother-to-child HIV transmission despite antiretroviral therapy in the ANRS French perinatal cohort. AIDS 2008;22(2): 289–99.

8. Mirochnick M, Siminski S, Fenton T, et al. Nevirapine pharmacokinetics in pregnant women and in their infants after in utero exposure. Pediatr Infect Dis J 2001;20(8):803–5.

9. Mirochnick M, Thomas T, Capparelli E, et al. Antiretroviral concentrations in breast-feeding infants of mothers receiving highly active antiretroviral therapy. Antimicrob Agents Chemother 2009;53(3):1170–6.

10. Gingelmaier A, Kurowski M, Kastner R, et al. Placental transfer and pharmacokinetics of lopinavir and other protease inhibitors in combination with nevirapine at delivery. AIDS 2006;20(13):1737–43.

11. Bauer GR, Welles SL, Colgrove RR, et al. Zidovudine resistance phenotype and risk of perinatal HIV-1 transmission in zidovudine monotherapy-treated mothers with moderately advanced disease. J Acquir Immune Defic Syndr 2003;34(3):312–9.

12. Soto-Ramirez LE, Rodriguez-Diaz R, Duran AS, et al. Antiretroviral resistance among HIV type 1-infected women first exposed to antiretrovirals during pregnancy: plasma versus PBMCs. AIDS Res Hum Retroviruses 2008;24(6):797–804.

13. Muro E, Droste JA, Hofstede HT, et al. Nevirapine plasma concentrations are still detectable after more than 2 weeks in the majority of women receiving single-dose nevirapine: implications for intervention studies. J Acquir Immune Defic Syndr 2005;39(4):419–21.

14. Delaugerre C, Chaix ML, Blanche S, et al. Perinatal acquisition of drug-resistant HIV-1 infection: mechanisms and long-term outcome. Retrovirology 2009;6:85.

15. Frenkel LM, Wagner LE, Demeter LM, et al. Effects of zidovudine use during pregnancy on resistance and vertical transmission of human immunodeficiency virus type 1. Clin Infect Dis 1995;20(5):1321–6.

16. Persaud D, Palumbo P, Ziemniak C, et al. Early archiving and predominance of nonnucleoside reverse transcriptase inhibitor-resistant HIV-1 among recently infected infants born in the United States. J Infect Dis 2007;195(10):1402–10.

17. Karchava M, Pulver W, Smith L, et al. Prevalence of drug-resistance mutations and non-subtype B strains among HIV-infected infants from New York state. J Acquir Immune Defic Syndr 2006;42(5):614–9.

18. Parker MM, Wade N, Lloyd RM Jr, et al. Prevalence of genotypic drug resistance among a cohort of HIV-infected newborns. J Acquir Immune Defic Syndr 2003; 32(3):292–7.

19. Cunningham CK, Chaix ML, Rekacewicz C, et al. Development of resistance mutations in women receiving standard antiretroviral therapy who received intrapartum nevirapine to prevent perinatal human immunodeficiency virus type 1 transmission: a substudy of pediatric AIDS clinical trials group protocol 316. J Infect Dis 2002;186(2):181–8.

20. Paredes R, Cheng I, Kuritzkes DR, et al. High prevalence of primary lamivudine and nelfinavir resistance in HIV-1-infected pregnant women in the United States, 1998-2004. AIDS 2007;21(15):2103–6.

21. Paredes R, Cheng I, Kuritzkes DR, et al. Postpartum antiretroviral drug resistance in HIV-1-infected women receiving pregnancy-limited antiretroviral therapy. AIDS 2010;24(1):45–53.

22. Shah SS, Crane M, Monaghan K, et al. Genotypic resistance testing in HIV-infected pregnant women in an urban setting. Int J STD AIDS 2004;15(6):384–7.

23. Weinberg A, Forster-Harwood J, McFarland EJ, et al. Resistance to antiretrovirals in HIV-infected pregnant women. J Clin Virol 2009;45(1):39–42.
24. Welles SL, Bauer GR, LaRussa PS, et al. Time trends for HIV-1 antiretroviral resistance among antiretroviral-experienced and naive pregnant women in New York City during 1991 to early 2001. J Acquir Immune Defic Syndr 2007;44(3):329–35.
25. Eastman PS, Shapiro DE, Coombs RW, et al. Maternal viral genotypic zidovudine resistance and infrequent failure of zidovudine therapy to prevent perinatal transmission of human immunodeficiency virus type 1 in pediatric AIDS clinical trials group protocol 076. J Infect Dis 1998;177(3):557–64.
26. Mandelbrot L, Landreau-Mascaro A, Rekacewicz C, et al. Lamivudine-zidovudine combination for prevention of maternal-infant transmission of HIV-1. JAMA 2001; 285(16):2083–93.
27. Palumbo P, Holland B, Dobbs T, et al. Antiretroviral resistance mutations among pregnant human immunodeficiency virus type 1-infected women and their newborns in the United States: vertical transmission and clades. J Infect Dis 2001;184(9):1120–6.
28. Welles SL, Pitt J, Colgrove R, et al. HIV-1 genotypic zidovudine drug resistance and the risk of maternal–infant transmission in the women and infants transmission study. The Women and Infants Transmission Study Group. AIDS 2000; 14(3):263–71.
29. Lyons FE, Coughlan S, Byrne CM, et al. Emergence of antiretroviral resistance in HIV-positive women receiving combination antiretroviral therapy in pregnancy. AIDS 2005;19(1):63–7.
30. Clarke JR, Braganza R, Mirza A, et al. Rapid development of genotypic resistance to lamivudine when combined with zidovudine in pregnancy. J Med Virol 1999;59(3):364–8.
31. Tubiana R, Le CJ, Rouzioux C, et al. Factors associated with mother-to-child transmission of HIV-1 despite a maternal viral load <500 copies/ml at delivery: a case-control study nested in the French perinatal cohort (EPF-ANRS CO1). Clin Infect Dis 2010;50(4):585–96.
32. World Health Organization, UNICEF, UNAIDS. Towards universal access: scaling up priority HIV/AIDS interventions in the health sector. September 2009 progress report. Geneva (Switzerland): World Health Organization; 2009. p. 1–162.
33. Bardeguez AD, Shapiro DE, Mofenson LM, et al. Effect of cessation of zidovudine prophylaxis to reduce vertical transmission on maternal HIV disease progression and survival. J Acquir Immune Defic Syndr 2003;32(2):170–81.
34. Eshleman SH, Mracna M, Guay LA, et al. Selection and fading of resistance mutations in women and infants receiving nevirapine to prevent HIV-1 vertical transmission (HIVNET 012). AIDS 2001;15(15):1951–7.
35. Eshleman SH, Jackson JB. Nevirapine resistance after single dose prophylaxis. AIDS Rev 2002;4(2):59–63.
36. Flys T, Nissley DV, Claasen CW, et al. Sensitive drug-resistance assays reveal long-term persistence of HIV-1 variants with the K103N nevirapine (NVP) resistance mutation in some women and infants after the administration of single-dose NVP: HIVNET 012. J Infect Dis 2005;192(1):24–9.
37. Flys TS, Donnell D, Mwatha A, et al. Persistence of K103N-containing HIV-1 variants after single-dose nevirapine for prevention of HIV-1 mother-to-child transmission. J Infect Dis 2007;195(5):711–5.
38. Lallemant M, Jourdain G, Le CS, et al. Single-dose perinatal nevirapine plus standard zidovudine to prevent mother-to-child transmission of HIV-1 in Thailand. N Engl J Med 2004;351(3):217–28.

39. Lockman S, Shapiro RL, Smeaton LM, et al. Response to antiretroviral therapy after a single, peripartum dose of nevirapine. N Engl J Med 2007;356(2): 135–47.

40. Stringer JS, McConnell MS, Kiarie J, et al. Effectiveness of non-nucleoside reverse-transcriptase inhibitor-based antiretroviral therapy in women previously exposed to a single intrapartum dose of nevirapine: a multi-country, prospective cohort study. PLoS Med 2010;7(2):e1000233.

41. Chi BH, Sinkala M, Mbewe F, et al. Single-dose tenofovir and emtricitabine for reduction of viral resistance to non-nucleoside reverse transcriptase inhibitor drugs in women given intrapartum nevirapine for perinatal HIV prevention: an open-label randomised trial. Lancet 2007;370(9600):1698–705.

42. McIntyre JA, Hopley M, Moodley D, et al. Efficacy of short-course AZT plus 3TC to reduce nevirapine resistance in the prevention of mother-to-child HIV transmission: a randomized clinical trial. PLoS Med 2009;6(10):e1000172.

43. World Health Organization. Rapid advice: antiretroviral therapy for HIV infection in adults and adolescents. World Health Organization. Geneva (Switzerland): WHO Press; November 2009. p. 1–26.

44. Eshleman SH, Hoover DR, Chen S, et al. Resistance after single-dose nevirapine prophylaxis emerges in a high proportion of Malawian newborns. AIDS 2005; 19(18):2167–9.

45. Guay LA, Musoke P, Fleming T, et al. Intrapartum and neonatal single-dose nevirapine compared with zidovudine for prevention of mother-to-child transmission of HIV-1 in Kampala, Uganda: HIVNET 012 randomised trial. Lancet 1999; 354(9181):795–802.

46. Arrive E, Newell ML, Ekouevi DK, et al. Prevalence of resistance to nevirapine in mothers and children after single-dose exposure to prevent vertical transmission of HIV-1: a meta-analysis. Int J Epidemiol 2007;36(5):1009–21.

47. Bedri A, Gudetta B, Isehak A, et al. Extended-dose nevirapine to 6 weeks of age for infants to prevent HIV transmission via breastfeeding in Ethiopia, India, and Uganda: an analysis of three randomised controlled trials. Lancet 2008; 372(9635):300–13.

48. Kumwenda NI, Hoover DR, Mofenson LM, et al. Extended antiretroviral prophylaxis to reduce breast-milk HIV-1 transmission. N Engl J Med 2008; 359(2):119–29.

49. Kafulafula G, Hoover DR, Taha TE, et al. Frequency of gastroenteritis and gastroenteritis-associated mortality with early weaning in HIV-1-uninfected children born to HIV-infected women in Malawi. J Acquir Immune Defic Syndr 2010; 53(1):6–13.

50. Coovadia HM, Rollins NC, Bland RM, et al. Mother-to-child transmission of HIV-1 infection during exclusive breastfeeding in the first 6 months of life: an intervention cohort study. Lancet 2007;369(9567):1107–16.

51. Hudelson SE, McConnell MS, Bagenda D, et al. Emergence and persistence of nevirapine resistance in breast milk after single-dose nevirapine administration. AIDS 2010;24(4):557–61.

52. Thomas T, Masaba R, Ndivo R, et al. Prevention of mother-to-child transmission of HIV-1 among breastfeeding mother in Kisumu, Kenya using highly active antiretroviral therapy: the Kisumu breastfeeding study [abstract]. In: 15th Conference on Retroviruses and Opportunistic Infectious (CROI) 2008.

53. Colebunders R, Hodossy B, Burger D, et al. The effect of highly active antiretroviral treatment on viral load and antiretroviral drug levels in breast milk. AIDS 2005;19(16):1912–5.

54. Shapiro RL, Holland DT, Capparelli E, et al. Antiretroviral concentrations in breast-feeding infants of women in Botswana receiving antiretroviral treatment. J Infect Dis 2005;192(5):720–7.
55. Bulterys M, Weidle PJ, Abrams EJ, et al. Combination antiretroviral therapy in African nursing mothers and drug exposure in their infants: new pharmacokinetic and virologic findings. J Infect Dis 2005;192(5):709–12.
56. Zeh C, Weidle PJ, Nafisa L, et al. Emergence of HIV-1 drug resistance among breastfeeding infants born to HIV-infected mothers taking antiretrovirals for prevention of mother-to-child transmission of HIV: the Kisumu breastfeeding study, Kenya [abstract]. In: 15th Conference on Retroviruses and Opportunistic Infections 2010.
57. Macleod IJ, Rowley CF, Thior I, et al. Minor resistant variants in nevirapine-exposed infants may predict virologic failure on nevirapine-containing ART. J Clin Virol 2010;48(2):162–7.
58. Kully C, Yerly S, Erb P, et al. Codon 215 mutations in human immunodeficiency virus-infected pregnant women. Swiss Collaborative 'HIV and Pregnancy' Study. J Infect Dis 1999;179(3):705–8.
59. Juethner SN, Williamson C, Ristig MB, et al. Nonnucleoside reverse transcriptase inhibitor resistance among antiretroviral-naive HIV-positive pregnant women. J Acquir Immune Defic Syndr 2003;32(2):153–6.
60. Masquelier B, Chaix ML, Burgard M, et al. Zidovudine genotypic resistance in HIV-1-infected newborns in the French perinatal cohort. J Acquir Immune Defic Syndr 2001;27(2):99–104.
61. Fiscus SA, Adimora AA, Schoenbach VJ, et al. Trends in human immunodeficiency virus (HIV) counseling, testing, and antiretroviral treatment of HIV-infected women and perinatal transmission in North Carolina. J Infect Dis 1999;180(1):99–105.
62. Delaugerre C, Chaix ML, Warszawski J, et al. [HIV-1 drug resistance in French infected-children: from newborn to adolescent]. Arch Pediatr 2007;14(3):298–302.

Survival and Health Benefits of Breastfeeding Versus Artificial Feeding in Infants of HIV-Infected Women: Developing Versus Developed World

Louise Kuhn, PhD[a,b,]*, Grace Aldrovandi, MD[c]

KEYWORDS

- Breastfeeding • HIV transmission • Artificial feeding
- Mother-to-child transmission

Artificial feeding has been recommended for HIV-infected women in the developed world since 1985 after an occurrence of HIV transmission through breastfeeding was first described.[1] When the World Health Organization (WHO) initially recommended that HIV-infected women in the developing world continue to breastfeed (1992),[2] the guidance was criticized by some as upholding a double standard. Twenty-five years later, with an HIV epidemic that has established itself with a vengeance in some of the poorest and most vulnerable communities of the developing world, the international community still grapples with this complex issue. There are now considerably more empirical data to inform this dilemma as well as the possibility of antiretroviral and behavioral interventions that change the terms of this debate. This

---

The authors have nothing to disclose.
This article was supported by the National Institutes of Child Health and Human Development (HD 57161, HD 39611, and HD 40777).
[a] Gertrude H. Sergievsky Center, College of Physicians and Surgeons, Columbia University, 630 West 168th Street, New York, NY 10032, USA
[b] Department of Epidemiology, Mailman School of Public Health, Columbia University, 722 West 168th Street, New York, NY 10032, USA
[c] Department of Pediatrics, Children's Hospital Los Angeles, University of Southern California, 4650 Sunset Boulevard, Los Angeles, CA 90027, USA
* Corresponding author. Gertrude H. Sergievsky Center, College of Physicians and Surgeons, Columbia University, 630 West 168th Street, New York, NY 10032.
E-mail address: lk24@columbia.edu

Clin Perinatol 37 (2010) 843–862
doi:10.1016/j.clp.2010.08.011
0095-5108/10/$ – see front matter **perinatology.theclinics.com**

review summarizes the data describing the survival and health benefits of breastfeeding versus artificial feeding for infants and young children born to HIV-infected women. The authors conclude that context matters. For most of the developing world, the health and survival benefits of breastfeeding exceed the risks of HIV transmission, especially when antiretroviral interventions are provided.

HIV TRANSMISSION THROUGH BREASTFEEDING

It is now well established that HIV is transmitted throughout the duration of breastfeeding.[3–5] Thus, the major health benefit of artificial feeding in both developed and developing countries is that postnatal HIV transmission is avoided. Pregnancy and delivery transmission cannot be so easily avoided and in the absence of antiretroviral drugs approximately 20% of HIV-infected women transmit the virus via these two routes.[6] Breastfeeding adds further infections with the cumulative rate of breastfeeding-associated infection determined by the nature of breastfeeding practices and the duration of all breast milk exposure. Unqualified statements that breastfeeding adds an additional transmission rate of 14%[3,7] neglect the variability of normative infant feeding practices across communities and across women within communities. It is logical that the postnatal transmission rate increases with breastfeeding duration because infections accumulate with each month of additional exposure.[8] It is more difficult, however, to quantify the instantaneous hazard or force of infection during early or later periods of breastfeeding. A combined analysis of selected studies concluded that hazards were constant over time.[8] But several cohort studies with tighter intervals for determining the timing of transmission have reported declining hazards as a child becomes older.[4,5,9] Estimates of whether or not most transmission occurs early or late depend on the instantaneous hazards and the duration of breastfeeding.

A further complexity in quantifying the magnitude of postnatal HIV transmission is that although breastfeeding is a biologic process, it is also a cultural practice.[10] What is healthiest and what is normative do not necessarily coincide. For example, colostrum is a fluid rich in immunologically active components capable of protecting newborns over the most vulnerable period immediately after delivery. Yet in some societies, colostrum is considered dirty and is discarded.[11] Cultural practices that displace breastfeeding are detrimental to mothers and infants. Non-nutritive herbal supplements deprive infants of essential nutrition as well as the immunologic protection afforded by milk. Inconsistent breastfeeding predisposes women to mastitis and hastens the return to menses, increasing the risk of postpartum anemia as well as pregnancy.[12–14] Yet in some societies, introduction of non-nutritive herbal supplements that displace breast milk is considered essential to infant health.[15]

Quantifying rates of postnatal transmission have to take these cultural variations into account. One parameter that has emerged as a strong influence on the extent of postnatal transmission during the first few months of life is the quality of breastfeeding ascertained by the extent of exclusive breastfeeding.[9,16–18] When breastfeeding occurs without the addition of formula, other nonhuman milks, non-nutritive liquids, and solids and semisolid foods, transmission is lower than when breastfeeding is inclusive of these unnecessary supplements.[9,16–18] Estimates of postnatal transmission gathered from settings where support of exclusive breastfeeding is lacking or in communities with poor uptake of recommendations to breastfeed exclusively are likely to differ from settings more favorable to exclusive breastfeeding. Almost all of these data carefully clarifying risks of transmission under these different circumstances come from studies conducted in developing countries.

SURVIVAL AND HEALTH BENEFITS OF BREASTFEEDING

The harms of artificial feeding were brought to the attention of the international community most strongly after the deaths that resulted when Nestlé and other formula companies began marketing their products in developing countries in the 1970s.[19] Thereafter, strict controls on marketing of formula in developing countries and public health programs supporting breastfeeding were largely successful in re-establishing breastfeeding as the almost universal mode of infant feeding in most developing countries in the pre-HIV era. For example, in the1980s, uptake of breastfeeding in Zambia was close to 100% with a median duration of 24 months.[20] In the meantime, in developed countries, as infant mortality rates continued to decline through health service interventions and rising standards of living, breastfeeding practices deteriorated. In 1990, in the United States, uptake of breastfeeding was a mere 51%.[21] Moreover, among the poorest sectors of wealthier countries, breastfeeding uptake was even worse.[21] As the HIV epidemic in women in the United States has differentially affected impoverished minority communities, artificial feeding was already the norm in many of the communities most affected by HIV, independent of any recommendations. In the United States, where racial disparities in infant health are of grave concern, lower uptake and duration of breastfeeding in socioeconomically disadvantaged populations is one of the factors that account for poorer perinatal health outcomes in African American women.[22-24]

As the defining characteristic of mammalian reproduction, it is challenging to approach study of the benefits of breastfeeding with evidence-based medicine's reliance on the randomized clinical trial. There are few circumstances in which randomization of an intimate personal behavior, widely considered healthiest for mothers and infants, can be considered ethical. There are also practical constraints. Even the most persuasive investigator faces limitations in enticing mothers and infants to obey their assigned practice. So, for obvious reasons, data demonstrating survival and health advantages of breastfeeding largely come from epidemiologic studies.

The results of epidemiologic studies are remarkably consistent. Breastfeeding is a significant protector against diarrheal disease, respiratory disease, and other infections.[25-28] Breastfeeding tends to result in better nutritional outcomes, including protecting against obesity in overfed populations and against wasting in underfed populations.[29-32] It has beneficial effects on cognitive functioning and psychosocial development.[33-35] This is a large body of literature. There are reviews,[25,26,36-38] and reviews of reviews,[39,40] and even a long report from the Agency for Healthcare Research and Quality of studies only in developed countries.[41] What is particularly striking is that the conclusions are consistent regardless of whether or not the studies are from the developing or the developed world. Breastfeeding protects infants not only in Bangladesh[42] but also in Boston,[43] not only in historical times[44] but also in the new millennium.[45]

To understand why artificial feeding can be recommended for HIV-infected women in developed countries despite the known risks associated with this practice, it is important to make the distinction between an absolute risk and a relative risk. An absolute risk is the frequency with which an event occurs in the population (eg, an infant mortality rate might be 10 deaths per 1000 live births). A relative risk requires a comparison. For example, it might said that an infant mortality rate is 10/1000 live births if women breastfeed but 20/1000 live births if women avoid all breastfeeding (ie, a 2-fold increased risk). The ratio of rates in the two groups is referred to as the relative risk. Studies show that the relative risk associated with artificial feeding is elevated in all populations, but what makes developed countries different is that the absolute rates of morbidity and mortality are generally low. Moreover, breastfeeding may protect against morbidity, but because most morbidity in these settings is not fatal, arguably the benefits can be ignored.

STRENGTHS AND WEAKNESSES OF USING HIV-FREE SURVIVAL AS AN OUTCOME

In the spectrum of possible benefits of breastfeeding that could be weighed against the risks of HIV transmission, the field has tended to focus on only one, namely, the benefits of breastfeeding for infant survival. The concept of HIV-free survival, which refers to the absence of a combined outcome of either (1) HIV infection or (2) death before HIV infection, has emerged as a consensus outcome to evaluate strategies. The advantage of this approach is that it is a reminder that some of the strategies proposed to prevent HIV transmission, such as abstinence from breastfeeding or early weaning, also carry a cost in terms of lives of uninfected infants. The disadvantage of the approach is that it counts an HIV infection as equivalent to a death, a pessimistic approach and one that is out of date now that pediatric HIV infection can be success-fully treated. It also stacks the deck in favor of interventions that prevent HIV transmis-sion and neglects the range of other nonfatal, but potentially serious, adverse outcomes associated with limiting breastfeeding.

MECHANISMS BY WHICH BREASTFEEDING PROTECTS

To appreciate the reasons for differential infant feeding recommendations in different circumstances, it is helpful to consider the potential mechanisms whereby breastfeed-ing protects infants' health. For heuristic purposes, this article separates the biologic basis for the benefits of breastfeeding into three overarching mechanisms (**Fig. 1**): (1) contamination (ie, artificial feeding places infants at risk through introducing environ-mental contaminants and creating a less hygienic feeding method); (2) poor nutrition (ie, abstinence from breastfeeding could compromise an infant's nutritional status if formula is not mixed correctly or not given in appropriate quantities); and (3) absence of immune protection.

Contamination

It is perhaps no surprise that studies have shown that it is difficult for women to prepare formula hygienically in resource-poor settings.[46,47] In a study conducted in KwaZulu-Natal, South Africa, approximately 80% of formula mothers prepared at home after instructions from the counselors were contaminated with fecal bacteria.[48] Approximately 20% of the samples that the counselors prepared at the clinic while showing the mothers how to do everything correctly were also contaminated.[48] The

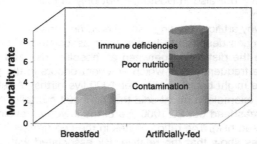

Fig. 1. Theoretic mechanisms by which artificial feeding increases the risk of infant and young child death.

dramatic epidemic of diarrhea-related deaths that occurred in Botswana in formula-fed infants after severe flooding affected urban areas is another example of the dangers of contaminated water.[49–51] Contaminated water is a major threat to child health and the provision of a sustained supply of adequate clean water at the point of use in the household is a major priority for public health.[52] But is it enough?

Infant formula is not the only source of exposure to pathogens, especially in contaminated environments. Despite their parents' best efforts, children do not live in aseptic environments. They explore their world with their hands and mouths. Breast milk has evolved to protect children from these pathogens. Diarrhea morbidity and mortality are significantly reduced even when breastfeeding is not exclusive[53] and even in young children when consuming relatively small quantities of breast milk.[54] Also, breastfeeding reduces the risk of respiratory illness, an outcome where contaminated water plays little to no role.[42,43,55,56] Breastfeeding also protects against severe infectious disease in settings with a predominantly safe water supply.[28,43,45]

An exemplary demonstration of the multifactorial source of breastfeeding's benefits came from a confluence of circumstances in a clinical study in rural Kenya. As part of an evaluation of the effects of extending antiretroviral therapy during lactation on reduction in postnatal HIV transmission, HIV-infected women were encouraged to stop all breastfeeding by 6 months (the duration of the antiretroviral therapy). Elevated diarrhea morbidity was coincident with weaning and the study was temporarily suspended while the investigators considered what to do.[57] The investigators elected to introduce a state-of-the-art home water quality-improvement program that had been found effective in other settings. When they introduced this intervention, diarrhea was reduced in breastfed infants but there was no effect on weaning-related diarrhea.[58] Contamination plays a role in exaggerating the risks of artificial feeding[59] but clean water is insufficient to mitigate artificial feeding's risks.

Poor Nutrition

Infant formula is specifically developed to mirror the nutritional composition of breast milk as closely as possible but falls short in several respects. Breast milk is exquisitely regulated such that the content varies from the beginning to the end of the feed so that a child can be most quickly satiated even with a short feed but can continue to feed for comfort and not become overfed on longer feeds.[60] The composition of human milk also varies based on the amount the child consumes and over time is regulated to adapt to the unique needs of a specific child.[61] This individualization cannot be achieved with formula but, if given in correct volumes and frequencies, should be nutritionally adequate. The primary concern related to poor nutrition of formula-fed infants is incorrect mixing and overdilution. A related health systems concern is sustained supply and the problem of stockouts.

In situations of scarcity, infant formula is usually perceived as valuable or precious by members of the community. In most developing countries, the costs of formula make it prohibitive for all but a small minority unless it subsidized or provided free by a health service. Provision of free or subsidized formula poses complex ethical challenges.[62,63] Qualitative research has highlighted the coercive dynamics of free formula and there are several examples of confusion and misinformation that may result in suboptimal practices.[47,64–67] For example, in a study of three sites in South Africa, a surprising pattern was noted of inadequate use of the formula that was provided by the health service. Mothers were not giving their infants formula in sufficient quantities. Rather, they were avoiding breastfeeding, were giving some formula, and were also providing a substantial proportion of the infants' diet with nutritionally inadequate foods and liquids.[68] Audits of the South African national formula program have noted serious gaps in supply to both urban and rural clinics.[69] Population mobility introduces further complications for sustained access.

Absence of Immune Protection

During pregnancy, maternal antibodies are transported across the placenta to protect infants whose immune system is not fully mature at the time of birth. This process is referred to as passive immunity because the child is reliant on the mother's antibodies. This process continues during breastfeeding.[70,71] Other than antibodies, breast milk contains many immunomodulatory components that bolster a child's immune system and protect against disease.[38,70,71] The recent introduction of long chain fatty acids and probiotics into infant formula demonstrates the awareness that formula companies have of the deficiencies of their product.[72–74] It might have been expected that because HIV has so many immunologic effects that the quality of breast milk might be compromised. A study from Botswana, however, showed that HIV-infected and uninfected women had similar quantities of the immunologic components that they measured.[75]

DANGERS OF EXTRAPOLATING FROM CLINICAL STUDIES

Several factors combine to create the beneficial effects of breastfeeding. Theoretically, a strong public health program may be able to minimize risks of environmental contamination and poor nutrition associated with artificial feeding but can do nothing to mitigate the risks conferred by the absence of the immunologically active components of breast milk. The fact that breastfeeding continues to confer benefits to infant health even in developed countries, such as the United States and the United Kingdom,[43,45] suggests that there is a biologic threshold below which it is not possible to go even with the strongest programs.

Caution is required in extrapolating results on the risks of artificial feeding from clinical studies (**Fig. 2**). In most clinical studies, participants are highly motivated, receive the best possible educational interventions, and are provided with close monitoring and a health service safety set. Yet even in this protected environment, only one study in Nairobi, Kenya, has been able to demonstrate a net benefit for HIV-free survival of

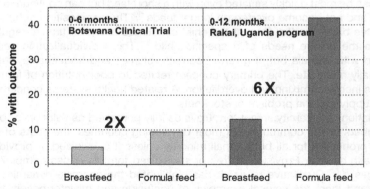

Fig. 2. The magnitude of adverse effects of artificial feeding differs across settings. In this example, effects were stronger in a program in rural Uganda than in a clinical trial in urban Botswana. (*Data from* Thior I, Lockman S, Smeaton LM, et al. Breastfeeding plus infant zidovudine prophylaxis for 6 months vs formula feeding plus infant zidovudine for 1 month to reduce mother-to-child HIV transmission in Botswana: a randomized trial: the Mashi Study. JAMA 2006;296:794–805; and Kagaayi J, Gray RH, Brahmbhatt H, et al. Survival of infants born to HIV-positive mothers by feeding modality in Rakai, Uganda. PLoS One 2008;3:e3877.)

artificial feeding.[3] The study's strict inclusion criteria limit its relevance to the majority of HIV-infected. In a somewhat more generalizable but an otherwise equally thoroughly supervised and monitored population in Botswana, HIV-exposed, uninfected infants randomized to infant formula from birth had a 2-fold increase in mortality compared with those randomized to breastfeeding.[76] These results are contrasted with reports from programs in Uganda where infant mortality was increased more than 6-fold in women who chose formula feeding.[77,78] Thus, in the best-case scenario, when infant formula is provided under carefully monitored conditions with adequate access to medical care, sufficient education and support, and optimal selection of women considered to have adequate personal resources to safely formula feed, the mortality risks of artificial feeding are approximately 2-fold. In programmatic settings, the risks of death are much greater.

LEARNING FROM HISTORY

Current international guidelines for the general population recommend that breast milk alone be given for the first 6 months of a child's life (exclusive breastfeeding) and that complementary foods be introduced at approximately 6 months of age with continued breastfeeding to 24 months or longer.[79] The word, complementary, is preferred because it refers to foods given to complement the nutrients in and immunologic and other components of breast milk. Replacement food usually is used to refer to foods given to replace breast milk in a nonbreastfed child.[80] Between 6 and 24 months, the proportion of nutrients a young child receives from breast milk gradually declines whereas the proportion the child receives from breast milk substitutes and complementary foods gradually increases. Thus, weaning extends over a period of a year or more. A child is referred to as fully weaned once no breast milk is given at all and the child is fully supported on non–breast milk foods and liquids. This pattern of breastfeeding extending into the second year of life is well established as the healthiest for infants in low-resource settings[79] and is recommended for the general population in developed countries as well.

Over the past 10 years, complex advice given to HIV-infected women in developing countries has led to shifts away from breastfeeding and to generally shorter durations of breastfeeding than usual in these communities. A dubious positive upshot of these changes is that they introduce greater heterogeneity into infant feeding practices than usually observed, allowing for epidemiologic analysis of the effects of these behavioral shifts.[81] One group who initially theorized that shifts away from breastfeeding simply to avoid HIV would not result in adverse health outcomes[82] observed in their own program substantial elevations in mortality in women who elected not to breastfeed.[77] This is consistent with what has been observed in other programs, which, even after the benefits of HIV prevention are taken into account, observed worse or, at best, no benefit of artificial feeding.[77,78,83–85]

Four separate cohorts (two in Malawi, one in Kenya, and one in Uganda), all recommending to women enrolled in their trials to wean early, reported elevated morbidity and mortality associated with diarrheal disease at approximately the time of weaning (**Table 1**).[57,86–88] All of these studies included close monitoring and follow-up and education/counseling, which were expected by the investigators to make early weaning safe. Two of the studies were interrupted by their data safety and monitoring boards, which noticed the elevations in morbidity after weaning. Subsequent comparisons with historical cohorts at the same sites revealed worse outcomes in the more recent eras,[89,90] which is surprising because access to antiretroviral therapy and prophylaxis as well as other child-related services had mostly improved over time.

Table 1
Studies on the effects of artificial feeding on HIV transmission and mortality among infants born to HIV-infected mothers in developing countries

	Study Design	Comparisons	Uninfected or all Cause Child Mortality/Morbidity	HIV-free Survival
Randomized trials				
Nairobi, Kenya[3]	Randomized trial (n = 401)	BF versus FF from birth	Trend toward higher 2-year mortality (24%) in FF than in BF (20%) group	Net benefit in FF group
Botswana (MASHI)[76]	Randomized trial (n = 1200)	BF for 6 months versus FF	Significantly higher mortality at 7 months in FF (9.3%) versus BF (4.9%)	No net benefit of FF
Lusaka, Zambia (ZEBS)[92–94]	Randomized trial (n = 958)	16 Months of BF versus early weaning at 4 months	2- to 4-Fold increase in uninfected child mortality due to weaning	No net benefit of early weaning
Historical controls				
Kampala, Uganda[88,90]	Observations during a trial versus previous study (n = 1307)	BF then weaning at median 4 months versus median 9 months	Peak of diarrhea post weaning. Trend toward higher diarrhea-related and all cause mortality in cohort encouraged to wean earlier	Not reported
Malawi[86,89]	Comparison to prior trial with longer BF (n = 3845)	BF >24 months versus weaning at approximately 6 months	Significantly higher rate of diarrhea-related morbidity and mortality and all cause mortality in cohort encouraged to wean at 6 months	Not reported
Kisumu, Kenya[57,58]	Comparison to prior study with longer BF (n = 491)	Wean at 6 months versus BF >12 months	Significantly higher rate of diarrhea hospitalizations post weaning Water safety intervention ineffective	Not reported

Epidemiologic studies

Study	Design	BF versus FF adjusted for socioeconomic factors	Outcome	Conclusion
South Africa[99]	Program evaluation	BF versus FF adjusted for socioeconomic factors	Both BF and FF had higher rates of adverse outcomes if poor socioeconomic status relative to FF and good socioeconomic status	No net benefit of FF if poor socioeconomic status
Côte d'Ivoire[98]	Self-selected feeding choice (n = 557)	Exclusive BF plus early weaning at 4 months versus FF	No increase in mortality or morbidity in either group	No net benefit of FF
Malawi[91]	Combined studies (n = 2000)	Multivariate analysis of actual feeding practices	Significant reduction (hazard ratio = 0.44) in mortality if breastfed (both infected and uninfected children)	Not reported
Rakai, Uganda[77]	Program evaluation (n = 182)	BF versus FF	6-Fold increase in mortality if FF	Nonsignificant trend to worse outcomes if FF
Rwanda[83]	Self-selected feeding choice (n = 532)	BF, then early weaning at 6 months or FF	Nonsignificant trend toward higher mortality in FF (5.6%) than BF (3.3%)	No net benefit of FF
Pune, India[85]	Program evaluation (n = 148)	BF versus FF	Significantly elevated risks of hospitalization if FF	Not reported
Rural Uganda[78]	Self-selected feeding practices (n = 109)	Wean before 6 months versus wean after 6 months	6-Fold increase in death if wean before 6 months	Not reported
Western Kenya[84]	Self-selected feeding practices (n = 2477 but high dropout)	BF with weaning at 3–4 months versus FF	Not reported	No net benefit of FF
Botswana[49,51]	Public health outbreak investigation in emergency rooms after severe floods	BF versus not BF	25-Fold increase in diarrhea deaths if not breastfed	Not reported

Abbreviations: BF, any duration breastfeeding; FF, formula feeding from birth.

Epidemiologic analyses of mortality in breastfed and nonbreastfed infants and young children between birth and 24 months in two trials in Malawi revealed that breastfeeding was associated with a 2.9-fold lower risk of mortality in exposed-uninfected infants after adjustment for confounders.[91]

The observational data are consistent with the findings from the authors' trial in Zambia in which women were randomized to either stop breastfeeding at 4 months or to continue breastfeeding for their own preferred duration. Women in the intervention group were provided with infant formula and a specially developed, fortified weaning cereal for their infants. Because the cereal required cooking, contamination of the water source would, theoretically, be less of a concern. Infants from both groups were weighed regularly and were provided with food supplements if there was any evidence of failure to thrive. Children in both groups also received cotrimoxazole as well as routine childhood interventions (vaccines, vitamin A, and so forth). Counseling and education, including about safe water and hygiene, was intensive, and monitoring and follow-up were close.[92] Because early weaning was not well accepted by the study population, the authors have analyzed the effects of noncompliance. Infants born to women who adhered to their assignment to the early weaning group and weaned early as instructed had worse outcomes than those whose mothers who ignored their random assignment and continued breastfeeding, as did infants born to women who refused to adhere to their assignment to the control group and weaned early.[93] Benefits of breastfeeding on infant and young child survival persisted into the second year of life to approximately 18 months.[94] Benefits of continued breastfeeding were also observed for child growth[95] and for diarrheal morbidity and mortality.[96]

SPECIAL NEEDS OF HIV-INFECTED CHILDREN

HIV-infected children who are formula fed or who are weaned off breast milk early are at high risk of dying prematurely.[76,91,92] The decision to formula feed is usually made during pregnancy or soon after delivery. At that time, infant HIV status, even in the most well-organized programs, is unknown and remains unknown for weeks. HIV testing is rarely done at birth and, when done at 6 weeks, results are usually not available for 2 weeks. Early infant testing programs have been difficult to establish for multiple reasons and, even when the laboratory capacity is in place, tend to identify only a small proportion of HIV-infected children. Once identified as HIV-infected, there are also major logistic challenges and delays in entering pediatric HIV care and treatment programs. Rapid progression of HIV infection in infants means that delays in identifying children and delays in starting therapy can lead to death.[97] Thus, any means of slowing the progression of HIV infection is particularly important for HIV-infected infants if they are to benefit from antiretroviral therapy.

CAN THE RISKS OF ARTIFICIAL FEEDING BE JUSTIFIED?

The increased risks of mortality in HIV-exposed, uninfected infants due to artificial feeding might be justifiable if a net benefit in terms of HIV-free survival could be accomplished. Other than in the original study in Nairobi, Kenya,[3] however, in which no antiretroviral prophylaxis or treatment was available, this is not what has been found (see **Table 1**). In the clinical trial in Botswana (discussed previously), there was no net benefit of artificial feeding on HIV-free survival. The reduced risk of HIV transmission as a result of formula feeding was outweighed by the increased risk of mortality in uninfected children[76] nor was there a net benefit for HIV-free survival of artificial feeding from birth versus short breastfeeding in a study in Côte d'Ivoire.[98] At best, artificial feeding results in no improvements in health status. When implemented under real-world conditions, HIV-free survival has generally been worse, as shown in programs from South Africa and Uganda.[77,99] For example, in an evaluation of the South African national program, women's infant feeding choices bore little relation to their living circumstances. For women who lived in two of the poorer urban and rural sites, both HIV infection and death was increased in women who opted for formula feeding.[99]

For early weaning, the net benefit for HIV prevention is less. The older the child when all breastfeeding ends, the less there is to gain. In essence, the horse is already out of the barn. Because there is less to gain by early weaning, the risks take on greater weight. Even a small increase in mortality can offset a small benefit of HIV prevented. The authors' primary intent-to-treat analysis trial in Lusaka, Zambia, reported no benefit of cessation of breastfeeding at 4 months for the combined outcome of HIV infection or death (HIV-free survival) compared with standard practice of breastfeeding for an unrestricted duration which in this study population was for a median of 16 months.[92] Further analysis of the actual practices of the study population revealed that the magnitude of benefit (ie, the amount of HIV prevented) was almost the same as the magnitude of the harm (ie, the numbers of deaths caused in the population overall).[93] Overall in the study population, women who stopped breastfeeding by 5 months added an HIV transmission rate of 1.1% after 4 months and a mortality rate in the uninfected children of 17.4%. Women who continued breastfeeding for 18 months added a transmission rate of 11.2% of late postnatal transmission and a mortality rate of 9.7% (**Fig. 3**).[93]

These data are in the absence of either maternal antiretroviral treatment or extended antiretroviral regimens that continue during breastfeeding. Because these interventions reduce postnatal transmission considerably, it can be extrapolated from these results that the magnitude of mortality caused by artificial feeding will be larger than the magnitude of HIV transmission prevented. In the authors' trial, among women who were not yet at an advanced enough disease stage to require antiretroviral therapy for their own health, stopping breastfeeding at 4 months led to a 3-fold increase in the combined outcome of HIV infection or death occurring between 4 and 24 months.[93]

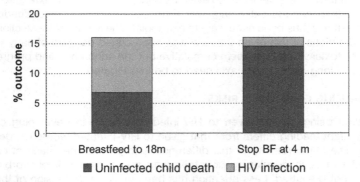

Fig. 3. Benefits of early weaning for HIV prevention are counterbalanced by risks of uninfected mortality in resource-poor countries. Hence, there is no benefit for HIV-free survival of early weaning in such settings. (*Data from* Kuhn L, Aldrovandi G, Sinkala M, et al. Effects of early, abrupt cessation of breastfeeding on HIV-free survival of children in Zambia. N Eng J Med 2008;359:130–41; Kuhn L, Aldrovandi GM, Sinkala M, et al. Differential effects of early weaning for HIV-free survival of children born to HIV-infected mothers by severity of maternal disease. PLoS One 2009;4:e6059.)

BETTER WAYS TO PREVENT HIV TRANSMISSION

There have been important scientific breakthroughs in recent years informing how best to use antiretroviral drugs during the breastfeeding period.[100] It is helpful to make the distinction between using antiretroviral drugs primarily to treat maternal HIV infection and improve the health of the mother (therapeutic regimens), with prevention of transmission as a beneficial side effect, versus using antiretroviral drugs primarily for preventing transmission (prophylaxis regimens to either mother or child). The new WHO guidelines[101] that expand treatment criteria to include all pregnant women with CD4 counts less than 350 cells/µL go a long way to also reduce postnatal transmission. Programs that have proactively initiated treatment in pregnant women with low CD4 counts have also consistently reported low rates of postnatal transmission as well.[102] This is even in the absence of providing additional interventions for women and/or infants born to women with higher CD4 counts. This is because, like morbidity in the mother, transmission is strongly concentrated in women with low CD4 counts.[103] Studies in Mozambique, Tanzania, Kenya, Botswana, and Côte d'Ivoire have all observed low rates (<5%) of HIV transmission (via all routes combined [ie, intrauterine, intrapartum, and postpartum]) in breastfeeding women receiving therapeutic regimens initiated during pregnancy and then continued thereafter.[83,102,104–109] For women who meet clinical criteria, treatment has to continue indefinitely and thus can protect infants throughout the course of breastfeeding.

For women who do not require therapy for their own health, some of the short-course regimens currently recommended for prophylaxis, including single-dose nevirapine and nevirapine combined with short-course zidovudine, seem to reduce the risk of early postnatal transmission during the first weeks of life.[110] In addition, three clinical trials, one multicountry study in Ethiopia, Uganda, and India[111] and two in Malawi,[112,113] have demonstrated that extended infant prophylaxis with nevirapine can significantly reduce postnatal HIV transmission. Lamivudine given to infants during breastfeeding also seems to reduce transmission[114] but zidovudine does not.[76] In the first nevirapine study, prophylaxis was continued for only 6 weeks, in the second for only 14 weeks, and in the third for 24 weeks. Benefits were observed when prophylaxis was given and stopped once the drug was withdrawn.[115] With the wisdom of hindsight, the decisions to evaluate only short periods of extended prophylaxis rather than periods extending over a normal duration of breastfeeding were unfortunate. It has thus been necessary to extrapolate the results of these clinical trials to longer durations of use given the now well-appreciated dangers of early weaning. Fortunately, toxicity does not seem cumulative but the adherence and programmatic challenges of long-term prophylaxis need to be investigated.

INDIVIDUALIZING COMMUNITY RISKS

For the time being, advice given to HIV-infected women in developing countries regarding infant feeding differs from that given to HIV-infected women in developed countries. The prime reason for this difference is to protect the health of exposed-uninfected infants in developing countries who are at high risk of morbidity and mortality if not breastfed. Less attention has been given to discussion of the infant-feeding policies for HIV-infected women in developed countries, in part because background rates of mortality are low and in part because the numbers of women and infants affected is so much lower. Nevertheless, debates around this issue in the developing world may be beginning to spill over to developed countries. With growing appreciation of the effectiveness of antiretrovirals, some have argued for less zealous promotion of artificial feeding for HIV-infected women in developed countries.[116] A more complex issue is the heterogeneity of socioeconomic status between the many countries that fall within the general category of developing and the heterogeneity within developing countries. Previous WHO guidelines attempted to individualize choice, introducing the concept that artificial feeding should be recommended when women meet certain personal criteria, making artificial feeding affordable, feasible, acceptable, sustainable, and safe (AFASS).[117,118] These attempts have largely failed in practice[66,67,69] and programs continue to struggle with how to support individual freedoms without compromising the health of infants. New WHO guidelines attempt to bring greater attention to community-level parameters, including background rates of infectious diseases and the adequacy of child health services in making recommendations for infant feeding practices.[119]

SUMMARY

The gross economic inequalities between the developed and the developing world create global inequities in health status that are ethically unacceptable and should be tackled at every level. The unreflective desire to simply enforce the same programs in vastly different circumstances, however, does nothing to address these inequalities and has been shown in the field of infant feeding and HIV to do considerable harm. Antiretroviral drugs markedly reduce all forms of mother-to-child HIV transmission and culturally appropriate counseling programs can improve the quality of breastfeeding and thereby reduce HIV transmission and improve child survival. Therefore, the time has come to implement these programs in the developing countries where they are most needed. Effective use of antiretroviral drugs can now reduce transmission to such low levels that there are few circumstances in developing countries where artificial feeding can be justified.

REFERENCES

1. Centers for Disease Control and Prevention. Recommendations for assisting in the prevention of perinatal transmission of human T-lymphotropic virus type III/lymphadenopathy-associated virus and acquired immunodeficiency syndrome. MMWR Morb Mortal Wkly Rep 1985;34:721–6, 731–2.
2. World Health Organization Global Programme on AIDS. Consensus statement from the WHO/UNICEF consultation on HIV transmission and breastfeeding. Geneva (Switzerland): WHO; 1992. Report No WHO/GAPA/INF/92 1.
3. Nduati R, John G, Mbori-Ngacha D, et al. Effect of breastfeeding and formula feeding on transmission of HIV-1: a randomized clinical trial. JAMA 2000;283:1167–74.
4. Miotti PG, Taha TE, Kumwenda NI, et al. HIV transmission through breast feeding: a study in Malawi. JAMA 1999;282:744–9.
5. Fawzi W, Msamanga G, Spiegelman D, et al. Transmission of HIV-1 through breastfeeding among women in Dar es Salaam, Tanzania. J Acquir Immune Defic Syndr 2002;31:331–8.
6. Connor EM, Sperling RS, Gelber R, et al. Reduction of maternal-infant transmission of human immunodeficiency virus type 1 with zidovudine treatment. N Engl J Med 1994;331:1173–80.
7. Dunn DT, Newell ML, Ades AE, et al. Risk of human immunodeficiency virus type 1 transmission through breastfeeding. Lancet 1992;340:585–8.
8. Breastfeeding and HIV International Transmission Study Group. Late postnatal transmission of HIV-1 in breast-fed children: an individual patient data meta-analysis. J Infect Dis 2004;189:2154–66.

9. Kuhn L, Sinkala M, Kankasa C, et al. High uptake of exclusive breastfeeding and reduced early post-natal HIV transmission. PLoS One 2007;2(12): e1363.
10. Pak-Gorstein S, Haq A, Graham EA. Cultural influences on infant feeding practices. Pediatr Rev 2009;30:e11–21.
11. Kumar D, Goel NK, Mittal PC, et al. Influence of infant-feeding practices on nutritional status of under-five children. Indian J Pediatr 2006;73:417–21.
12. Fewtrell MS, Morgan JB, Duggan C, et al. Optimal duration of exclusive breastfeeding: what is the evidence to support current recommendations? Am J Clin Nutr 2007;85(Suppl):635S–8S.
13. Flores M, Filteau S. Effect of lactation counselling on subclinical mastitis among Bangladeshi women. Ann Trop Paediatr 2002;22:85–8.
14. Kramer MS, Kakuma R. The optimal duration of exclusive breastfeeding: a systematic review. Adv Exp Med Biol 2004;554:63–77.
15. Fjeld E, Siziya S, Katepa-Bwalya M, et al. 'No sister, the breast alone is not enough for my baby' a qualitative assessment of potentials and barriers in the promotion of exclusive breastfeeding in southern Zambia. Int Breastfeed J 2008;3:26.
16. Coutsoudis A, Pillay K, Kuhn L, et al. Method of feeding and transmission of HIV-1 from mothers to children by 15 months of age: prospective cohort study from Durban, South Africa. AIDS 2001;15:379–87.
17. Coovadia HM, Rollins NC, Bland RM, et al. Mother-to-child transmission of HIV-1 infection during exclusive breastfeeding in the first 6 months of life: an intervention cohort study. Lancet 2007;369:1107–16.
18. Iliff P, Piwoz E, Tavengwa N, et al. Early exclusive breastfeeding reduces the risk of postnatal HIV-1 transmission and increases HIV-free survival. AIDS 2005;19: 699–708.
19. Jelliffe DB, Jelliffe EF. Human milk in the modern world. New York: Oxford University Press; 1978.
20. Ng'andu NH, Watts TE. Child growth and duration of breast feeding in urban Zambia. J Epidemiol Community Health 1990;44:281–5.
21. Grummer-Strawn LM, Shealy KR. Progress in protecting, promoting, and supporting breastfeeding: 1984–2009. Breastfeed Med 2009;4(Suppl 1):S31–9.
22. Chen A, Rogan WJ. Breastfeeding and the risk of postneonatal death in the United States. Pediatrics 2004;113:e435.
23. Forste R, Weiss J, Lippincott E. The decision to breastfeed in the United States: does race matter? Pediatrics 2001;108:291–6.
24. Bartick M, Reinhold A. The burden of suboptimal breastfeeding in the United States: a pediatric cost analysis. Pediatrics 2010;125:e1048–56.
25. Feachem RG, Koblinsky MA. Interventions for the control of diarrhoeal diseases among young children: promotion of breast-feeding. Bull World Health Organ 1984;62:271–91.
26. Habicht JP, DaVanzo J, Butz WP. Does breastfeeding really save lives, or are apparent benefits due to biases? Am J Epidemiol 1986;123:279–90.
27. WHO Collaborative Study Team on the Role of Breastfeeding on the Prevention of Infant Mortality. Effect of breastfeeding on infant and child mortality due to infectious diseases in less developed countries: a pooled analysis. Lancet 2000;355:451–5.
28. Kramer MS, Chalmers B, Hodnett E, et al. Promotion of Breastfeeding Intervention Trial (PROBIT) a randomized trial in the Republic of Belarus. JAMA 2001; 285:413–20.

29. Hummel S, Pfluger M, Kreichauf S, et al. Predictors of overweight during child-hood in offspring of parents with type 1 diabetes. Diabetes Care 2009;32:921–5.
30. Koletzko B, von Kries R, Monasterolo RC, et al. Can infant feeding choices modulate later obesity risk? Am J Clin Nutr 2009;89:1502S–8S.
31. Owen CG, Martin RM, Whincup PH, et al. The effect of breastfeeding on mean body mass index throughout life: a quantitative review of published and unpub-lished observational evidence. Am J Clin Nutr 2005;82:1298–307.
32. Owen CG, Whincup PH, Kaye SJ, et al. Does initial breastfeeding lead to lower blood cholesterol in adult life? A quantitative review of the evidence. Am J Clin Nutr 2008;88:305–14.
33. Mortensen EL, Michaelsen KF, Sanders SA, et al. The association between dura-tion of breastfeeding and adult intelligence. JAMA 2007;18:2365–71.
34. Kramer MS, Aboud F, Mironova E, et al. Breastfeeding and child cognitive devel-opment: new evidence from a large randomized trial. Arch Gen Psychiatry 2008; 65:578–84.
35. Caspi A, Williams B, Kim-Cohen J, et al. Moderation of breastfeeding effects on the IQ by genetic variation in fatty acid metabolism. Proc Natl Acad Sci U S A 2007;104:18860–5.
36. Cunningham AS, Jelliffe DB, Jelliffe EF. Breast-feeding and health in the 1980s: a global epidemiologic review. J Pediatr 1991;118:659–66.
37. Jason JM, Nieburg P, Marks JS. Mortality and infectious disease associated with infant feeding practices in developing countries. Pediatrics 1984;74:702–27.
38. Morrow AL, Rangel JM. Human milk protection against infectious diarrhea: impli-cations for prevention and clinical care. Semin Pediatr Infect Dis 2004;15:221–8.
39. American Academy of Pediatrics. Breast feeding and the use of human milk. Pediatrics 1997;100:1035–9.
40. American Academy of Pediatrics. Policy Statement. Section on Breastfeeding. Breastfeeding and the use of human milk. Pediatrics 2005;115:496–506.
41. Ip S, Chung M, Raman G, et al. A summary of the Agency for Healthcare Research and Quality's evidence report on breastfeeding in developed coun-tries. Breastfeed Med 2009;4(Suppl 1):S17–30.
42. Arifeen S, Black RE, Antelman G, et al. Exclusive breastfeeding reduces acute respiratory infection and diarrhea deaths among infants in Dhaka slums. Pediat-rics 2001;108:E67.
43. Chantry CJ, Howard CR, Auinger P. Full breastfeeding duration and associated decrease in respiratory tract infection in US children. Pediatrics 2006;117:425–32.
44. Dunn PM. Sir Hans Sloane (1660–1753) and the value of breast milk. Arch Dis Child Fetal Neonatal Ed 2001;85:F73–4.
45. Quigley MA, Kelly YJ, Sacker A. Breastfeeding and hospitalization for diarrheal and respiratory infection in the United Kingdom Millennium Cohort Study. Pedi-atrics 2007;119:e837–42.
46. Dunne EF, Angoran-Benie H, Kamelan-Tano A, et al. Is drinking water in Abidjan, Cote d'Ivoire, safe for infant formula? J Acquir Immune Defic Syndr 2001;28: 393–8.
47. Doherty T, Chopra M, Nkonki L, et al. Effect of the HIV epidemic on infant feeding in South Africa: "when they see me coming with the tins they laugh at me". Bull World Health Organ 2006;84:90–6.
48. Andresen E, Rollins NC, Sturm AW, et al. Bacterial contamination and over-dilu-tion of commercial infant formula prepared by HIV-infected mothers in a preven-tion of mother-to-child transmission (PMTCT) programme in South Africa. J Trop Pediatr 2007;53:410–4.

49. Creek T, Arvelo W, Kim A, et al. Role of infant feeding and HIV in a severe outbreak of diarrhea and malnutrition among young children, Botswana, 2006 [abstract # 770]. In: 14th Conference on Retroviruses and Opportunistic Infections. Los Angeles (CA), February 25–28; 2007.

50. Mach O, Lu L, Creek T, et al. Population-based study of a widespread outbreak of diarrhea associated with increased mortality and malnutrition in Botswana, January-March, 2006. Am J Trop Med Hyg 2009;80:812–8.

51. Creek TL, Kim A, Lu L, et al. Hospitalization and mortality among primarily non-breastfed children during a large outbreak of diarrhea and malnutrition in Botswana, 2006. J Acquir Immune Defic Syndr 2010;53:14–9.

52. Marino DD. Water and food safety in the developing world: global implications for health and nutrition of infants and young children. J Am Diet Assoc 2007; 107:1930–4.

53. Victora CG, Smith PG, Vaughan JP, et al. Evidence for protection by breast-feeding against infant deaths from infectious diseases in Brazil. Lancet 1987; 2:319–22.

54. Brown KH, Black RE, Lopez de Romana G, et al. Infant-feeding practices and their relationship with diarrheal and other diseases in Huascar (Lima) Peru. Pediatrics 1989;83:31–40.

55. Cesar JA, Victora CG, Barros FC, et al. Impact of breast feeding on admission for pneumonia during the postnatal period in Brazil: nested case-control study. BMJ 1999;318:1316–20.

56. Bahl R, Frost C, Kirkwood BR, et al. Infant feeding patterns and risks of death and hospitalization in the first half of infancy: multicentre cohort study. Bull World Health Organ 2005;83:418–26.

57. Thomas T, Masaba R, van Eijk A, et al. Rates of diarrhea associated with early weaning among infants in Kisumu, Kenya [abstract # 774]. In: 14th Conference on Retroviruses and Opportunistic Infections. Los Angeles (CA): 25–28 February; 2007.

58. Harris JR, Greene SK, Thomas TK, et al. Effect of a point-of-use water treatment and safe water storage intervention on diarrhea in infants of HIV-infected mothers. J Infect Dis 2009;200:1186–93.

59. Habicht JP, DaVanzo J, Butz WP. Mother's milk and sewage: their interactive effects on infant mortality. Pediatrics 1988;81:456–61.

60. Neville MC. Determinants of milk volume and composition. In: Jensen RG, editor. Handbook of milk composition. San Diego (CA): Academic Press; 1995. p. 87–114.

61. Neville MC, Keller RP, Seacat J, et al. Studies on human lactation. I. Within-feed and between-breast variation in selected components of human milk. Am J Clin Nutr 1984;40:635–46.

62. Coutsoudis A, Goga AE, Rollins N, et al. Free formula milk for infants of HIV-infected women: blessing or curse? Health Policy Plan 2002;17:154–60.

63. Coutsoudis A, Coovadia HM, Wilfert CM. HIV, infant feeding and more perils for poor people: new WHO guidelines encourage review of formula milk policies. Bull World Health Organ 2008;86:210–4.

64. Sibeko L, Coutsoudis A, Nzuza S, et al. Mothers' infant feeding experiences: constraints and supports for optimal feeding in an HIV-impacted urban community in South Africa. Public Health Nutr 2009;10:1–8.

65. Bland RM, Rollins NC, Coovadia HM, et al. Infant feeding counselling for HIV-infected and unifnected women: appropriateness of choice and practice. Bull World Health Organ 2007;85:289–96.

66. Doherty T, Chopra M, Nkonki L, et al. A longitudinal qualitative study of infant-feeding decision making and practices among HIV-positive women in South Africa. J Nutr 2006;136:2421–6.
67. Desclaux A, Alfieri C. Counseling and choosing between infant-feeding options: overall limits and local interpretations by health care providers and women living with HIV in resource-poor countries (Burkina Faso, Cambodia, Cameroon). Soc Sci Med 2009;69:821–9.
68. Goga A, Colvin M, Doherty T, et al. How do routine PMTCT programmes influence infant feeding practices and infant outcome? Results from an observational cohort study, South Africa, submitted for publication.
69. Chopra M, Rollins N. Infant feeding in the time of HIV: rapid assessment of infant feeding policy and programmes in four African countries scaling up prevention of mother to child transmission programmes. Arch Dis Child 2008;93:288–91.
70. Goldman AS. The immune system of human milk: antimicrobial, antiinflammatory and immunomodulating properties. Pediatr Infect Dis J 1993;12:664–71.
71. Labbok MH, Clark D, Goldman AS. Breastfeeding: maintaining an irreplaceable immunological resource. Nat Rev Immunol 2004;4:565–72.
72. Lonnerdal B. Personalizing nutrient intakes of formula-fed infants: breast milk as a model. Nestle Nutr Workshop Ser Pediatr Program 2008;62:189–98 [discussion: 198–203].
73. Heird WC. Progress in promoting breast-feeding, combating malnutrition, and composition and use of infant formula, 1981–2006. J Nutr 2007;137:499S–502S.
74. Koletzko B, Baker S, Cleghorn G, et al. Global standard for the composition of infant formula: recommendations of an ESPGHAN coordinated international expert group. J Pediatr Gastroenterol Nutr 2005;41:584–99.
75. Shapiro RL, Lockman S, Kim S, et al. Infant morbidity, mortality, and breast milk immunologic profiles among breast-feeding HIV-infected and HIV-uninfected women in Botswana. J Infect Dis 2007;196:562–5.
76. Thior I, Lockman S, Smeaton LM, et al. Breastfeeding plus infant zidovudine prophylaxis for 6 months vs formula feeding plus infant zidovudine for 1 month to reduce mother-to-child HIV transmission in Botswana: a randomized trial: the Mashi Study. JAMA 2006;296:794–805.
77. Kagaayi J, Gray RH, Brahmbhatt H, et al. Survival of infants born to HIV-positive mothers by feeding modality in Rakai, Uganda. PLoS One 2008;3:e3877.
78. Homsy J, Moore D, Barasa A, et al. Breastfeeding, mother-to-child HIV transmission, and mortality among infants born to HIV-Infected women on highly active antiretroviral therapy in rural Uganda. J Acquir Immune Defic Syndr 2010;53:28–35.
79. World Health Organization. Planning guide for national implementation of the global strategy for infant and young child feeding. 2007. Available at: http://www.who.int/nutrition/publications/infantfeeding/9789241595193/en/. Accessed September 20, 2010.
80. Greiner T. The concept of weaning: definitions and their implications. Commentary. J Hum Lact 1996;12:123–8.
81. Simondon KB. Early breast-feeding cessation and infant mortality in low-income countries: workshop summary. Adv Exp Med Biol 2009;639:319–29.
82. Brahmbhatt H, Gray RH. Child mortality associated with reasons for non-breastfeeding and weaning: is breastfeeding best for HIV-positive mothers? AIDS 2003;17:879–85.
83. Peltier CA, Ndayisaba GF, Lepage P, et al. Breastfeeding with maternal antiretroviral therapy or formula feeding to prevent HIV postnatal mother-to-child transmission in Rwanda. AIDS 2009;23:2415–23.

84. Nyandiko WM, Otieno-Nyunya B, Musick B, et al. Outcomes of HIV-exposed children in western Kenya: efficacy of prevention of mother to child transmission in a resource-constrained setting. J Acquir Immune Defic Syndr 2010;54:42–50.
85. Phadke MA, Gadgil B, Bharucha KE, et al. Replacement-fed infants born to HIV-infected mothers in India have a high early postpartum rate of hospitalization. J Nutr 2003;133:3153–7.
86. Kafulafula G, Thigpen M, Hoover DR, et al. Post-weaning gastroenteritis and mortality in HIV-uninfected African infants receiving antiretroviral prophylaxis to prevent MTCT of HIV-1 [abstract # 773]. In: 14th Conference on Retroviruses and Opportunistic Infections. Los Angeles (CA), February 25–28, 2007.
87. Kourtis AP, Fitzgerald D, Hyde L. et al. Diarrhea in uninfected infants of HIV-infected mothers who stop breastfeeding at 6 months: the BAN study experience [abstract # 772]. In: 14th Conference on Retroviruses and Opportunistic Infections. Los Angeles (CA), February 25–28, 2007.
88. Onyango C, Mmiro F, Bagenda D et al. Early breastfeeding cessation among HIV-exposed negative infants and risk of serious gastroenteritis: findings from a perinatal prevention trial in Kampala, Uganda [abstract # 775]. In: 14th Conference on Retorviruses and Opportunistic Infections. Los Angeles (CA), February 25–28, 2007.
89. Kafulafula G, Hoover DR, Taha TE, et al. Frequency of gastroenteritis and gastroenteritis-associated mortality with early weaning in HIV-1-uninfected children born to HIV-infected women in Malawi. J Acquir Immune Defic Syndr 2010; 53:6–13.
90. Onyango-Makumbi C, Bagenda D, Mwatha A, et al. Early weaning of HIV-exposed uninfected infants and risk of serious gastroenteritis: findings from two perinatal HIV prevention trials in Kampala, Uganda. J Acquir Immune Defic Syndr 2010;53:20–7.
91. Taha TE, Kumwenda NI, Hoover DR, et al. The impact of breastfeeding on the health of HIV-positive mothers and their children in sub-Saharan Africa. Bull World Health Organ 2006;84:546–54.
92. Kuhn L, Aldrovandi GM, Sinkala M, et al. Effects of early, abrupt cessation of breastfeeding on HIV-free survival of children in Zambia. N Engl J Med 2008; 359:130–41.
93. Kuhn L, Aldrovandi GM, Sinkala M, et al. Differential effects of early weaning for HIV-free survival of children born to HIV-infected mothers by severity of maternal disease. PLoS One 2009;4:e6059.
94. Kuhn L, Sinkala M, Semrau K, et al. Elevations in mortality due to weaning persist into the second year of life among uninfected children born to HIV-infected mothers. Clin Infect Dis 2010;54:437–44.
95. Arpadi SM, Fawzy A, Aldrovandi GM, et al. Growth faltering due to breastfeeding cessation among uninfected children born to HIV-infected mothers in Zambia. Am J Clin Nutr 2009;90:344–50.
96. Fawzy A, Arpadi S, Aldrovandi GM, et al. Diarrhea morbidity and mortality increases with weaning prior to 6 months among uninfected infants born to HIV-infected mothers in Zambia. In: International AIDS Society Conference in Cape Town, July 19–22, 2009; TUAC104.
97. Violari A, Cotton MF, Gibb DM, et al. Early antiretroviral therapy and mortality among HIV-infected infants. N Engl J Med 2008;359:2233–44.
98. Becquet R, Bequet L, Ekouevi DK, et al. Two-year morbidity-mortality and alternatives to prolonged breastfeeding among children born to HIV-infected mothers in Cote d'Ivoire. PLoS Med 2007;4:e17.

99. Doherty T, Chopra M, Jackson D, et al. Effectiveness of the WHO/UNICEF guidelines on infant feeding for HIV-positive women: results from a prospective cohort study in South Africa. AIDS 2007;21:1791–7.
100. Bulterys M, Wilfert C. HAART during pregnancy and during breastfeeding among HIV-infected women in the developing world: has the time come? AIDS 2009;23:2473–7.
101. World Health Organization. Antiretroviral therapy for HIV infection in adults and adolescents. Geneva (Switzerland). 2009. Available at:http://www.who.int/hiv/pub/arv/rapid_advice_art.pdf. Accessed September 20, 2010.
102. Tonwe-Gold B, Ekouevi DK, Viho I, et al. Antiretroviral treatment and prevention of peripartum and postnatal HIV transmission in West Africa: evaluation of a two-tiered approach. PLoS Med. 2007;4:e257.
103. Kuhn L, Aldrovandi GM, Sinkala M, et al. Potential impact of new World Health Organization criteria for antiretroviral treatment for prevention of mother-to-child HIV transmission. AIDS 2010;24:1374–7.
104. Thomas T, Masaba R, Ndivo R, et al. Prevention of mother-to-child transmission of HIV-1 among breastfeeding mothers using HAART: The Kisumu Breastfeeding Study, Kisumu, Kenya, 2003–2007 [abstract 45aLB]. In: 15th Conference of Retrovirus and Opportunistic Infections. Boston, USA, February 3–6, 2008.
105. Palombi L, Marazzi MC, Voetberg A, et al. Treatment acceleration program and the experience of the DREAM program in prevention of mother-to-child transmission of HIV. AIDS 2007;21(Suppl 4):S65–71.
106. de Vincenzi I, The Kesho Bora Study Group. HIV-free survival at 12 months among children born to HIV-infected women receiving antiretrovirals from 34 to 36 weeks of pregnancy [abstract 638]. In: 15th Conference of Retrovirus and Opportunistic Infections. Boston (MA), USA, February 3–6, 2008.
107. Kilewo C, Karlsson K, Ngarina M, et al. Prevention of mother-to-child transmission of HIV-1 through breastfeeding by treating mothers with triple antiretroviral therapy in Dar es Salaam, Tanzania: the Mitra Plus study. J Acquir Immune Defic Syndr 2009;52:406–16.
108. Shapiro RL, Hughes M, Ogwu A. A randomized trial comparing highly active antiretroviral therapy regimens for virologic effiacy and the prevention of mother-to-child transmission among breastfeeding women in Botswana (The Mma Bana Study). In: 5th IAS Conference on HIV Pathogenesis, Treatment and Prevention. WELBB101, Cape Town, July 19–22, 2009.
109. Marazzi MC, Nielsen-Saines K, Buonomo E, et al. Increased infant human immunodeficiency virus-type one free survival at one year of age in sub-saharan Africa with maternal use of highly active antiretroviral therapy during breastfeeding. Pediatr Infect Dis J 2009;28:483–7.
110. Chung MH, Kiarie JN, Richardson BA, et al. Breast milk HIV-1 suppression and decreased transmission: a randomized trial comparing HIVNET 012 nevirapine versus short-course zidovudine. AIDS 2005;19:1415–22.
111. Six Week Extended-Dose Nevirapine (SWEN) Study Team. Extended-dose nevirapine to 6 weeks of age for infants to prevent HIV transmission via breastfeeding in Ethiopia, India, and Uganda: an analysis of three randomised controlled trials. Lancet 2008;372:300–13.
112. Kumwenda NI, Hoover DR, Mofenson LM, et al. Extended antiretroviral prophylaxis to reduce breast-milk HIV-1 transmission. N Engl J Med 2008;359:119–29.
113. Chasela C, Hudgens M, Jamieson DJ. Both maternal HAART and daily infant nevirapine (NVP) are effective in reducing HIV-1 transmission during breastfeeding in a randomized trial in Malawi: 28 week results of the Breastfeeding,

Antiretroviral and Nutrition (BAN) Study. In: 5th IAS Conference on HIV Pathogenesis, Treatment and Prevention. WELBC103, Cape Town, July 19–22, 2009.

114. Kilewo C, Karlsson K, Massawe A, et al. Prevention of mother-to-child transmission of HIV-1 through breast-feeding by treating infants prophylactically with lamivudine in Dar es Salaam, Tanzania: the Mitra Study. J Acquir Immune Defic Syndr 2008;48:315–23.

115. Taha TE, Kumwenda J, Cole SR, et al. Postnatal HIV-1 transmission after cessation of infant extended antiretroviral prophylaxis and effect of maternal highly active antiretroviral therapy. J Infect Dis 2009;200:1490–7.

116. Tudor-Williams G. Changing UK practice: influence from resource-poor setting, including new infant feeding guidance. In: Second Joint Conference of the British HIV Association (BHIVA) and the British Association for Sexual Health and HIV (BASHI) Plenary Session 3. April 20–23, 2010: Imperial College London-Manchester Central Convention Complex.

117. World Health Organization. New data on the prevention of mother-to-child transmission of HIV and their policy implications. Conclusions and recommendations. WHO technical consultation on behalf of the UNFPA/UNICEF/WHO/UNAIDS Inter-agency Task Team on Mother-to-child Transmission of HIV. October 11–13, 2000. Available at: http://whqlibdoc.who.int/hq/2001/WHO_RHR_01.28.pdf. Accessed September 20, 2010.

118. World Health Organization. HIV and infant feeding. Guidelines for decision-makers. Geneva (Switzerland). Available at: http://whqlibdoc.who.int/hq/2003/9241591226.pdf. Accessed September 20, 2010.

119. World Health Organization. HIV and infant feeding: revised principles and recommendations: rapid advice. November 2009. Available at: http://www.hqlibdocwhoint/publications/2009/9789241598873_eng.pdf. Accessed April 1, 2010.

Clinical Care of the Exposed Infants of HIV-Infected Mothers

Lisa-Gaye E. Robinson, MD*, Aracelis D. Fernandez, MD

KEYWORDS

- Pediatric HIV • Pediatric AIDS • Perinatal transmission of HIV
- HIV-exposed infant

Clinical care of the human immunodeficiency virus (HIV)-exposed infant involves important management considerations that are intended to reduce the risk of transmission of HIV infection from mother to child. To obtain the maximal reduction in transmission, care for the HIV-exposed infant should begin well before delivery. Ideally, a woman who intends to get pregnant should know her HIV status before conception. Thereafter, those who are identified as HIV negative can be counseled on how to remain HIV uninfected during the pregnancy. Those who are identified as HIV infected can receive state-of-the-art care that can almost eliminate the risk of transmission of HIV from the mother to the child. Care of the HIV-exposed newborn must then focus on reducing the risk of infection with postexposure prophylaxis, monitoring for signs and symptoms of HIV infection, and following the recommended testing schedule to confirm the absence of infection in the vast majority of infants or confirm infection and begin treatment as soon as possible in the small percentage of infants who continue to be diagnosed with perinatal HIV infection in the United States.

MOTHER-TO-CHILD TRANSMISSION OF HIV
Epidemiology

At the end of 2008, it was estimated that there were 33.4 million people living with HIV worldwide.[1] Of those, 2.7 million were new infections, 430,000 of which were in children younger than 15 years.[1] Most of these infections were the result of mother-to-child transmissions occurring during the pregnancy, during labor and delivery, or

The authors have nothing to disclose.

Department of Pediatrics, Columbia University, The Affiliation at Harlem Hospital, 506 Lenox Avenue, MLK 16-119, New York, NY 10037, USA

* Corresponding author.

E-mail address: lr2043@columbia.edu

Clin Perinatol 37 (2010) 863–872

doi:10.1016/j.clp.2010.08.008

0095-5108/10/$ – see front matter

postpartum, primarily through breastfeeding.[2] In resource-limited settings, more than 21% of the new infections occurred through mother-to-child transmission, whereas in resource-abundant settings, this transmission risk accounted for less than 1% of new infections.[1]

In the absence of interventions to reduce mother-to-child transmission, transmission rates range from 13% to 42%, with most US studies reporting rates of approximately 25%.[3-5] A variety of independent risk factors have been demonstrated to affect the transmission rates. These include, but are not limited to, high maternal viral load, low maternal CD4+ cell count, advanced disease in mother, prematurity, prolonged rupture of membranes, mode of delivery, primary maternal HIV infection, receipt of antiretrovirals (ARVs) in mother and child, and breastfeeding and premastication of food in the postnatal period.[6-8] Interventions that improve maternal HIV disease, decrease exposure to cervicovaginal secretions, particularly in women with high viral loads, offer postexposure prophylaxis to the infants, and allow for safe infant feeding reduce transmission to less than 2%.[9]

Prevention of Mother-to-Child Transmission of HIV

The AIDS Clinical Trial Group-076 Protocol published in 1994 was the seminal study that demonstrated the efficacy of the ARV zidovudine to reduce mother-to-child transmission of HIV.[5] This multicenter, randomized, double-blind, placebo-controlled trial demonstrated that when women received oral zidovudine during their pregnancy and intravenous zidovudine during labor and their formula-fed infants received oral zidovudine for 6 weeks, the transmission rate of HIV to the infant decreased from 25.5% in the placebo group to 8.3% in the treatment group.[5] The US Public Health Service released guidelines that same year to offer zidovudine to HIV-infected pregnant women to reduce transmission of HIV from the mother to the child.[10] To offer zidovudine to HIV-infected women, providers must know that the pregnant woman is HIV infected. In 1995, the Centers for Disease Control and Prevention (CDC) recommended universal routine HIV counseling and voluntary prenatal HIV testing.[11] Precipitous falls in the estimated numbers of perinatally acquired pediatric AIDS cases followed. Thereafter, with the introduction of potent combination ARV therapies that achieve viral suppression in the pregnant woman and with cesarean section in women whose HIV viral loads remain greater than 1000 copies/mL close to delivery, transmission rates of less than 2% are now common in resource-abundant settings.[9]

Zidovudine reduces mother-to-child transmission of HIV by a variety of mechanisms. Prenatal exposure decreases maternal viral load in the blood and genital secretions.[12-14] Zidovudine administered prenatally and intrapartum crosses the placenta, leading to systemic drug levels in the infant, which is protective at delivery, a time of significant exposure to infected maternal blood and maternal genital tract virus. Postexposure prophylaxis in the infant protects the infant from virus that may have gained access to the fetal/infant circulation through maternal-fetal transfusion, mucosal exposure (including the infant's gastrointestinal tract from swallowed blood/secretions) or obstetric monitoring/delivery procedures.[6,8] To achieve the maximal reduction in transmission, antepartum, intrapartum, and postpartum prophylaxis to the infant is recommended.[5,9,15]

Simplified, short-course, and cost-effective regimens have been found to be efficacious in resource-limited settings.[16,17] However, these regimens do not achieve the vanishing transmission rates experienced in resource-abundant settings. Postnatal exposure to breast milk from an HIV-infected woman and solid food premasticated by an HIV-infected caregiver can transmit HIV.[18,19] Consequently, breastfeeding is not recommended in the United States because safe and affordable alternatives are readily available for all women and free for women in need. Moreover, all HIV caregivers must be counseled against the practice of premasticating food for infants.

Although the mother-to-child transmission rates of HIV in the United States have plummeted and there are means to potentially eliminate it, transmission of HIV from the mother to the child continues to occur. The annual number of perinatal HIV infections in the United States decreased from a peak of 1650 infections in 1991 to at least 182 cases in 2008.[20,21] Missed opportunities to interrupt infection stem from poor access to care and low maintenance in care for some subpopulations.[22] The HIV status of some women remains unknown during their pregnancy. The CDC recommendations on HIV testing were updated in 2006 to an opt out screening approach. HIV screening is recommended as soon as pregnancy is confirmed, and after confirmation the patient is notified that testing will be performed unless the patient declines.[23] Testing is repeated in the high-risk populations in the third trimester to identify new infections.[23] A case for repeating testing in all pregnant women in the third trimester was described by Wallihan and colleagues[24] who reported 3 infants whose mothers tested HIV negative early in pregnancy but were not re-tested in the third trimester because they did not fall into any of the designated CDC risk groups. All 3 infants presented with AIDS-defining illnesses by 5 months of age. Third-trimester HIV testing in the mothers may have identified maternal infection, allowed for implementation of prevention strategies, and decreased the morbidities in the infants.

Determination of the HIV Status of the HIV-Exposed Infant

HIV diagnostic testing in infants and children younger than 18 months requires the use of virological assays. Antibody testing cannot be used to determine the infection status of an infant because maternal HIV antibodies transferred across the placenta in the third trimester do not decay completely from the bloodstream of some infants until 18 months of age.[25,26] A positive HIV antibody test result in an infant only definitively identifies exposure to HIV, that is, maternal infection. The 2 most common virological tests used in the United States are nucleic acid amplification tests, HIV-1 DNA polymerase chain reaction (PCR) and HIV-1 RNA PCR. The HIV-1 DNA PCR assay detects cell-associated proviral DNA. The HIV-1 RNA PCR assay detects plasma viral RNA. Both these assays have high sensitivity and specificity by the first 4 to 6 weeks of age.[26] It does not appear that the 6 weeks of zidovudine recommended for the HIV-exposed infant delays HIV diagnosis via HIV-1 DNA PCR.[5,27] However, it is unknown how potent ARV therapy in the mother or child might affect the sensitivity of both of these tests.

Until HIV infection in the infant is determined to be presumptively or definitively excluded, the HIV status of the infant is considered to be indeterminate. HIV infection can be presumptively excluded with 2 negative virological tests, with one at 2 or more weeks of age and the second at 1 or more months of age.[28] HIV infection can be definitively excluded with 2 negative virological tests, with one at 1 or more months of age and the second at 4 or more months of age. No further virological testing is needed thereafter.[28] The infant is not HIV infected *jiroveci* pneumonia (PCP) prophylaxis can be discontinued when HIV infection has been excluded.[15]

HIV-1 is the predominant HIV infection in the United States and worldwide, but in this era of globalization, it is important to mention that the less-virulent HIV-2 infection prevalent in West Africa can be transmitted from mother to child.[29,30] Unlike HIV-1, without any medical interventions, the HIV-2 perinatal transmission rates are very low (<2%).[29,30] Nonetheless, HIV-2–infected pregnant women as well as their exposed infants should receive ARVs for prevention of mother-to-child transmission. The HIV-2–exposed infant should be tested specifically for HIV-2.[30]

CARE OF THE HIV-EXPOSED INFANT

Optimal care of the HIV-exposed infant involves first identifying that the infant has in fact been exposed to HIV. Once exposure has been reasonably established, subsequent management considerations aim to reduce the transmission of HIV from the mother to the child and eventually determine the HIV status of the exposed infant. Prenatally, the HIV-infected mother should receive specialty prenatal care that includes the receipt of potent combination ARV therapy. She should be monitored closely throughout the pregnancy, and cesarean section is recommended if her viral load is greater than 1000 copies/mL in the weeks before delivery.[15] Postnatally, a thorough maternal and delivery history taking helps establish the level of risk of transmission for the infant. The physical examination in the newborn may not be revealing for stigmata of HIV. Prophylaxis against HIV should be started immediately after birth, followed by prophylaxis for P jiroveci at 6 weeks of age, as recommended by current national guidelines.[15] A recommended HIV testing schedule excludes or identifies HIV infection in the infant. Anticipatory guidance around efforts to reduce transmission of HIV infection determine the HIV status of the exposed infant and necessary subsequent follow-ups must be provided. Table 1 provides a summary of the clinical care of the HIV-exposed infant. The National Perinatal HIV Hotline (1-888-448-8765) that provides free consultation on care of the HIV-exposed infant is also available.

History

The pertinent history of a newborn is the maternal history. For HIV-exposed infants, the maternal history helps establish whether the transmission risk is high and close to the natural transmission rates for mother-baby dyads who received no intervention or approaches the low transmission rate for mother-baby dyads who received all recommended interventions to reduce transmission. The history should include obstetric history, sexually transmitted disease history, date of maternal HIV diagnosis, timing of initiation of ARVs in the mother, maternal ARV regimen, adherence to regimen, resistance testing of maternal HIV virus, maternal viral load (particularly close to the time of delivery), maternal CD4[+] count, maternal clinical status, prematurity, mode of delivery, length of rupture of membranes, and use of intrapartum monitoring that may have breeched the newborn's skin. In most cases, recommended prenatal HIV testing that identified infant exposure to HIV would have been determined by the provider of the infected mother. However, if during acquisition of the maternal history for any newborn it is determined that prenatal HIV testing has not been done or third trimester re-testing in recommended populations has not been done, a rapid HIV antibody testing of the mother and/or infant is recommended as soon after birth as possible.[15] It is important that all providers remain cognizant of the HIV confidentiality laws and obtain the maternal history in a confidential manner to avoid an unplanned disclosure.

Physical Examination

The physical examination of an HIV-exposed newborn is most commonly unremarkable.[31] Only a small percentage of exposed infants who are eventually identified as HIV infected are born with physical examination findings typical in the HIV-infected infant.[31] The most common physical examination findings include lymphadenopathy, splenomegaly, and hepatomegaly, with an initial age of onset at about 3 months.[31] Failure to thrive and neurodevelopmental delays are common in the first year of

Table 1
Clinical care of the HIV-exposed infant

Age	Birth	1 wk	2 wk	3 wk	4 wk	6 wk	2 mo	4 mo	6 mo	9 mo	12 mo	15mo	18 mo
PPHC visit[a]	✓	✓	✓	✓	✓	✓	✓	✓	✓	✓	✓	✓	✓
HIV exposure prophylaxis[b]	⟵————— start through discontinuation of drug —————⟶ (Birth to 6 wk)												
PCP prophylaxis[c]						⟵————— start through discontinuation of drug —————⟶ (6 wk to 6 mo)							
Laboratory tests[d] HIV PCR[e]			⟺	⟺			⟺	⟺	⟺				
CBC with differential[f]	✓										✓		
HIV antibody[g]													✓
Immunizations	The recommended immunizations for the HIV-exposed infant are the same as those recommended by the Advisory Committee on Immunizations Practices for the well infant. Although live vaccines are not recommended for HIV-infected children who are severely immunocompromised, the Advisory Committee on Immunization Practices supports the administration of the live Rotavirus vaccine to HIV-indeterminate and HIV-infected infants because the infant's infection may not be determined before the time for first vaccine dose and benefits outweigh the potential risks.												

The National Perinatal HIV Hotline (1-888-448-8765), a free, federally funded consult line, provides free consultation on care of the HIV-exposed infant.

Key: ✓, perform at this time; ⟵———⟶, start through discontinuation of drug; ⟺, perform test during this period.

[a] PPHC, Pediatric Preventive Healthcare. This includes all the components of a well-child visit, history, growth and development, physical examination, recommended screenings, immunizations, and anticipatory guidance. The frequency of the visits for the first 2 months should be individualized as per the psychosocial issues that may affect the caregiver's ability to adhere to the treatment plan.

[b] Zidovudine prophylaxis should be started as close to delivery as possible, within 12 hours of birth. Some experts recommend starting additional antiretrovirals in certain situations (see the section ARV Prophylaxis). This administration should be done in consultation with a pediatric HIV specialist. Prophylaxis should be discontinued immediately if the result of an HIV PCR is positive.

[c] Trimethoprim-sulfamethoxazole should be started at 6 weeks if the status of the infant is indeterminate at that time. PCP prophylaxis need not be started or can be discontinued if the infant is presumptively or definitively uninfected but continued through the infant's first year of life if infant is HIV infected.

[d] Additional laboratory tests, including serum chemistries and liver function tests, may be considered at birth and while the infant is receiving prophylaxis for those prescribed multiple antiretrovirals. A lactate level test should be considered for infants who develop severe clinical symptoms suggestive of lactic acidosis.

[e] HIV RNA PCR and HIV DNA PCR are both acceptable diagnostic assays. Some experts recommend an HIV PCR at birth in infants whose mothers did not receive antepartum antiretrovirals. A positive test should be repeated immediately.

[f] A follow-up complete blood count could be considered at 4 weeks and should be done in any infant who presents with signs and symptoms of severe anemia. A decision to shorten the length of or discontinue antiretroviral prophylaxis secondary to laboratory abnormalities should be made in consultation with a pediatric HIV specialist.

[g] HIV antibody testing at this time in infants who are already determined to be definitively HIV uninfected is to simply confirm the loss of passively transferred maternal antibody.

life.[31] It is important to closely monitor the growth and development and physical examination findings at each clinical visit because these factors may serve as clues to the HIV status of the infant before definitive laboratory results.

ARV Prophylaxis

All HIV-exposed infants should receive postnatal zidovudine to reduce the transmission of perinatal HIV infection. For the maximal effect, zidovudine should be started as close to birth as possible but certainly within 12 hours of birth.[15] Zidovudine should be continued through day 42 of life (6 weeks). The dose for full-term infants is 2 mg/kg/dose by mouth every 6 hours. Premature infants require less frequent dosing because their immature hepatic clearance slows the elimination of the drug. Intravenous zidovudine, 1.5 mg/kg/dose, should be used in infants who are clinically unable to take the zidovudine by mouth.[15] **Table 2** outlines zidovudine dosing by gestational age. Infants born to mothers with resistant virus or mothers who did not receive the antenatal and/or intrapartum components of zidovudine to reduce transmission are at higher risk of HIV infection. These infants may theoretically benefit from combination ARV prophylaxis[15]; however, there are no clinical data to support this practice. Evaluation of such an infant should be done in consultation with a pediatric HIV specialist. **Table 3** outlines dosing of other ARVs commonly used in these situations.

The primary toxicity of zidovudine is anemia, but neutropenia and hepatic enzyme elevations can also occur.[5] A baseline evaluation of the complete blood count (CBC) is prudent before starting zidovudine, but it is not necessary to wait for the results before the administration of the first dose of zidovudine. A follow-up CBC during the zidovudine course should be considered, particularly if there is clinical evidence of severe anemia.[15] A decision to discontinue ARV prophylaxis before the recommended 6-week course secondary to laboratory abnormalities should be done in consultation with a pediatric HIV specialist.

ARV prophylaxis should be discontinued immediately if any of the newborn's PCR results are positive, and these infants should be referred to a pediatric HIV specialist for ARV therapy. Continuing ARV monotherapy in an HIV-infected infant leads to the development of resistance.

HIV-exposed infants who present for initial care more than 48 hours after birth would not benefit from postexposure prophylaxis.[32]

P jiroveci Prophylaxis

HIV-infected infants are at high risk for acquiring PCP.[33] The peak incidence of this opportunistic infection is between 3 to 6 months of age.[33] The mortality associated

Table 2	
Neonatal dose of zidovudine to prevent perinatal transmission of HIV[a]	
Gestational Age (wk)	**Dose**
>35	2 mg/kg/dose po q 6 h or 1.5 mg /kg/dose IV q 6 h if unable to take po
>30 and <35	2 mg/kg/dose po or 1.5 mg/kg/dose IV q 12 h, advancing to q 8 h at 2 wk of life
<30	2 mg/kg/dose po or 1.5 mg/kg/dose IV q 12 h, advancing to q 8 h at 4 wk of life

Abbreviation: IV, intravenous.
[a] All infants born to HIV-infected mothers should be given zidovudine preferably as soon as after birth, but certainly within the first 12 hours of life, and for 6 weeks. For HIV-exposed infants not recognized as being HIV-exposed at birth or immediately after, zidovudine should be administered as soon as exposure is identified provided that the newborn is younger than 48 hours.

Table 3
Neonatal dosing of other antiretrovirals to be used only in selected circumstances to prevent perinatal transmission of HIV and after discussion with a pediatric HIV specialist[a]

Antiretroviral Drug	Dose	Duration
Nevirapine	2 mg/kg/dose po as single dose	If mother did not receive a dose of nevirapine[b] or if it was given to her at 2 h or less before delivery, then the infant dose should be administered as soon as possible after birth, otherwise between birth and 72 h of life
Lamivudine (in combination with zidovudine to decrease the development of nevirapine resistance after single-dose nevirapine administration)	2 mg/kg/dose po bid	1 wk

[a] All babies born to HIV-infected mothers should receive zidovudine either alone or as part of a combination regimen to prevent perinatal transmission. In circumstances in which combination of antiretrovirals are being considered, the decision must be made after consultation with a pediatric HIV specialist.
[b] Some experts would give a second dose of nevirapine at 48 to 72 hours if the mother did not receive a dose at time of delivery. The National Perinatal HIV Hotline (1-888-448-8765) provides free consultation on care of the HIV-exposed infant.

with this infection is extremely high in the infants.[33] HIV infection in some HIV-exposed infants may not be excluded by the age of the peak incidence of this devastating infection. Consequently, it is recommended that PCP prophylaxis with trimethoprim-sulfamethoxazole begins at 6 weeks of age if the status of the infant is indeterminate at that time. PCP prophylaxis need not be started or can be discontinued when HIV infection in the infant is presumptively or definitively excluded.[34]

HIV Testing

HIV testing in HIV-exposed infants requires repeated virological testing over several months to definitively exclude infection. Virological testing should be performed at 14 to 21 days of life, 1 to 2 months, and 4 to 6 months.[15,25,26] A virological test should be performed at birth if the HIV-infected pregnant mother did not have good virological control during the pregnancy; if there are concerns of unrecognized maternal primary HIV infection during the pregnancy, increasing the risk of in utero infection; or if the physical examination of the newborn is remarkable for signs of HIV infection, suggesting in utero transmission.[15] A positive virological test should be repeated immediately and usually indicates infection in the infant. The infant ARV prophylaxis should be discontinued once the first positive test result is available to avoid monotherapy of HIV with subsequent development of resistant virus. Two positive virological tests confirm HIV infection in the infant.[15] For infants in whom HIV infection has been excluded virologically, some experts confirm the loss of maternal HIV antibody with an HIV antibody test at 18 months of age.[15]

Feeding Practices

Breastfeeding by HIV-infected mothers is not recommended in the United States because safe and affordable alternatives are readily available for all women and free for women in need.[15] It is important to discuss this with the HIV-infected mother at every encounter in the first several weeks of the infant's life. There may be infants born to women who come from cultures in which breastfeeding is expected, and if the woman is not seen breastfeeding by family members, she may be ridiculed or assumptions may be made about her HIV status of which others were not aware. It is important that the provider discuss the psychosocial ramifications of abstaining from breastfeeding with the mother and work with her to be able to justify her decision at home. HIV-infected caregivers must be counseled against the practice of premasticating food for infants as transmission via this route has been demonstrated in 3 infants.[19]

Anticipatory Guidance

In addition to the routine age-appropriate anticipatory guidance provided for non–HIV-exposed infants, mothers and caregivers of HIV-exposed infants should receive anticipatory guidance around all components of care for the HIV-exposed infant. The caregiver needs education on the HIV testing schedule and must be advised that the HIV status of the baby may remain unknown for several months. This delay in diagnosis can create a great deal of anxiety for some families and supportive care should be offered. Every visit must include a discussion about the importance of giving the infant ARV drugs as prescribed to prevent perinatal transmission and the administration of trimethoprim-sulfamethoxazole to prevent PCP if necessary.

In the United States, breastfeeding by HIV-infected mothers is not recommended and mothers should be repeatedly counseled against this before delivery and during the initial outpatient visits. In addition, HIV-infected caregivers should be advised against premastication of food for older infants.

In the United States, HIV-exposed infants should receive the same routine vaccines given to their non–HIV-exposed peers and the same schedule should be followed.[35] These exposed infants should receive hepatitis B vaccine, diphtheria and tetanus toxoids and acellular pertussis vaccine, inactivated poliovirus vaccine, pneumococcal conjugate vaccine 13, *Haemophilus influenzae* type b vaccine, and Rotavirus vaccine. Caregivers of HIV-exposed but uninfected infants should be made aware that the perinatal HIV exposure and ARV use or exposure of the infant are important medical history. This history should remain a part of the infant's medical record for life because the long-term consequences of these exposures are yet unknown.

Mothers and caregivers should receive education on the modes of HIV transmission. The discussion should also underscore how HIV is not transmitted and provide reassurance that touching, hugging, or kissing their infants is safe.

SUMMARY

Clinical care of the HIV-exposed infant requires knowledge of the unique management considerations specific to these infants. All HIV-exposed infants should be administered postexposure prophylaxis with ARVs immediately after birth. A 6-week course of ARV prophylaxis is recommended. Knowledge of the associated drug toxicities and signs and symptoms of HIV disease are required to conduct appropriate monitoring of the infant. Determination of the HIV status of the infant requires serial HIV PCR testing that confirms or excludes infection within the first 4 months of life.

REFERENCES

1. Joint United Nations Programme on HIV/AIDS and World Health Organization. AIDS epidemic update 2009. Available at: www.unaids.org/pub/report/2009/JC1700_Epi_Update_2009_en.pdf. Accessed June 13, 2010.

2. Kourtis AP, Bulterys M, Nesheim S, et al. Understanding the timing of HIV transmission from mother to child. JAMA 2001;285(6):709–12.
3. Working Group on Mother-to-child transmission of HIV. Rate of mother-to-child transmission of HIV-1 in Africa, America and Europe. J Acquir Immune Defic Syndr Hum Retrovirol 1995;8:506–10.
4. De Cock KM, Fowler MG, Mercier E, et al. Prevention of mother-to-child HIV transmission in resource poor countries. JAMA 2000;283:1175–82.
5. Connor EM, Sperling RS, Gelber R, et al. Reduction of maternal-infant transmission of human immunodeficiency virus type 1 with zidovudine treatment. Pediatric AIDS Clinical Trial Group Protocol 076 Study Group. N Engl J Med 1994;331:1173–80.
6. The European Collaborative Study. Vertical transmission of HIV-1: maternal immune status and obstetric factors. AIDS 1996;10:1675–81.
7. Burns DN, Landesman S, Muenz LR, et al. Cigarette smoking, premature rupture of membranes, and vertical transmission of HIV-1 among women with low CD4$^+$ levels. J Acquir Immune Defic Syndr 1994;7:718–26.
8. Mofenson LM, Lambert JS, Stiehm ER, et al. Risk factors for perinatal transmission of human immunodeficiency virus type 1 in women treated with zidovudine. N Engl J Med 1999;341:385–93.
9. Cooper ER, Charurat M, Mofenson L, et al. Combination antiretroviral strategies for the treatment of pregnant HIV-1 infected women and prevention of perinatal HIV-1 transmission. Women and Infants' Transmission Study Group. J Acquir Immune Defic Syndr 2002;29:484–94.
10. Centers for Disease Control and Prevention. Recommendations of the US Public Health Services Task Force on the use of zidovudine to reduce perinatal transmission of human immunodeficiency virus. MMWR Morb Mortal Wkly Rep 1994;43:1–20.
11. Centers for Disease Control and Prevention. U.S. Public Health Service recommendations for human immunodeficiency virus counseling and voluntary testing for pregnant women. MMWR Recomm Rep 1995;44:1–15.
12. Sperling RS, Shapiro DE, Coombs RW, et al. Maternal viral load, zidovudine treatment, and the risk of transmission of human immunodeficiency virus type 1 from mother to infant. N Engl J Med 1996;335:1621–9.
13. Chuachoowong R, Shaffer N, Siriwasin W, et al. Short course antenatal zidovudine reduces both cervicovaginal HIV-1 RNA levels and risk of perinatal transmission. J Infect Dis 2000;181:99–106.
14. Su-Win S, Caliendo AM, Reinert S. Effect of highly active antiretroviral therapy on cervicovaginal HIV-1 RNA. AIDS 2000;14:415–21.
15. Panel on Treatment of HIV-Infected Pregnant Women and Prevention of Perinatal Transmission. Recommendations for use of antiretroviral drugs in pregnant HIV-1-infected women for maternal health and interventions to reduce perinatal HIV transmission in the United States. May 24, 2010. p. 1–17. Available at: http://aidsinfo.nih.gov/ContentFiles/PerinatalGL.pdf. Accessed June 13, 2010.
16. Jackson JB, Musoke P, Fleming T, et al. Intrapartum and neonatal single-dose nevirapine compared with zidovudine for prevention of mother-to-child transmission of HIV-1 in Kampala, Uganda: 18-month follow-up of the HIVNET 012 randomised trial. Lancet 2003;362(9387):859–68.
17. Petra Study Team. Efficacy of three short-course regimens of zidovudine and lamivudine in preventing early and late transmission of HIV-1 from mother to child in Tanzania, South Africa, and Uganda (Petra study): a randomised, double-blind, placebo-controlled trial. Lancet 2002;359(9313):1178–86.
18. Miotti PG, Taha TE, Kumwenda NI, et al. HIV transmission through breastfeeding: a study in Malawi. JAMA 1999;282:744–9.

19. Gaur A, Dominguez KL, Kalish ML, et al. Practice of feeding premasticated food to infants: a potential risk factor for HIV transmission. Pediatrics 2009;124: 658–66.
20. Lindegren ML, Byers RH Jr, Thomas P, et al. Trends in perinatal transmission of HIV/AIDS in the United States. JAMA 1999;282:531–8.
21. Centers for Disease Control and Prevention. HIV/AIDS surveillance report, 2008. Available at: www.cdc.gov/hiv/surveillance/resources/reports/2008report/table5a. htm. Accessed June 13, 2010.
22. Peters V, Liu K, Dominguez K, et al. Missed opportunities for perinatal HIV prevention among HIV-exposed infants born 1996–2000, pediatric spectrum of HIV disease cohort. Pediatrics 2003;111(5):1186–91.
23. Branson BM, Handsfield HH, Lampe MA, et al. Revised recommendations for HIV testing of adults, adolescents, and pregnant women in health-care settings. MMWR Recomm Rep 2006;55:1–17.
24. Wallihan R, Koranyi K, Brady M. Perinatally human immunodeficiency virus-1 infected children born to low risk mothers who tested antibody negative during pregnancy. Pediatr Infect Dis J 2010;29(3):274–5.
25. Committee on Pediatric AIDS. HIV testing and prophylaxis to prevent mother-to-child transmission in the United States. Pediatrics 2008;122:1127–34.
26. Read JS. Diagnosis of HIV-1 infection in children younger than 18 months in the United States. Pediatrics 2007;120:e1547–62.
27. Kovacs A, Xu J, Rasheed S, et al. Comparison of a rapid nonisotopic polymerase chain reaction assay with four commonly used methods for the early diagnosis of human immunodeficiency virus type 1 infection in neonates and children. Pediatr Infect Dis J 1995;14(11):948–54.
28. Centers for Disease Control and Prevention (CDC). Revised surveillance case definitions for HIV infection among adults, adolescents, and children aged <18 months and for HIV infection and AIDS among children aged 18 months to <13 years—United States, 2008. MMWR Recomm Rep 2008;57(RR-10):1–12.
29. Adjorlolo-Johnson G, De Cock KM, Ekpini E, et al. Prospective comparison of mother-to-child transmission of HIV-1 and HIV-2 in Abidjan, Ivory Coast. JAMA 1994;272(6):462–6.
30. Padua E, Almeida C, Nunes B, et al. Assessment of mother-to-child HIV-1 and HIV-2 transmission: an AIDS reference laboratory collaborative study. HIV Med 2009;10(3):182–90.
31. Galli L, de Martino M, Tovo P, et al. Onset of clinical signs in children with HIV-1 perinatal infection. AIDS 1995;9:455–61.
32. Wade NA, Birkhead GS, Warren BL, et al. Abbreviated regimens of zidovudine prophylaxis and perinatal transmission of the human immunodeficiency virus. N Engl J Med 1998;339(20):1409–14.
33. Simonds RJ, Oxtoby MJ, Caldwell MB, et al. Pneumocystis carinii pneumonia among US children with perinatally acquired HIV infection. JAMA 1993;270: 470–3.
34. Centers for Disease Control and Prevention. Guidelines for the Prevention and Treatment of Opportunistic Infections Among HIV-Exposed and HIV-Infected Children. MMWR Recomm Rep 2009;58(No. RR11):45–50.
35. Centers for Disease Control and Prevention. Recommended Immunization schedule for persons aged 0 through 6 years—United States 2010. Available at: www.cdc.gov/vaccines/rec/acip. Accessed June 13, 2010.

The Clinical Care of the HIV-1–Infected Infant

Andres F. Camacho-Gonzalez, MD, Allison C. Ross, MD,
Rana Chakraborty, MD, PhD*

KEYWORDS

• HIV-1 • Perinatal transmission • Infants • Children

Interventions to prevent the mother-to-child transmission (MTCT) of human immuno-deficiency virus (HIV) 1 infection were first documented with the landmark Pediatric AIDS Clinical Trials Group (PACTG) 076 trial conducted 16 years ago.[1] Despite well-established studies since that time and strategies to decrease MTCT risk to less than 2%,[2] new perinatal infections continue to occur. This article focuses on the recommendations for the management of HIV-1–infected infants in environments with good access to health care, where replacement of breastfeeding is safely indicated and antiretroviral medications are widely available.

THE GLOBAL EPIDEMIOLOGY OF MTCT OF HIV-1

Only 28% to 65% of pregnant women residing in low-to-middle-income countries are tested for HIV-1. Only 45% of women who are tested and are HIV-1 seropositive and 32% of their HIV-exposed infants receive antiretrovirals for prophylaxis.[3] As a possible consequence, there were approximately 430,000 new HIV-1 infections worldwide among children aged 0 to 14 years reported in 2008, with 280,000 deaths from HIV/AIDS complications. In contrast, there has been a 90% decrease in the MTCT of HIV-1 in North America and Western Europe since the early 1990s, reflecting increased awareness and improved testing during pregnancy (approximately 83%–93% of pregnant women are tested at least once during their pregnancy) with the implementation of interventions to offset the MTCT of HIV-1.[4] However, there is still an unacceptable annual rate of newly diagnosed HIV-1 infection among infants,

Disclosures: The authors receive research support from Bristol-Myers Squibb (A.F.C.); Bristol-Myers Squibb, Cubist Pharmaceuticals, and GlaxoSmithKline (A.C.R.); and Emory Center for AIDS Research (P30 AI050409) (R.C.).
Division of Pediatric Infectious Diseases, Department of Pediatrics, Children's Healthcare of Atlanta, Emory University, 2015 Uppergate Drive, Suite 500, Atlanta, GA 30322, USA
* Corresponding author.
E-mail address: rchakr5@emory.edu

Clin Perinatol 37 (2010) 873–885
doi:10.1016/j.clp.2010.08.002   **perinatology.theclinics.com**

with marked racial disparities in the United States (an MTCT rate of 12.3 per 100,000 among African American vs 0.5 per 100,000 in whites during the last reported period, 2004–2007).[5] Preventive efforts need to improve and target high-risk populations to further decrease transmission rates.

THE PREVENTION OF MTCT OF HIV-1

Implementing successful strategies consistently and universally can prevent perinatal HIV-1 infection. Comprehensive programs to prevent the MTCT of HIV-1 have decreased the transmission to less than 2% in most states in the United States. These interventions should be initiated as early as possible in a woman's pregnancy and include measures taken during pregnancy, labor, and delivery as well as postpartum infant prophylaxis.[6] In an effort to minimize missed opportunities for intervention before delivery, a greater emphasis has been placed on maternal HIV-1 testing and treatment throughout pregnancy in association with rapid testing during labor.[7] Once the infant is born, the addition of postpartum prophylaxis and complete avoidance of breastfeeding for the infant should close the cycle of preventive measures.[8–12] More extensive discussions on the prevention of MTCT are found in articles elsewhere in this issue.

THE HIV-1–INFECTED INFANT
The Diagnosis of HIV-1 Infection in the Exposed Infant

The use of a specific diagnostic method for HIV-1 detection in infants after perinatal exposure depends on the age of the subject. Serologic testing should be avoided in children younger than 18 months because the potential detection of transplacentally acquired maternal antibodies is likely. Instead, polymerase chain reaction (PCR) should be done to detect HIV-1 DNA or RNA in this age group. Testing is recommended after the first 2 weeks of life, because the sensitivity of PCR for detecting either HIV-1 DNA or RNA increases after this age. Approximately 93% of infected infants have detectable HIV-1 DNA by 2 weeks of age, and approximately 95% of HIV-1–infected infants have a positive HIV-1 DNA PCR result by 1 month of age. A single HIV-1 DNA PCR assay has a sensitivity of 95% and a specificity of 97% for samples collected from infected infants aged 1 to 36 months. After testing infants by PCR in the first 2 weeks of life, the evaluation should continue, with PCR done again at the ages 1 to 2 months and 4 to 6 months (**Fig. 1**). The diagnosis of HIV in infants and children younger than 18 months is established with 2 positive virologic test results at different times. If older than 18 months, a positive HIV-1 antibody test result with a confirmatory Western blot confirms HIV infection.[13] The definitive exclusion of perinatal HIV-1 infection in nonbreastfed infants can be made when the infant has (1) 2 negative PCR results by 6 months of age or (2) a negative PCR result when the infant is older than 1 month and another negative PCR result when older than 4 months. The presumptive exclusion of HIV-1 infection can be made when the infant has (1) a negative PCR result after 14 days of life and a second negative PCR result when aged 1 month or older or (2) 1 negative PCR result when aged 2 months or older. Confirmatory testing can be done by serologic methods after 18 months of age.[14]

Management of the HIV-1–Infected Infant

Once the diagnosis of HIV-1 infection has been established, transition of care to a multidisciplinary pediatric HIV clinic is recommended.

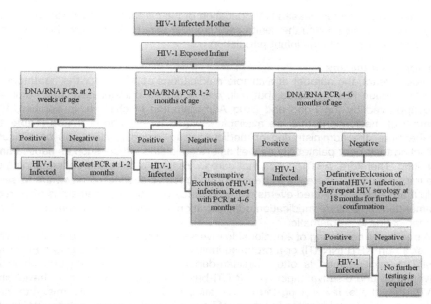

Fig. 1. Algorithm for HIV-1 testing and diagnosis in an exposed infant.

Disease progression and initiation of therapy

Multiple risk factors have been associated with more rapid disease progression in HIV-infected infants and children, including intrauterine transmission, specific HLA genotypes (HLA-DR3, C4A, and DQB1*0604), presence and maintenance of HIV-1–specific CD4 responses, higher HIV-1 RNA concentrations in infants, thymic dysfunction, lack of perinatal zidovudine (AZT) prophylaxis, enhanced viral fitness, and poorer maternal health.[15–21]

HIV-1–infected infants constitute possibly the only age group in which there is a generalized consensus among HIV experts that early initiation of antiretroviral therapy (ART) (before 12 weeks of age) rather than deferring it decreases the disease progression and mortality. In a phase 3 randomized controlled trial of 377 HIV-1–infected infants with a $CD4^+$ T-cell percentage greater than 25%, progression to AIDS in the early treatment group (therapy started at a median age of 7 weeks) was 6.3% compared with 25.6% in the deferred-therapy group (ART initiated when CD4 percentage decreased to <20%, or <25% if the infant was <1 year of age) [$P<.001$]. In addition, there was a 76% reduction in early mortality in the early treatment group compared with the deferred therapy group.[22] This study provided strong support for the Department of Health and Human Services' recommendation of initiating ART in children younger than 12 months, irrespective of the $CD4^+$ T-cell count, CD4 percentage, HIV-1 RNA plasma concentration, or clinical presentation.

Despite these recommendations, there are important factors that should be considered before starting therapy. The administration of antiretrovirals, and therefore the success of treatment in the infected infant, depends solely on the caregiver. Factors such as the caregiver's perception of the disease, level of education, infant antiretroviral regimen (doses per day, palatability), and social circumstances, such as interference with family dynamics and fear of social disclosure, greatly affect the ability of the caregiver to adhere to the infant's regimen.[23–26] Studies have shown adherence rates in children between 40% and 70%.[24] A better understanding of adherence-related factors as well as an increased HIV education of the caregiver in association with an improved relationship with the health care provider may be key factors in increasing the adherence rates in the infant population.

Antiretroviral therapy

In recent years, the number of available medications approved for the treatment of HIV-1 infection has increased, but still, only a limited number have been studied and approved by the Food and Drug Administration in children. In addition, the number of medications that are available in liquid formulation is limited (**Table 1**). Furthermore, the administration of medications to young children can be difficult, reflecting their poor palatability as well as systemic side effects such as nausea and vomiting. Therefore, ART requires that caregivers have a complete understanding of the importance of adherence to treatment and receive counseling on where to seek help if adverse ART-related events occur. Gastrostomy tube placement is often recommended to facilitate medication administration in some infants when acceptance of medication is problematic.

A backbone consisting of 2 nucleoside reverse transcriptase inhibitors (NRTIs) with either a non-NRTI (NNRTI) or a protease inhibitor (PI) is indicated. Using a PI- or an NNRTI-based regimen is often clinician-dependent, because both options have advantages and disadvantages. An NNRTI-based regimen in the form of nevirapine (NVP) may have fewer long-term side effects, such as dyslipidemia, but has a decreased threshold for the induction of key viral mutations, with resistance developing rapidly with monotherapy or incomplete adherence to treatment. In contrast, the development of multiple key viral mutations to confer resistance to lopinavir/ritonavir (LPV/r), the most commonly used PI in infants, often reflects poor adherence to this medication over a prolonged period. However, LPV/r is associated with more long-term side effects including dyslipidemia, abnormal fat distribution including lipoatrophy and lipohypertrophy, and insulin resistance.

The NRTI backbone should be composed of either zidovudine/lamivudine or abacavir (ABC)/lamivudine. The use of ABC has been associated with a hypersensitivity reaction in 5% to 8% of treated patients.[27] It has been shown that the presence of HLA-B5701 is a strong predictor of this reaction, increasing the chances of developing the reaction by more than 70%.[28] Genetic testing is indicated, specifically evaluating

Table 1
Commonly used antiretroviral drugs administered to HIV-infected infants

Antiretroviral Drug	Dose and Route of Administration	Interval
AZT	12 m/kg/dose (4 kg–<9 kg) 9 mg/kg/dose (9 kg-30 kg)	Twice a day
3TC	2 mg/kg/dose po (<1 mo) 4 mg/kg/dose po (>1 mo)	Twice a day
ABC	8 mg/kg/dose po	Twice a day
DDI	50 mg/m^2/dose (2 weeks to 3 months) 100 mg/m^2/dose (>3 months)	Twice a day
NVP	200 mg/m^2/dose	Once a day for the first 14 d, then twice a day
LPV/r	12 mg/kg/dose of LPV + 3 mg/kg/dose of RTV	Twice a day

Abbreviations: 3TC, lamivudine; ABC, abacavir; DDI, didanosine; LPV/r, ritonavir booster lopinavir; NVP, nevirapine; RTV, ritonavir.

for the presence or absence of this allele in the infant before administration of this medication. Didanosine offers another option, although it requires an empty stomach, which may further complicate its administration to infants and young children.

Potential toxicities from NRTIs result from the inhibition of polymerase-γ, blocking the synthesis of mitochondrial DNA. The mechanisms of inhibition can be secondary to chain termination by incorporation of the nucleoside analogue during mitochondrial DNA synthesis, direct inhibition of polymerase-γ without incorporation, inhibition of DNA polymerase-γ exonuclease activity, or alteration of the fidelity of mitochondrial DNA synthesis by polymerase-γ.[29–31] Besides the antiretroviral properties of these mechanisms, impairment of the aerobic metabolism and ATP production can lead to rare but serious reactions.[31,32] Clinical manifestations vary depending on the degree of mitochondrial damage[30] and include lactic acidosis, hepatic steatosis, pancreatitis, muscular weakness and rhabdomyolysis, peripheral neuropathies, lipodystrophy, nephrotoxicity, central nervous system dysfunction, osteopenia, and myopathies.[14] In several studies, perinatal NRTI exposure has been implicated in asymptomatic hyperlactatemia ranging from 13.1% to 50%.[33–36] Symptomatic disease was seen in 12 of 2644 patients in a French cohort, presenting mainly with motor and cognitive delays and seizures.[37] Other symptoms may include weight loss, fatigue, abdominal pain, tachycardia, tachypnea, and liver failure.[38,39] Patients with symptomatic hyperlactatemia should stop ART and start supportive measures aiming to reverse the metabolic acidosis, which may include fluid and electrolyte corrections, ventilatory support, and dialysis if needed. Once the acidosis resolves, ART may be resumed with an NRTI-sparing regimen if possible, but if needed, a different NRTI backbone with a lower risk of mitochondrial toxicity may be considered.[40]

Monitoring

Pre-ART All HIV-1–infected infants should undergo routine laboratory monitoring to assess disease progression as well as drug efficacy and toxicity. It has been well documented that children younger than 12 months have higher mortality than older children[41–43]; therefore, monitoring should begin as soon as the diagnosis is made and before the initiation of ART. Monitoring should include baseline enumeration of CD4$^+$ T-cell count and percentage, HIV-1 RNA plasma quantification, determination of the presence or absence of the HLA-B5701 allele, complete blood cell count (CBC) with differential, complete metabolic panel (CMP), and viral genotyping. An important fact to remember is that children younger than 5 years have a greater degree of variation in their absolute CD4$^+$ T-cell count, and therefore, the CD4$^+$ percentage is more useful for monitoring the immune status.[41,42]

On-ART After the initiation of ART, infants and children should undergo routine blood testing to assess medication compliance and evaluate for drug toxicity. The ultimate goals of the therapy are to decrease morbidity and mortality, achieve undetectable levels of HIV-1 in the blood with the least toxicity possible, and restore immune function. Infants tend to have higher viral loads than older children, and reaching undetectable levels may be more challenging.[21] Monitoring should be done at 1 to 2 weeks and 4 to 8 weeks after initiation of the therapy and include CBC, CMP, CD4 cell count, and HIV-1 RNA quantification. Once an undetectable level of HIV-1 has been established, monitoring can be spaced out to every 2 to 3 months with the same investigations.

Failure to respond to therapy Failure to respond to therapy, which can be defined on immunologic, virologic, or clinical grounds, requires immediate attention and evaluation of the possible causes. Immunologic failure should be considered when the

CD4 percentage does not increase by 5% or more than the baseline in the first year after initiation of the ART or if there is a 5% or more sustained decline in the CD4 percentage; virologic failure occurs when the decrease in HIV-1 RNA level is less than 1 log after 8 to 12 weeks of therapy or more than 400 copies/mL after 6 months of ART. Clinical failure occurs when opportunistic or severe infections continue to occur or if there is progressive neurodevelopmental deterioration or growth failure despite ART. In any of these cases, a thorough evaluation by the clinician is warranted. Caregivers should be questioned about medication compliance and intolerance,[44] and appropriate dosing adjustments should be made by the clinician not only because of frequent weight changes but also because of possible differences in pharmacokinetic variables during these initial years of life.[45,46] Pharmacokinetic determination of serum concentrations of NNRTIs including NVP and PIs such as lopinavir may be done at some centers and can be a useful tool to evaluate the adherence to ART.

Resistance genotypic testing should be considered in cases in which despite the aforementioned considerations there is persistent uncontrolled viral replication and poor immune recovery. Transmission of the resistant virus from the mother to the infant has been documented in 12% to 19% of infants,[47,48] but development of de novo resistance in the infant is also possible. Regardless of the case, an alternative ART regimen may be required and consultation with a pediatric HIV specialist is warranted.

Drug toxicities Besides appropriately monitoring the therapeutic response, the clinician needs to be alert to the signs and symptoms of medication toxicity. As described earlier, these signs may include mitochondrial toxicity and hyperlactatemia as well as lipodystrophy syndrome, lipid metabolism abnormalities, hepatic toxicity, hematologic disturbances, insulin resistance, cardiovascular problems, hypersensitivity reactions, and metabolic bone problems. Most complications can be adequately monitored with the baseline laboratory testing done every 3 to 4 months, but occasionally, certain medications may have toxicities requiring specific testing and follow-up. In addition, testing for 25-hydroxyvitamin D levels, dual energy X-ray absorptiometry scans, and lipoprotein profiles may need to be obtained every 6 to 12 months, depending on the specific medications used.[14] Drug toxicities may necessitate a change in the ART regimen with the removal of the offending agent; this change is best managed in consultation with a pediatric HIV specialist.

Pneumocystis pneumonia prophylaxis

Pneumocystis pneumonia (PCP) is a common asymptomatic or mild infection in humans, with antibodies found in about 80% of children by 13 years of age.[49] In contrast, infection in an HIV-1–infected infant can result in a severe lower respiratory tract infection usually in the first 6 months of life with significant respiratory distress including tachypnea and hypoxia.[50] This AIDS-defining illness is associated with a high mortality rate in infants.[51] Prevention of PCP is essential and highly effective. Prophylaxis should be initiated in all children younger than 12 months irrespective of the CD4+ T-cell count between 4 and 6 weeks of age and continued for the first year of life.

For children older than 1 year, the CD4+ T-cell count or percentage can guide the need for PCP prophylaxis. Children aged between 1 and 5 years should receive prophylaxis when the CD4+ T-cell count or percentage decreases below either 500 cells/mm^3 or 15%; children aged 6 years or older should receive prophylaxis when the CD4+ T-cell count is less than 200 cells/mm^3.[14] PCP prophylaxis in these age groups can be discontinued after immunologic reconstitution with ART if CD4+ T-cell counts or percentages increase above these values.

Children with an indeterminate HIV-1 status should receive prophylaxis from 4 to 6 weeks of life until their status is defined as presumptively or definitely negative. Trimethoprim-sulfamethoxazole (TMP-SMX) is the drug of choice for prophylaxis at doses of TMP, 150 mg/m²/d, and SMX, 750 mg/m²/d, in a once daily dose or in divided doses twice per day given for 3 consecutive or alternate days per week. Alternatives to TMP-SMX include atovaquone (30 mg/kg/d until 3 months of age and 45 mg/kg/d thereafter) and dapsone, 2 mg/kg/d (maximum 100 mg/d). Aerosolized pentamidine, although effective, may be difficult to administer in children younger than 1 year.[52]

Vaccination of HIV-1–infected infants

The use of vaccines is an important means of disease prevention in all HIV-1–infected individuals. This importance is highlighted by evidence documenting that HIV-1–infected individuals have a 20- to 40-fold increased risk of developing invasive pneumococcal disease.[53] Routine immunization recommendations for HIV-1–infected children are essentially similar to those for uninfected children, but certain considerations are important to review.

First, the immunologic response of the HIV-1–infected infant may be less robust, requiring revaccination.[54,55] T- and B-cell responses, despite immunologic reconstitution after ART, may be attenuated and suboptimal, which may affect individual responses to vaccine antigens.[56] For example, Siriaksorn and colleagues[57] showed that only 1% of their vaccinated population had protective antibodies against hepatitis B after the recommended primary series. Therefore, revaccination for hepatitis B with a second 3-dose series is recommended in patients with levels of protective antibodies lower than 10 mIU/mL, with retesting for protective antibodies 1 to 2 months after revaccination.[58] Second, live virus vaccines, except bacille Calmette-Guérin (BCG) and rotavirus vaccines, are generally recommended for infants who are HIV-1–infected and have asymptomatic infection. The use of rotavirus vaccine seems to be safe, but larger studies are needed in HIV-infected patients before routinely recommending its use.[59] Infants in whom HIV-1 has been presumptively excluded (those who have [1] a negative HIV-1 DNA PCR result after 14 days of life and a second negative PCR result when aged 1 month or older or [2] a negative PCR result when aged 2 months or older) may receive this vaccine as recommended by the American Academy of Pediatrics (AAP) and the Centers for Disease Control and Prevention (CDC).[52,60] The use of BCG vaccine in HIV-1–exposed infants is determined by the risk of acquiring tuberculosis infection. If the risk is high, BCG vaccine is recommended at birth, but if the risk is low, vaccination may be deferred.[61] BCG vaccine administration in infants with progressive disease and/or advancing immunosuppression significantly increases the risk for regional lymphadenitis and disseminated BCG infection.[62] BCG is not recommended during childhood in the United States but is frequently used in other countries. Yearly influenza immunization, with the inactivated vaccine, is recommended in all patients aged 6 months or older.

Growth and development

At the time of birth, most HIV-infected infants have anthropometric measurements similar to their uninfected counterparts. This similarity may be explained by the fact that most of the infections are acquired around the time of birth.[63] With time, HIV-1–infected children have progressive decreases in both height and weight velocity when compared with uninfected children. Although the cause is usually multifactorial, HIV infection itself seems to be an independent factor.[64] A longitudinal prospective study in England showed that uninfected children were 22% heavier and 5.6% taller than HIV-1–infected children after 10 years of follow-up.[65] Similar trends were seen in underdeveloped countries.[66,67] The use of ART has been associated with the recovery of the patient's nutritional status, with better outcomes obtained with earlier initiation of therapy.[68]

In a similar way, HIV-infected infants have poorer developmental staging scores when compared with uninfected infants. When appropriate ART is started early, most of these patients have an accelerated development and can either overcome or limit the amount of delay. Van Rie and colleagues[69] showed that HIV-infected children have lower mean scores for both cognitive and motor skills at baseline but after 1 year of therapy the mean scores were similar to exposed but uninfected children.

Breastfeeding

After the first reported case of HIV-1 transmission through breastfeeding, the CDC and AAP recommended that HIV-1–infected mothers in the United States avoid breastfeeding.[8,9,11] Current World Health Organization guidelines also encourage replacement feeding methods if safe and sustainable alternatives are available. However, even in areas where safe replacement feeding methods are available, cultural sensitivities and fear of HIV stigmatization may prevent infant formula feeding.[70] A significant amount of research has been done aimed at preventing HIV transmission through breastfeeding. In resource-limited countries, where avoidance of breastfeeding is not possible and formula feeding has been shown to significantly decrease survival rates, decreasing HIV transmission through breastfeeding is the most logical approach. Recently, observational studies as well as clinical trials have suggested that giving prolonged postpartum ART to breastfeeding mothers decreases HIV-1 transmission to levels comparable to those from developed countries. Although promising, more studies are needed on the development of high-level ART resistance in infants who become infected despite prophylaxis as well as the consequences of potential treatment interruptions in women who received medication only for prevention of an MTCT.[71–74] Further details in breastfeeding and HIV transmission are discussed elsewhere in this issue.

SUMMARY

Although significant progress has been made, more is needed to further decrease the rates of MTCT of HIV-1. Once the infection has been established, early initiation of ART with PCP prophylaxis is paramount, together with the administration of routine infant vaccinations. The importance of compliance and close follow-up with a comprehensive pediatric HIV center should be stressed to caregivers because the development of a resistant virus will adversely affect an infant's subsequent ART options.

REFERENCES

1. Connor EM, Sperling RS, Gelber R, et al. Reduction of maternal-infant transmission of human immunodeficiency virus type 1 with zidovudine treatment. Pediatric AIDS Clinical Trials Group Protocol 076 Study Group. N Engl J Med 1994;331(18): 1173–80.
2. Cooper ER, Charurat M, Mofenson L, et al. Combination antiretroviral strategies for the treatment of pregnant HIV-1-infected women and prevention of perinatal HIV-1 transmission. J Acquir Immune Defic Syndr 2002;29(5):484–94.
3. UNAIDS/WHO. AIDS epidemic update. Available at: http://data.unaids.org:80/pub/Report/2009/JC1700_Epi_Update_2009_en.pdf. Accessed November 21, 2009.

4. From the Centers for Disease Control and Prevention. HIV testing among pregnant women–United States and Canada, 1998–2001. JAMA 2002;288(21): 2679–80.
5. Centers for Disease Control and Prevention (CDC). Racial/ethnic disparities among children with diagnoses of perinatal HIV infection–34 states, 2004–2007. MMWR Morb Mortal Wkly Rep 2010;59(4):97–101.
6. Wade NA, Birkhead GS, Warren BL, et al. Abbreviated regimens of zidovudine prophylaxis and perinatal transmission of the human immunodeficiency virus. N Engl J Med 1998;339(20):1409–14.
7. Branson BM, Handsfield HH, Lampe MA, et al. Revised recommendations for HIV testing of adults, adolescents, and pregnant women in health-care settings. MMWR Recomm Rep 2006;55(RR-14):1–17 [quiz: CE1–4].
8. Centers for Disease Control (CDC). Recommendations for assisting in the prevention of perinatal transmission of human T-lymphotropic virus type III/lymphadenopathy-associated virus and acquired immunodeficiency syndrome. MMWR Morb Mortal Wkly Rep 1985;34(48):721–6, 31–2.
9. Human milk, breastfeeding, and transmission of human immunodeficiency virus in the United States. American Academy of Pediatrics Committee on Pediatric AIDS. Pediatrics 1995;96(5 Pt 1):977–9.
10. Perinatal HIV Guidelines Working Group. Public Health Service Task Force recommendations for use of antiretroviral drugs in pregnant HIV-1 infected women for maternal health and interventions to reduce perinatal HIV transmission in the United States. Available at: http://aidsinfoniggov/ContentFiles/PerinatalGLpdf. Accessed May 16, 2010.
11. Read JS. Human milk, breastfeeding, and transmission of human immunodeficiency virus type 1 in the United States. American Academy of Pediatrics Committee on pediatric AIDS. Pediatrics 2003;112(5):1196–205.
12. Ziegler JB, Cooper DA, Johnson RO, et al. Postnatal transmission of AIDS-associated retrovirus from mother to infant. Lancet 1985;1(8434):896–8.
13. Centers for Disease Control and Prevention. Revised recommendations for HIV screening of pregnant women. MMWR Recomm Rep 2001;50(RR-19):63–85; quiz CE1-19a2–CE6-a2.
14. Working Group on Antiretroviral Therapy and Medical Management of HIV-Infected Children. Guidelines for the use of antiretroviral agents in pediatric HIV infection. Available at: http://aidsinfo.nih.gov/ContentFiles/PediatricGuidelines. pdf. Accessed February 23, 2009.
15. Chakraborty R, Morel AS, Sutton JK, et al. Correlates of delayed disease progression in HIV-1-infected Kenyan children. J Immunol 2005;174(12):8191–9.
16. Blanche S, Mayaux MJ, Rouzioux C, et al. Relation of the course of HIV infection in children to the severity of the disease in their mothers at delivery. N Engl J Med 1994;330(5):308–12.
17. Just JJ, Abrams E, Louie LG, et al. Influence of host genotype on progression to acquired immunodeficiency syndrome among children infected with human immunodeficiency virus type 1. J Pediatr 1995;127(4):544–9.
18. Kourtis AP, Ibegbu C, Nahmias AJ, et al. Early progression of disease in HIV-infected infants with thymus dysfunction. N Engl J Med 1996;335(19): 1431–6.
19. Kuhn L, Abrams EJ, Weedon J, et al. Disease progression and early viral dynamics in human immunodeficiency virus-infected children exposed to zidovudine during prenatal and perinatal periods. J Infect Dis 2000;182(1): 104–11.

20. Kuhn L, Steketee RW, Weedon J, et al. Distinct risk factors for intrauterine and intrapartum human immunodeficiency virus transmission and consequences for disease progression in infected children. Perinatal AIDS Collaborative Transmission Study. J Infect Dis 1999;179(1):52–8.

21. Shearer WT, Quinn TC, LaRussa P, et al. Viral load and disease progression in infants infected with human immunodeficiency virus type 1. Women and Infants Transmission Study Group. N Engl J Med 1997;336(19):1337–42.

22. Violari A, Cotton MF, Gibb DM, et al. Early antiretroviral therapy and mortality among HIV-infected infants. N Engl J Med 2008;359(21):2233–44.

23. Steele RG, Anderson B, Rindel B, et al. Adherence to antiretroviral therapy among HIV-positive children: examination of the role of caregiver health beliefs. AIDS Care 2001;13(5):617–29.

24. Nicholson O, Mellins C, Dolezal C, et al. HIV treatment-related knowledge and self-efficacy among caregivers of HIV-infected children. Patient Educ Couns 2006;61(3):405–10.

25. Watson DC, Farley JJ. Efficacy of and adherence to highly active antiretroviral therapy in children infected with human immunodeficiency virus type 1. Pediatr Infect Dis J 1999;18(8):682–9.

26. Gibb DM, Goodall RL, Giacomet V, et al. Adherence to prescribed antiretroviral therapy in human immunodeficiency virus-infected children in the PENTA 5 trial. Pediatr Infect Dis J 2003;22(1):56–62.

27. Lucas A, Nolan D, Mallal S. HLA-B*5701 screening for susceptibility to abacavir hypersensitivity. J Antimicrob Chemother 2007;59(4):591–3.

28. Mallal S, Nolan D, Witt C, et al. Association between presence of HLA-B*5701, HLA-DR7, and HLA-DQ3 and hypersensitivity to HIV-1 reverse-transcriptase inhibitor abacavir. Lancet 2002;359(9308):727–32.

29. White AJ. Mitochondrial toxicity and HIV therapy. Sex Transm Infect 2001;77(3): 158–73.

30. Kakuda TN. Pharmacology of nucleoside and nucleotide reverse transcriptase inhibitor-induced mitochondrial toxicity. Clin Ther 2000;22(6):685–708.

31. Brinkman K, ter Hofstede HJ, Burger DM, et al. Adverse effects of reverse transcriptase inhibitors: mitochondrial toxicity as common pathway. AIDS 1998; 12(14):1735–44.

32. Lewis W, Kohler JJ, Hosseini SH, et al. Antiretroviral nucleosides, deoxynucleotide carrier and mitochondrial DNA: evidence supporting the DNA pol gamma hypothesis. AIDS 2006;20(5):675–84.

33. Noguera A, Fortuny C, Munoz-Almagro C, et al. Hyperlactatemia in human immunodeficiency virus-uninfected infants who are exposed to antiretrovirals. Pediatrics 2004;114(5):e598–603.

34. Ekouevi DK, Toure R, Becquet R, et al. Serum lactate levels in infants exposed peripartum to antiretroviral agents to prevent mother-to-child transmission of HIV: Agence Nationale de Recherches Sur le SIDA et les Hepatites Virales 1209 Study, Abidjan, Ivory Coast. Pediatrics 2006;118(4):e1071–7.

35. Desai N, Mathur M, Weedon J. Lactate levels in children with HIV/AIDS on highly active antiretroviral therapy. AIDS 2003;17(10):1565–8.

36. Noguera A, Fortuny C, Sanchez E, et al. Hyperlactatemia in human immunodeficiency virus-infected children receiving antiretroviral treatment. Pediatr Infect Dis J 2003;22(9):778–82.

37. Barret B, Tardieu M, Rustin P, et al. Persistent mitochondrial dysfunction in HIV-1-exposed but uninfected infants: clinical screening in a large prospective cohort. AIDS 2003;17(12):1769–85.

38. Brinkman K. Editorial response: hyperlactatemia and hepatic steatosis as features of mitochondrial toxicity of nucleoside analogue reverse transcriptase inhibitors. Clin Infect Dis 2000;31(1):167–9.

39. Falco V, Rodriguez D, Ribera E, et al. Severe nucleoside-associated lactic acidosis in human immunodeficiency virus-infected patients: report of 12 cases and review of the literature. Clin Infect Dis 2002;34(6):838–46.

40. Lonergan JT, Barber RE, Mathews WC. Safety and efficacy of switching to alternative nucleoside analogues following symptomatic hyperlactatemia and lactic acidosis. AIDS 2003;17(17):2495–9.

41. Dunn D. Short-term risk of disease progression in HIV-1-infected children receiving no antiretroviral therapy or zidovudine monotherapy: a meta-analysis. Lancet 2003;362(9396):1605–11.

42. HIV Paediatric Prognostic Markers Collaborative Study. Predictive value of absolute CD4 cell count for disease progression in untreated HIV-1-infected children. AIDS 2006;20(9):1289–94.

43. Dunn D, Woodburn P, Duong T, et al. Current CD4 cell count and the short-term risk of AIDS and death before the availability of effective antiretroviral therapy in HIV-infected children and adults. J Infect Dis 2008;197(3):398–404.

44. Van Dyke RB, Lee S, Johnson GM, et al. Reported adherence as a determinant of response to highly active antiretroviral therapy in children who have human immunodeficiency virus infection. Pediatrics 2002;109(4):e61.

45. Menson EN, Walker AS, Sharland M, et al. Underdosing of antiretrovirals in UK and Irish children with HIV as an example of problems in prescribing medicines to children, 1997–2005: cohort study. BMJ 2006;332(7551):1183–7.

46. Kearns GL, Abdel-Rahman SM, Alander SW, et al. Developmental pharmacology–drug disposition, action, and therapy in infants and children. N Engl J Med 2003;349(12):1157–67.

47. Karchava M, Pulver W, Smith L, et al. Prevalence of drug-resistance mutations and non-subtype B strains among HIV-infected infants from New York state. J Acquir Immune Defic Syndr 2006;42(5):614–9.

48. Parker MM, Wade N, Lloyd RM Jr, et al. Prevalence of genotypic drug resistance among a cohort of HIV-infected newborns. J Acquir Immune Defic Syndr 2003; 32(3):292–7.

49. Respaldiza N, Medrano FJ, Medrano AC, et al. High seroprevalence of pneumocystis infection in Spanish children. Clin Microbiol Infect 2004;10(11):1029–31.

50. Fatti GL, Zar HJ, Swingler GH. Clinical indicators of Pneumocystis jiroveci pneumonia (PCP) in South African children infected with the human immunodeficiency virus. Int J Infect Dis 2006;10(4):282–5.

51. Madhi SA, Cutland C, Ismail K, et al. Ineffectiveness of trimethoprim-sulfamethoxazole prophylaxis and the importance of bacterial and viral coinfections in African children with Pneumocystis carinii pneumonia. Clin Infect Dis 2002; 35(9):1120–6.

52. Mofenson LM, Brady MT, Danner SP, et al. Guidelines for the prevention and treatment of opportunistic infections among HIV-exposed and HIV-infected children: recommendations from CDC, the National Institutes of Health, the HIV Medicine Association of the Infectious Diseases Society of America, the Pediatric Infectious Diseases Society, and the American Academy of Pediatrics. MMWR Recomm Rep 2009;58(RR-11):1–166.

53. Madhi SA, Petersen K, Madhi A, et al. Impact of human immunodeficiency virus type 1 on the disease spectrum of Streptococcus pneumoniae in South African children. Pediatr Infect Dis J 2000;19(12):1141–7.

54. Aurpibul L, Puthanakit T, Sirisanthana T, et al. Response to measles, mumps, and rubella revaccination in HIV-infected children with immune recovery after highly active antiretroviral therapy. Clin Infect Dis 2007;45(5):637–42.

55. Lao-araya M, Puthanakit T, Aurpibul L, et al. Antibody response to hepatitis B revaccination in HIV-infected children with immune recovery on highly active antiretroviral therapy. Vaccine 2007;25(29):5324–9.

56. Madhi SA, Kuwanda L, Cutland C, et al. Quantitative and qualitative antibody response to pneumococcal conjugate vaccine among African human immunodeficiency virus-infected and uninfected children. Pediatr Infect Dis J 2005;24(5):410–6.

57. Siriaksorn S, Puthanakit T, Sirisanthana T, et al. Prevalence of protective antibody against hepatitis B virus in HIV-infected children with immune recovery after highly active antiretroviral therapy. Vaccine 2006;24(16):3095–9.

58. Mast EE, Margolis HS, Fiore AE, et al. A comprehensive immunization strategy to eliminate transmission of hepatitis B virus infection in the United States: recommendations of the Advisory Committee on Immunization Practices (ACIP) part 1: immunization of infants, children, and adolescents. MMWR Recomm Rep 2005;54(RR-16):1–31.

59. Steele AD, Cunliffe N, Tumbo J, et al. A review of rotavirus infection in and vaccination of human immunodeficiency virus-infected children. J Infect Dis 2009; 200(Suppl 1):S57–62.

60. Committee on Infectious Diseases, American Academy of Pediatrics. Prevention of rotavirus disease: updated guidelines for use of rotavirus vaccine. Pediatrics 2009;123(5):1412–20.

61. Moss WJ, Clements CJ, Halsey NA. Immunization of children at risk of infection with human immunodeficiency virus. Bull World Health Organ 2003;81(1):61–70.

62. Hesseling AC, Marais BJ, Gie RP, et al. The risk of disseminated Bacille Calmette-Guerin (BCG) disease in HIV-infected children. Vaccine 2007;25(1):14–8.

63. Mock PA, Shaffer N, Bhadrakom C, et al. Maternal viral load and timing of mother-to-child HIV transmission, Bangkok, Thailand. Bangkok Collaborative Perinatal HIV Transmission Study Group. AIDS 1999;13(3):407–14.

64. Miller TL. Nutritional aspects of HIV-infected children receiving highly active antiretroviral therapy. AIDS 2003;17(Suppl 1):S130–40.

65. Newell ML, Borja MC, Peckham C. Height, weight, and growth in children born to mothers with HIV-1 infection in Europe. Pediatrics 2003;111(1):e52–60.

66. Buonora S, Nogueira S, Pone MV, et al. Growth parameters in HIV-vertically-infected adolescents on antiretroviral therapy in Rio de Janeiro, Brazil. Ann Trop Paediatr 2008;28(1):59–64.

67. Villamor E, Fataki MR, Bosch RJ, et al. Human immunodeficiency virus infection, diarrheal disease and sociodemographic predictors of child growth. Acta Paediatr 2004;93(3):372–9.

68. Aurpibul L, Puthanakit T, Taecharoenkul S, et al. Reversal of growth failure in HIV-infected Thai children treated with non-nucleoside reverse transcriptase inhibitor-based antiretroviral therapy. AIDS Patient Care STDS 2009;23(12):1067–71.

69. Van Rie A, Harrington PR, Dow A, et al. Neurologic and neurodevelopmental manifestations of pediatric HIV/AIDS: a global perspective. Eur J Paediatr Neurol 2007;11(1):1–9.

70. Rankin WW, Brennan S, Schell E, et al. The stigma of being HIV-positive in Africa. PLoS Med 2005;2(8):e247.

71. Kilewo C, Karlsson K, Ngarina M, et al. Prevention of mother-to-child transmission of HIV-1 through breastfeeding by treating mothers with triple antiretroviral therapy in Dar es Salaam, Tanzania: the Mitra Plus Study. J Acquir Immune Defic Syndr 2009;52(3):406–16.
72. Palombi L, Marazzi MC, Voetberg A, et al. Treatment acceleration program and the experience of the DREAM program in prevention of mother-to-child transmission of HIV. AIDS 2007;21(Suppl 4):S65–71.
73. Shapiro RL, Hughes MD, Ogwu A, et al. Antiretroviral regimens in pregnancy and breast-feeding in Botswana. N Engl J Med 2010;362:2282–94.
74. Chasela C, Hudgens M, Jamieson DJ, et al. Maternal or infant antiretroviral drugs to reduce HIV-1 transmission. N Engl J Med 2010;362:2271–81.

Issues of Prematurity and HIV Infection

Julie Mirpuri, MD[a],*, Lucky Jain, MD, MBA[b]

KEYWORDS

- Premature infant • Preterm birth • Late preterm • HIV
- Perinatal transmission • Antiretroviral therapy
- Cesarean delivery

Despite significant advances in the management of HIV-infected women during pregnancy, labor, and delivery, mother-to-child transmission accounts for 92% of AIDS cases in children less than 13 years old in the United States.[1] Prematurity and HIV have a complex interaction; it is known that mothers with HIV are at increased risk for preterm delivery and the current approaches to reduce perinatal transmission can exacerbate risk.[2–4] This is particularly important in resource-poor countries, where high HIV prevalence rates may add to the burden of prematurity and strain the resource-strapped neonatal intensive care environment. Indeed, the last two decades have seen a steady rise in preterm birth rates, with the sharpest rise in late preterm (34 0/7 to 36 0/7) births. This is paralleled by an increase in medically indicated preterm births (inductions and cesarean sections).[5] It is common practice now to offer cesarean birth to HIV-infected mothers with an aim to reduce intrapartum transmission of the virus. However, this presents a bigger challenge in nations and populations with a high HIV rate, where poor recall of the date of the last menstrual period and lack of early prenatal care may result in unreliable gestational age assessment and the downstream risk of iatrogenic prematurity. This article discusses the impact of mother-to-child transmission of HIV in the United States, the factors that increase the risk of preterm delivery in HIV-infected mothers, and the management of preterm infants exposed to HIV.

EPIDEMIOLOGY

Transmission of HIV can occur during pregnancy, labor, delivery, or breastfeeding. Heterosexual women of childbearing age represent the fastest growing risk-group for HIV infection.[6] Changes in the management of HIV-infected women during

[a] Division of Neonatal-Perinatal Medicine, Department of Pediatrics, Emory University School of Medicine, 2015 Uppergate Drive, Atlanta, GA, USA
[b] Department of Pediatrics, Emory University School of Medicine, 2015 Uppergate Drive, Atlanta, GA, USA
* Corresponding author. UT Southwestern Medical Center, 5323 Harry Hines Boulevard, MC9063-Suite F3.302 East, Dallas, TX.
E-mail address: juliemir@gmail.com

Clin Perinatol 37 (2010) 887–905
doi:10.1016/j.clp.2010.08.012   **perinatology.theclinics.com**
0095-5108/10/$ – see front matter © 2010 Elsevier Inc. All rights reserved.

pregnancy have resulted in a significant decline in perinatal HIV infections. In the United States, the number of annual perinatal HIV infections peaked at 1650 in 1991,[7] but has since declined to an estimated range of 144 to 236 in 2002 as reported by the Centers for Disease Control and Prevention.[1] This rate has remained steady over the last several years, and there are now an estimated 2736 children in the United States living with HIV-AIDS in 2007 who were perinatally infected.[8]

The decline is largely attributed to increased HIV testing during pregnancy, the use of antiretroviral (ARV) drugs, avoidance of breastfeeding, and use of elective cesarean delivery when appropriate. These interventions, when successfully applied, reduce the risk of perinatal transmission to less than 2%[9] compared with transmission rates of 25% to 30% with no intervention.[10]

Maternal HIV infection increases the risk of several adverse perinatal outcomes, including spontaneous abortion, stillbirth, fetal and perinatal mortality, intrauterine growth retardation, low birthweight, and preterm delivery.[11] A total of 5% to 20% of infants born to mothers with HIV are born premature and 10% to 20% are low birthweight.[12–14] It is controversial whether this is related to HIV infection and its consequences, or to the fact that risk factors of preterm delivery are more prevalent in HIV-infected women.[12] There is a racial and ethnic disparity among infants infected with HIV in the United States, with an estimated 66% reported as black and 20% being Hispanic/Latino.[15,16]

PATHOPHYSIOLOGY OF PERINATAL HIV TRANSMISSION

HIV-1 is a *Lentivirus*, which belongs to a subgroup of retroviruses. The retrovirus family is known for latency, persistent viremia, infection of the nervous system, and weak host immune responses. $CD4^+$ T lymphocytes and monocytes have high affinity to HIV; when they bind, the virus becomes internalized and replicates itself by generating a DNA copy by reverse transcriptase. The viral DNA formed then becomes incorporated into the host DNA allowing further replication. HIV can be transmitted through sexual contact; parenteral transmission (occurs largely among intravenous drug users); transmission by contaminated blood products; and perinatal transmission. The hallmark of HIV infection is destruction of $CD4^+$ T cells.

Perinatal transmission of HIV is defined as HIV infection when a woman passes the virus to her baby either during pregnancy, labor, delivery, or breastfeeding. Without treatment, around 15% to 30% of babies born to HIV-positive women become infected with HIV during pregnancy and delivery with a further 5% to 20% becoming infected through breastfeeding.[17] The most important factor associated with perinatal transmission is the level of HIV viremia at the time of delivery. However, duration of rupture of membranes, use of any devices during delivery, cigarette smoking, concomitant genital tract infections, substance abuse, and unprotected sex with multiple partners during pregnancy have also been shown to be important.[18]

FACTORS AFFECTING PRETERM DELIVERY AND PERINATAL HIV TRANSMISSION
Early Detection and Treatment

One of the most important factors affecting perinatal transmission of HIV is the adequate identification of HIV-positive mothers and appropriate treatment of the mother and infant. Recent Centers for Disease Control and Prevention guidelines, adopted by the American College of Obstetrics and Gynecology (ACOG), recommend "opt-out" screening in the health care setting.[19] This allows HIV screening with the routine panel of prenatal screening tests for all pregnant women unless the patient explicitly declines. Repeat HIV screening in the third trimester is recommended among pregnant women in certain areas with elevated rates of HIV infection.[20]

With early identification, effective ARV therapy during gestation and intrapartum can be initiated, rupture of membranes can be limited, and postexposure prophylaxis and formula feeding of the newborn may be started.[21] Early initiation of ARV prophylaxis of the infant after birth has been shown to reduce the risk of perinatal HIV transmission.[10]

MATERNAL SIDE EFFECTS OF ARV THERAPY

Some, but not all, studies have shown an increased risk for maternal preeclampsia and premature labor with the use of ARV therapy during pregnancy. In a study of 8768 women delivering at a Spanish hospital between 2001 and 2003, 82 were HIV-infected on ARV therapy and had higher rates of preeclampsia (11% vs 2.8%) and fetal death (6.1% vs 0.5%) than HIV-negative women.[22] Analysis of all HIV-positive women delivering between 1985 and 2003 (N = 472) showed that although rates of mother-to-child transmission were markedly reduced, there was an increased risk of a poor pregnancy outcome (defined as an intrauterine death after 22 weeks) or preeclampsia with any form of highly active ARV therapy (HAART) taken prepregnancy (odds ratio [OR] 5.6; 95% confidence interval [CI], 1.7–17.9).[22]

Protease inhibitors (PIs) have also been reported to cause hyperglycemia, new-onset diabetes mellitus, exacerbation of existing diabetes mellitus, and diabetic ketoacidosis in patients infected with HIV.[23,24] One small retrospective study that examined 41 women on PI-based combination ARV therapy found an increased risk of glucose intolerance, but not gestational diabetes compared with zidovudine (ZDV) alone,[25] whereas two other retrospective studies failed to show an increased risk of glucose intolerance with PIs.[26,27] Some experts recommend earlier glucose screening in pregnant women with ongoing PI-based therapy initiated before pregnancy.[28] Nevertheless, these data encourage increased vigilance in preterm infants born to mothers infected with HIV who are on PIs to monitor for hyperinsulinemia and other complications related to being born to a mother with impaired glucose tolerance.

RISK OF PRETERM DELIVERY IN WOMEN INFECTED WITH HIV

Early observational studies reported a risk of preterm deliveries in women infected with HIV. Since then, there have been several large studies attempting to clarify this risk and its associated factors. In a cohort in the United Kingdom, women not on ARV therapy had lower rates of preeclampsia, but those on ARV therapy had rates similar to uninfected controls.[29] In a separate large European cohort (N = 3920), combination therapy with and without a PI was associated with an increased risk of preterm delivery (OR 2.6; 95% CI, 1.43–4.75) compared with no treatment. This study also found that women on combination therapy before pregnancy were more likely to deliver prematurely than those starting ARV therapy in the third trimester (OR 2.17; 95% CI, 1.03–4.58).[30] In several United States cohorts, however, although overall rate of premature delivery was about 17%, there was no significant difference in risk of preterm delivery between groups on ARV therapy, no ARV therapy, or when the combination therapy contained a PI.[31,32] In a meta-analysis by Kourtis and colleagues,[33] 13 prospective cohorts and one retrospective study investigating the risk of premature delivery and the use of ARV therapy in pregnant women infected with HIV were analyzed. The meta-analysis found that the use of ARV therapy was not associated with an increase in the risk of premature delivery (OR 1.01; 95% CI, 0.76–1.34). In subgroup analyses, neither monotherapy nor combination therapy when compared with no treatment resulted in a statistically significant increase in premature delivery (**Fig. 1**). However, the time of initiation of combination therapy seemed to be important, with an increase in preterm delivery when combination therapy was initiated before pregnancy or in the first trimester compared with initiation in the second trimester and beyond (**Fig. 2**).

In resource-limited countries, the contribution of HIV infection to preterm births may occur partly as a result of the need for elective cesarean sections in women with high viral loads.[34] The lack of availability of ARV therapy or ability to follow the viral load of women infected with HIV may result in an increased need for elective cesarean deliveries to reduce the risk of perinatal HIV transmission. This may lead to a corresponding increase in infants born prematurely. The likelihood of preterm delivery when elective cesarean sections are performed increases partly as a result of the inaccuracy of estimation of gestational age. In 2005, Barros and colleagues[35] reported an eightfold increase in cesarean sections in Brazil in the last 20 years, with a resulting threefold increase in the incidence of preterm births.

Data from the United States show similar trends with elective cesarean deliveries (**Fig. 3**). With guidelines from the National Institutes of Health recommending scheduled cesarean delivery at 38 weeks for women with HIV RNA levels of more than 1000 copies/mL or with unknown HIV levels, this contribution to premature births among HIV-infected women is likely significant and warrants further investigation. Although the panel acknowledged that delivery at 38 weeks or less results in an increased risk of adverse events, they state that for women infected with HIV the benefits of decreasing HIV transmission by planned delivery at 38 weeks outweigh the risks. The recommendations further discourage the use of amniocentesis to document lung maturity, which may result in an increase in late preterm infants with respiratory distress syndrome.[28]

NEONATAL SIDE EFFECTS OF ARV EXPOSURE

Newborn infants born to HIV-positive mothers are exposed to a growing variety of ARV drugs from conception, through fetal life, and continued as postexposure prophylaxis for 4 to 6 weeks following delivery. Nucleoside analogs may cause mitochondrial DNA depletion and have been implicated in the development of severe lactic acidosis, multisystem failure, and anemia in a small number of infants, all of whom recovered with supportive care.[36,37] Infants exposed to ARV therapy have been found to have elevated lactic acid levels.[38] Although the significance of this finding is as yet uncertain, the contribution of an elevated lactic acid level on decreased pH in blood gases and its effects on routine laboratory results should be considered. Lactic acidosis is thought to be potentially related to mitochondrial toxicity.[28]

The risk of mitochondrial dysfunction with the use of ARV therapy or prophylaxis has scientific plausibility and laboratory studies have confirmed the need for concern. Real-time polymerase chain reaction (PCR) quantification in the placenta and cord blood of HIV-infected women exposed to nucleoside reverse-transcriptase inhibitors (NRTI) in pregnancy has shown a statistically significant reduction in the mitochondrial DNA copy number compared with healthy controls,[39] and this was confirmed in another study by electron microscopy and quantification of mitochondrial DNA.[40] A prospective French cohort reported the death of two infants exposed to NRTI from encephalopathy and abnormalities in mitochondrial function.[41] A recent retrospective study in the United States concluded that ZDV and lamivudine in the third trimester may rarely be associated with the occurrence of possible mitochondrial dysfunction.[42]

The overall importance of these findings was evaluated in a larger cohort of 4392 HIV-exposed but uninfected children followed within the French Pediatric Cohort or identified within the French National Register. This study found that the 18-month incidence of clinical symptoms of mitochondrial dysfunction was 0.26% and mortality was 0.07%.[36] All the children in the study were exposed to ARV drugs; the risk was higher among infants exposed to combination ARV drugs. Studies in the United States and Europe have not been able to duplicate these results. The Perinatal Safety Review Working Group, a large retrospective review of deaths occurring among children born to mothers infected with HIV, found no deaths or clinical findings attributable to mitochondrial dysfunction.[43] However, this study must be interpreted with caution because most of the infants had been exposed to ZDV alone and only approximately 6% had been exposed to combination therapy.

Although the data are conflicting regarding whether mitochondrial dysfunction is associated with perinatal ARV exposure, this outcome seems to be extremely rare and the benefit of ARV prophylaxis outweighs the risk. It is important, however, for physicians to have a high index of suspicion when involved in the care of infants on ARVs, particularly in the preterm infant in the neonatal intensive care unit setting.

Neonatal anemia and neutropenia have been reported in infants exposed to NRTIs and there is evidence that this may be worse where there is exposure to combination therapy, or more prolonged therapy. A study of over 4000 infants has shown that perinatal ZDV may exert a small, but significant, negative effect on hematopoiesis up to the age of 18 months.[44] Neutropenia in the moderate to severe range has been shown to occur with increased incidence in infants exposed to ARV when compared with non–ARV-exposed children with long-lasting reduction until at least 8 months of age. Fortunately, in this study, there was no increase in infections or need for antibiotic treatment with lower absolute neutrophil counts.[45]

The preterm infant with HIV exposure in the neonatal intensive care unit warrants increased surveillance for hematopoietic complications when on ARV because they are at already increased risk for infection and hematopoiesis is less efficient.

Although there is a concern for teratogenic effects of first-trimester exposure to ARV therapy, none have been reported with the exception of efavirenz. Efavirenz has been associated with cases of neural tube defects and is contraindicated in women who wish to conceive and women who are in their first trimester of pregnancy. In pregnant women receiving ARV therapy reported to the ARV pregnancy registry, of the 1229 women enrolled, the overall prevalence of a congenital anomaly (per 100 live births) was 6.2, which is comparable with the rate in the general population (3%). Subanalysis showed the prevalence of birth defects after first-trimester exposure to ARV was similar to that after second- and third-trimester exposure.[46] Overall, there seemed to be no increased risk with first-trimester exposure; however, continued surveillance is needed.

HIV VIREMIA, PREMATURE RUPTURE OF MEMBRANES, AND MODE OF DELIVERY

Maternal plasma HIV-1 RNA viral load has an almost linear association with the risk of perinatal transmission.[47] With the introduction of HAART therapy, the need for cesarean delivery in women with low or undetectable viremia had been questioned. A meta-analysis of seven prospective trials (N = 1202) showed a transmission rate of 3.7% in women with plasma HIV RNA viral loads of less than 1000 copies/mL.[48] The Pediatric AIDS Clinical Trials Group showed no additional benefit of cesarean delivery for women (N = 1736) with HIV RNA viral loads less than 1000 copies/mL at their last antenatal visit. Current ACOG guidelines only recommend elective cesarean delivery at HIV RNA viral loads above 1000 copies/mL.[49] However, a prospective study of 1983 mother-infant pairs in

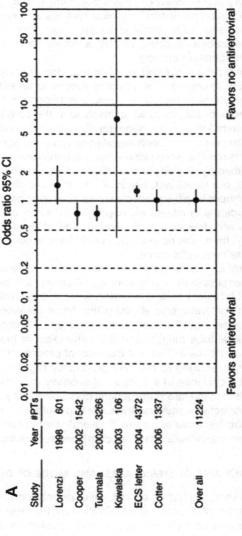

Fig. 1. Results of a meta-analysis of studies on the risk of preterm delivery in HIV-infected women on antiretroviral therapy. (*A*) Women who used antiretroviral therapy during pregnancy compared with those who did not use antiretroviral therapy. (*B*) Women who used monotherapy during pregnancy compared with those who used combination antiretroviral therapy. Each study is shown by name of first author, year, number of patients, point estimate, and 95% confidence intervals (CI) of odds ratios. Also shown are the pooled odds ratio and 95% CI by random-effects calculations. ECS, European Collaborative Study. (*From* Kourtis AP, Schmid CH, Jamieson DJ, et al. Use of antiretroviral therapy in pregnant HIV-infected women and the risk of premature delivery: a meta-analysis. *AIDS* 2007;21(5):607–15; with permission.)

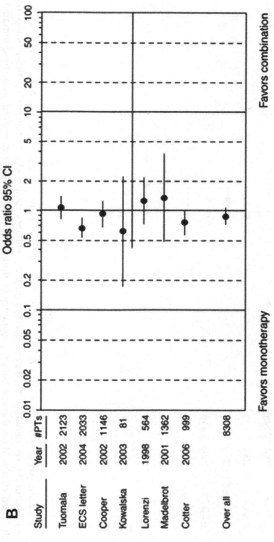

Fig. 1. (continued)

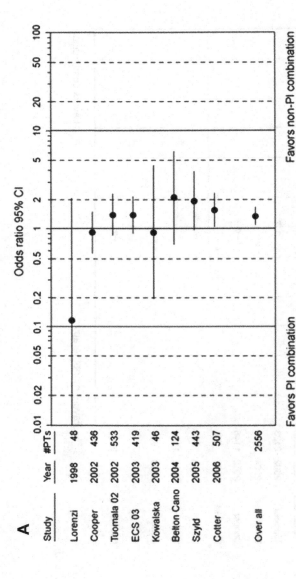

Fig. 2. Results of a meta-analysis of studies on the risk of preterm delivery among HIV-infected women on antiretroviral therapy. (*A*) HIV-infected women on protease inhibitor (PI)–containing antiretroviral therapy during pregnancy compared with other, non–PI-containing combination regimens and (*B*) women who used combination therapy before pregnancy or during the first trimester compared with those initiated during the second trimester and beyond. CI, confidence interval; ECS, European Collaborative Study. (*From* Kourtis AP, Schmid CH, Jamieson DJ, et al. Use of antiretroviral therapy in pregnant HIV-infected women and the risk of premature delivery: a meta-analysis. *AIDS* 2007;21(5):607–15; with permission.)

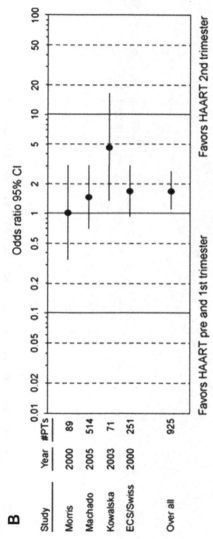

Fig. 2. (continued)

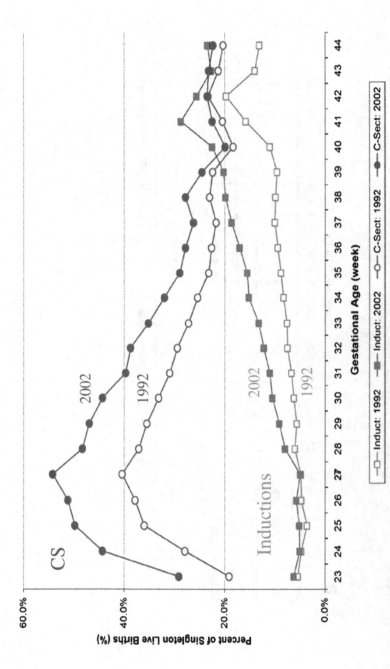

Fig. 3. Graph illustrates the increase in earlier gestation infants associated with elective cesarean sections. (*Data from* National Center for Health Statistics, final natality data; *Modified from* Davidoff MJ, Dias T, Damus K, et al. Changes in the gestational age distribution among U.S. singleton births: impact on rates of late preterm birth, 1992 to 2002. Semin Perinatol 2006;30(1):8–15; with permission.)

Europe between 1997 and 2004 showed reduction of transmission rates for HIV from 2.87% to 0.99% between 2001 and 2003 in mothers with low plasma viremia, suggesting possible continuing benefit of cesarean section.[50] With viral loads now approaching less than 50 or undetectable with effective HAART therapy, further studies are needed to assess whether there is any added benefit of operative delivery in these women.

In the United States, current ACOG recommendations are to offer patients vaginal delivery with viral counts of less than 1000 copies/mL after discussing the benefits of vaginal delivery and potential risk of operative delivery and perinatal transmission. Recent guidelines published by the National Institutes of Health have recommended scheduled cesarean delivery at 38 weeks gestation for women with RNA levels of more than 1000 copies/mL near the time of delivery and for women with unknown HIV RNA levels.[28] For women with HIV RNA levels less than 1000 copies/mL near the time of delivery the recommendations state that data are insufficient to make a recommendation and that decisions should be individualized based on discussion between the obstetrician and the mother. Most centers in the United States are counseling mothers with HIV viral loads of less than 1000 copies/mL and offering them a choice between cesarean section and vaginal delivery.

A meta-analysis of 15 prospective cohort studies showed that there was an increased risk of HIV transmission of 2% per hour of ruptured membranes up to 24 hours.[51] A retrospective study from Spain showed that duration of labor, duration of rupture of membranes, and use of invasive procedures significantly increased the risk of perinatal HIV transmission.[52]

These studies suggest that preterm premature rupture of membranes (PPROM) could increase the risk of mother-to-child HIV transmission. Although there are benefits of two doses of prenatal corticosteroids on the neonatal outcome of premature deliveries, this must be weighed against the increased risk of perinatal transmission in the background of PPROM. There are currently no clear guidelines for the management of PPROM occurring at less than or equal to 34 weeks of gestation in the presence of maternal HIV infection.

CONCOMITANT GENITAL TRACT INFECTIONS

Infection with herpes simplex virus type 2 (HSV2) is the most common cause of genital ulcer disease worldwide. Seroprevalence of HSV2 in people with HIV-1 may be as high as 70% to 90% in some populations.[53] It has been shown that plasma and genital HIV-1 concentrations increase during reactivation of HSV2, suggesting that herpes reactivation enhances HIV-1 replication and possibly increases the risk of transmission to the infant.[54–56] Control of HSV infection with acyclovir has been found to slow the rate of progression in HIV-infected patients.[57]

In a retrospective analysis of 402 HIV-infected pregnant women, Chen and colleagues[58] showed that a clinical diagnosis of genital HSV infection during pregnancy carried a significantly increased risk of perinatal HIV transmission (OR 3.4; 95% CI, 1.3–9.3), with this remaining a significant predictor of perinatal HIV transmission after controlling for lack of ZDV therapy during pregnancy, PROM, and preterm delivery. Mothers should be screened for other sexually transmitted diseases, including syphilis, and effective treatment initiated to reduce the risk of comorbidities in the background of HIV infection.

BREASTFEEDING

HIV-1 can be transmitted through breastfeeding with estimated transmission rates at approximately 16%, with prolonged feeding nearly doubling the overall rate of perinatal transmission. Mastitis, cracked nipples, lower maternal CD4 count, and higher plasma and breast milk HIV RNA viral loads increase the rate of HIV transmission by breastfeeding.[59] In the United States, where formula feeding is safe and affordable, the risk of HIV transmission by breastfeeding outweighs the benefits and breastfeeding should be completely avoided by HIV-infected women.[60] In preterm infants breastfeeding confers the added benefit of reduction in the risk of necrotizing enterocolitis and sepsis. Donor breast milk is an option that should be considered and offered to HIV-infected mothers of preterm infants if resources are available. The use of donor breast milk has been shown to reduce the incidence of necrotizing enterocolitis in preterm infants.[61]

Overall, even though risks from ARV therapy seem to be real, the benefits of HIV prevention for the infant continue to outweigh the risks of adverse outcomes. However, this warrants careful counseling with families during the planning and early part of pregnancy.

MANAGEMENT OF THE PRETERM INFANT AT RISK OF PERINATAL HIV TRANSMISSION
Testing of the Infant or Mother for HIV

If the mother's HIV status is unknown before delivery, then the mother or infant should have HIV-1 testing with maternal consent.[62] Some states mandate HIV-1 testing of all infants whose mothers' HIV-1 infection status is unknown. To allow appropriate treatment to be initiated within 24 hours, expedited testing using HIV-1 enzyme immunoassay or rapid testing kits should be used. The rapid test should then be confirmed by standard HIV-1 testing.[63] If the mother's HIV status is not known and the rapid test was not performed on the mother during labor, then the rapid test should be performed on the mother or infant as soon as possible after birth.[62] If the rapid test is positive, the confirmatory test should be sent and ARV infant prophylaxis be initiated as soon as possible after birth (before 24 hours).[60] Testing of the mother for co-infections, such as tuberculosis, congenital syphilis, hepatitis B or C, cytomegalovirus, or HSV, should be considered.[64]

ARV Therapy

The treatment of choice for infants born to mothers who have received prenatal and intrapartum maternal ARV therapy is oral ZDV, to be continued for 6 weeks.[65,66] This is the standard regimen in developed countries and ZDV is currently the only ARV drug available with preterm infant dosing (**Table 1**). In resource-limited countries, a single dose of nevirapine to the infant plus 1 week of infant ZDV and lamivudine is recommended for infants whose mothers did not receive ARV therapy during pregnancy or received only single-dose nevirapine during labor. Single-dose nevirapine and a week of lamivudine, in addition to the ZDV course, might also be considered in the United States if the mother had not received ARV antenatally or if she is known to harbor a ZDV-resistant virus. Prompt initiation of infant prophylaxis is critical, because animal studies have shown that ARV prophylaxis initiated 24 to 36 hours after exposure may not be effective in preventing infection.[67–69] Current guidelines recommend that prophylaxis be initiated within 6 to 12 hours of delivery.[28]

The safety of ARVs other than ZDV has not been adequately tested in term or preterm infants. Additionally, there is no standard dosing regimen for ARV drugs other than ZDV for preterm infants. Current recommendations state that the risk of perinatal transmission is increased in the following groups [28]: (1) infants born to mothers who received antepartum and intrapartum ARV but who had suboptimal viral suppression at delivery, particularly if delivered vaginally; (2) infants born to mothers who only

Table 1 Dosing regimen for zidovudine prophylaxis in term and preterm infants		
Gestational Age	**Oral Dose**	**IV Dose**
Term (>35 wk)	2 mg/kg/dose q 6 h for 6 wk	1.5 mg/kg/dose q 6 h for 6 wk
Preterm (<35 and >30 wk)	2 mg/kg/dose q 12 h for the first 2 wk, then increase to 2 mg/kg/dose q 8 h to complete a total of 6 wk	1.5 mg/kg/dose q 12 h for the first 2 wk, then increase to 1.5 mg/kg/dose q 8 h to complete a total of 6 wk
Preterm (<30 wk)	2 mg/kg/dose q 12 h for the first 4 wk, then increase to 2 mg/kg/dose q 8 h to complete a total of 6 wk	1.5 mg/kg/dose q 12 h for the first 4 wk, then increase to 1.5 mg/kg/dose q 8 h to complete a total of 6 wk

received ARV drugs intrapartum; (3) infants born to mothers who received no antepartum or intrapartum ARV drugs; and (4) infants born to mothers with known ARV drug-resistance virus.

In the previously mentioned situations, the recommendation is to approach each individual patient and assess other risk factors for the patient (ie, vaginal delivery, maternal viral load, and infant's gestational age at delivery) and consult an HIV specialist for further guidance. The risks and benefits should then be discussed with the mother of the baby to determine whether or not to initiate added ARV coverage.[28] Experience with lamivudine or nevirapine in preterm infants is extremely limited and any consideration of use should be made in consultation with a pediatric HIV specialist.

Determination of the HIV-1 Status of the Infant

HIV-1 DNA PCR is the preferred diagnostic test in North America. The specimen should not be obtained from cord-blood because this is associated with an unacceptably high rate of false-positive test results.[70] The HIV-1 DNA PCR should be performed at birth, 4 to 7 weeks of age, and 8 to 16 weeks of age.[60] If the mother is known to be infected with HIV-2 then specific request must be made for HIV-2 PCR testing. If the mother's HIV status is unknown, then rapid testing of the mother or infant should be performed as soon as possible after birth. HIV infection may be excluded with two or more negative tests with one at greater than or equal to 1 month and another at greater than or equal to 4 months of age. Many experts also confirm HIV-negative status at 12 to 18 months.

Special Clinical Considerations

The following clinical scenarios warrant special consideration (**Table 2**).

Lactic acidosis
ARVs are known occasionally to cause lactic acidosis. Acid-base status in the preterm infant should be closely monitored.

Anemia and neutropenia
ARVs can cause neutropenia in the mild to moderate range and delay in hematopoiesis. In the preterm population where anemia of prematurity is significant, close monitoring of hematocrit while on ARV therapy should be initiated. Neutropenia is also a side effect of therapy and in this population susceptible to infection, close monitoring for infection in the background of neutropenia is prudent. It is important for these reasons to obtain a baseline complete blood count with differential at birth before beginning ARV.

Table 2
Side effects of antiretroviral therapy and potential significance in preterm infants

Side Effect	Significance in Preterm Infants
Negative effect on hematopoiesis	May exacerbate anemia in the background of anemia of prematurity
Neutropenia	May increase risk of infection, evidence not clear
Lactic acidosis	Preterm infants prone to waste bicarbonate in the urine, may exacerbate acidosis
Mitochondrial dysfunction	Mitochondrial dysfunction may worsen neurodevelopmental status in population prone to worse neurodevelopmental outcomes
Teratogenic effects	In preterm infants, may slow growth and cause long-term worse outcome Long term follow-up is necessary

Breast milk
Breast milk from the mother should be avoided to prevent perinatal transmission. Where available, donor breast milk should be considered after counseling with the mother if benefits of breast milk are deemed desirable.

Congenital defects
Any congenital defects should be reported to the ARV pregnancy registry for surveillance data.

Follow-up
On discharge, appropriate follow-up of the infant and mother with a pediatric and adult HIV care provider should be arranged to ensure continuation of medication and follow-up testing for HIV status in the infant.

Immunizations
All routine immunizations may be given to infants exposed to HIV-1 unless HIV-1 infection is confirmed; then, guidelines for the child infected with HIV-1 should be followed.[71,72] All inactivated vaccines can be safely administered to infants exposed to HIV on ARV prophylaxis, including killed whole organism or recombinant, subunit, toxoid, polysaccharide, or polysaccharide protein-conjugate vaccines. These may be administered in the usual doses and schedules recommended. For live attenuated vaccines, further consideration of the level of immunosuppression needs to be considered. There are currently no safety or efficacy data related to the administration of rotavirus vaccine to infants infected with HIV and most likely the HIV diagnosis may not be established in infants born to mothers infected with HIV before the age of the first rotavirus dose. It is recommended that consultation with an immunologist or infectious disease specialist be obtained before administering the rotavirus vaccine in infants exposed to HIV. The varicella and mumps-measles-rubella vaccines can be considered in children infected with HIV who are not severely immunosuppressed (ie, those with age-specific CD4 cell percentages of $\geq 15\%$). Physicians taking care of preterm infants can administer inactivated vaccines starting at the chronologic age of 2 months at the recommended dosing.[71,72]

Counseling to caregivers
Counseling should be provided to parents and caregivers of infants exposed to HIV-1 about the infection and should include anticipatory guidance on the course of illness, infection-control measures, care of the infant, diagnostic tests, and potential drug toxicity.[60]

SUMMARY

With the availability of appropriate prenatal testing and ARV treatment, the incidence of perinatal transmission of HIV has been reduced significantly. Given that the number of child-bearing age women infected with HIV is increasing, the risk of mother-to-child transmission persists. With an increased rate of preterm delivery in this population of women, close monitoring and appropriate counseling should be provided. Care of the preterm infant in this setting warrants closer monitoring for potential side effects of ARV therapy and appropriate diagnosis and treatment of HIV infection. The social implications of HIV infection in the care of a preterm infant should also be considered.

REFERENCES

1. Achievements in public health. Reduction in perinatal transmission of HIV infection—United States, 1985–2005. MMWR Morb Mortal Wkly Rep 2006;55:592–7.
2. Kumar RM, Uduman SA, Khurranna AK. Impact of maternal HIV-1 infection on perinatal outcome. Int J Gynaecol Obstet 1995;49:137–43.
3. Leroy V, Ladner J, Nyiraziraje M, et al. Effect of HIV-1 infection on pregnancy outcome in women in Kigali, Rwanda, 1992–1994. Pregnancy and HIV Study Group. AIDS 1998;12:643–50.
4. Temmerman M, Chomba EN, Ndinya-Achola J, et al. Maternal human immunodeficiency virus-1 infection and pregnancy outcome. Obstet Gynecol 1994;83:495–501.
5. Ramachandrappa A, Jain L. Health issues of the late preterm infant. Pediatr Clin North Am 2009;56:565–77.
6. Aebi-Popp K, Lapaire O, Glass TR, et al. Pregnancy and delivery outcomes of HIV infected women in Switzerland 2003–2008. J Perinat Med 2010;38(4):353–8.
7. Lindegren ML, Byers RH Jr, Thomas P, et al. Trends in perinatal transmission of HIV/AIDS in the United States. JAMA 1999;282:531–8.
8. Centers for Disease Control and Prevention. Cases of HIV infection and AIDS in the United States and dependent areas, 2007. Available at: http://www.cdc.gov/hiv/surveillance/resources/reports/2007report/. Accessed August 18, 2010.
9. Cooper ER, Charurat M, Mofenson L, et al. Combination antiretroviral strategies for the treatment of pregnant HIV-1-infected women and prevention of perinatal HIV-1 transmission. J Acquir Immune Defic Syndr 2002;29:484–94.
10. Connor EM, Sperling RS, Gelber R, et al. Reduction of maternal-infant transmission of human immunodeficiency virus type 1 with zidovudine treatment. Pediatric AIDS Clinical Trials Group Protocol 076 Study Group. N Engl J Med 1994;331:1173–80.
11. Brocklehurst P, French R. The association between maternal HIV infection and perinatal outcome: a systematic review of the literature and meta-analysis. Br J Obstet Gynaecol 1998;105:836–48.
12. Traisathit P, Mary JY, Le Coeur S, et al. Risk factors of preterm delivery in HIV-infected pregnant women receiving zidovudine for the prevention of perinatal HIV. J Obstet Gynaecol Res 2009;35:225–33.
13. Tuntiseranee P, Olsen J, Chongsuvivatwong V, et al. Socioeconomic and work related determinants of pregnancy outcome in southern Thailand. J Epidemiol Community Health 1999;53:624–9.
14. Martin R, Boyer P, Hammill H, et al. Incidence of premature birth and neonatal respiratory disease in infants of HIV-positive mothers. The Pediatric Pulmonary and Cardiovascular Complications of Vertically Transmitted Human Immunodeficiency Virus Infection Study Group. J Pediatr 1997;131:851–6.

15. Racial/ethnic disparities in diagnoses of HIV/AIDS—33 states, 2001–2005. MMWR Morb Mortal Wkly Rep 2007;56:189–93.
16. Epidemiology of HIV/AIDS—United States, 1981–2005. MMWR Morb Mortal Wkly Rep 2006;55:589–92.
17. De Cock KM, Fowler MG, Mercier E, et al. Prevention of mother-to-child HIV transmission in resource-poor countries: translating research into policy and practice. JAMA 2000;283:1175–82.
18. Anderson BL, Cu-Uvin S. Pregnancy and optimal care of HIV-infected patients. Clin Infect Dis 2009;48:449–55.
19. Branson BM, Handsfield HH, Lampe MA, et al. Revised recommendations for HIV testing of adults, adolescents, and pregnant women in health-care settings. MMWR Recomm Rep 2006;55:1–17 [quiz: CE11–4].
20. Sansom SL, Jamieson DJ, Farnham PG, et al. Human immunodeficiency virus retesting during pregnancy: costs and effectiveness in preventing perinatal transmission. Obstet Gynecol 2003;102:782–90.
21. Nurutdinova D, Overton ET. A review of nucleoside reverse transcriptase inhibitor use to prevent perinatal transmission of HIV. Expert Opin Drug Saf 2009;8:683–94.
22. Suy A, Martinez E, Coll O, et al. Increased risk of pre-eclampsia and fetal death in HIV-infected pregnant women receiving highly active antiretroviral therapy. AIDS 2006;20:59–66.
23. Visnegarwala F, Krause KL, Musher DM. Severe diabetes associated with protease inhibitor therapy. Ann Intern Med 1997;127:947.
24. Eastone JA, Decker CF. New-onset diabetes mellitus associated with use of protease inhibitor. Ann Intern Med 1997;127:948.
25. Chmait R, Franklin P, Spector SA, et al. Protease inhibitors and decreased birth weight in HIV-infected pregnant women with impaired glucose tolerance. J Perinatol 2002;22:370–3.
26. Dinsmoor MJ, Forrest ST. Lack of an effect of protease inhibitor use on glucose tolerance during pregnancy. Infect Dis Obstet Gynecol 2002;10:187–91.
27. Tang JH, Sheffield JS, Grimes J, et al. Effect of protease inhibitor therapy on glucose intolerance in pregnancy. Obstet Gynecol 2006;107:1115–9.
28. Recommendations for use of antiretroviral drugs in pregnant HIV-1-Infected women for maternal health and Interventions to reduce perinatal HIV transmission in the United States. 2010. Available at: http://aidsinfo.nih.gov/contentfiles/PerinatalGL.pdf. Accessed August 18, 2010.
29. Wimalasundera RC, Larbalestier N, Smith JH, et al. Pre-eclampsia, antiretroviral therapy, and immune reconstitution. Lancet 2002;360:1152–4.
30. Combination antiretroviral therapy and duration of pregnancy. AIDS 2000;14:2913–20.
31. Tuomala RE, Shapiro DE, Mofenson LM, et al. Antiretroviral therapy during pregnancy and the risk of an adverse outcome. N Engl J Med 2002;346:1863–70.
32. Patel K, Shapiro DE, Brogly SB, et al. Prenatal protease inhibitor use and risk of preterm birth among HIV-infected women initiating antiretroviral drugs during pregnancy. J Infect Dis 2010;201:1035–44.
33. Kourtis AP, Schmid CH, Jamieson DJ, et al. Use of antiretroviral therapy in pregnant HIV-infected women and the risk of premature delivery: a meta-analysis. AIDS 2007;21:607–15.
34. Steer P. The epidemiology of preterm labor—a global perspective. J Perinat Med 2005;33:273–6.

35. Barros FC, Victora CG, Barros AJ, et al. The challenge of reducing neonatal mortality in middle-income countries: findings from three Brazilian birth cohorts in 1982, 1993, and 2004. Lancet 2005;365:847–54.
36. Barret B, Tardieu M, Rustin P, et al. Persistent mitochondrial dysfunction in HIV-1-exposed but uninfected infants: clinical screening in a large prospective cohort. AIDS 2003;17:1769–85.
37. Lewis W. Mitochondrial dysfunction and nucleoside reverse transcriptase inhibitor therapy: experimental clarifications and persistent clinical questions. Antiviral Res 2003;58:189–97.
38. Noguera A, Fortuny C, Munoz-Almagro C, et al. Hyperlactatemia in human immunodeficiency virus-uninfected infants who are exposed to antiretrovirals. Pediatrics 2004;114:e598–603.
39. Divi RL, Walker VE, Wade NA, et al. Mitochondrial damage and DNA depletion in cord blood and umbilical cord from infants exposed in utero to Combivir. AIDS 2004;18:1013–21.
40. Divi RL, Leonard SL, Kuo MM, et al. Transplacentally exposed human and monkey newborn infants show similar evidence of nucleoside reverse transcriptase inhibitor-induced mitochondrial toxicity. Environ Mol Mutagen 2007;48:201–9.
41. Blanche S, Tardieu M, Rustin P, et al. Persistent mitochondrial dysfunction and perinatal exposure to antiretroviral nucleoside analogues. Lancet 1999;354:1084–9.
42. Brogly SB, Ylitalo N, Mofenson LM, et al. In utero nucleoside reverse transcriptase inhibitor exposure and signs of possible mitochondrial dysfunction in HIV-uninfected children. AIDS 2007;21:929–38.
43. Poirier MC, Divi RL, Al-Harthi L, et al. Long-term mitochondrial toxicity in HIV-uninfected infants born to HIV-infected mothers. J Acquir Immune Defic Syndr 2003;33:175–83.
44. Le Chenadec J, Mayaux MJ, Guihenneuc-Jouyaux C, et al. Perinatal antiretroviral treatment and hematopoiesis in HIV-uninfected infants. AIDS 2003;17:2053–61.
45. Bunders MJ, Bekker V, Scherpbier HJ, et al. Haematological parameters of HIV-1-uninfected infants born to HIV-1-infected mothers. Acta Paediatr 2005;94:1571–7.
46. Joao EC, Calvet GA, Krauss MR, et al. Maternal antiretroviral use during pregnancy and infant congenital anomalies: the NISDI perinatal study. J Acquir Immune Defic Syndr 2010;53:176–85.
47. Garcia PM, Kalish LA, Pitt J, et al. Maternal levels of plasma human immunodeficiency virus type 1 RNA and the risk of perinatal transmission. Women and Infants Transmission Study Group. N Engl J Med 1999;341:394–402.
48. Ioannidis JP, Abrams EJ, Ammann A, et al. Perinatal transmission of human immunodeficiency virus type 1 by pregnant women with RNA virus loads <1000 copies/ml. J Infect Dis 2001;183:539–45.
49. ACOG committee opinion scheduled cesarean delivery and the prevention of vertical transmission of HIV infection. Number 234, May 2000 (replaces number 219, August 1999). Int J Gynaecol Obstet 2001;73:279–81.
50. European Collaborative Study Group. Mother-to-child transmission of HIV infection in the era of highly active antiretroviral therapy. Clin Infect Dis 2005;40:458–65.
51. International Perinatal HIV Group. Duration of ruptured membranes and vertical transmission of HIV-1: a meta-analysis from 15 prospective cohort studies. AIDS 2001;15:357–68.
52. Garcia-Tejedor A, Perales A, Maiques V. Duration of ruptured membranes and extended labor are risk factors for HIV transmission. Int J Gynaecol Obstet 2003;82:17–23.

53. Weiss H. Epidemiology of herpes simplex virus type 2 infection in the developing world. Herpes 2004;11(Suppl 1):24A–35A.
54. Baeten JM, McClelland RS, Corey L, et al. Vitamin A supplementation and genital shedding of herpes simplex virus among HIV-1-infected women: a randomized clinical trial. J Infect Dis 2004;189:1466–71.
55. Mbopi-Keou FX, Legoff J, Gresenguet G, et al. Genital shedding of herpes simplex virus-2 DNA and HIV-1 RNA and proviral DNA in HIV-1- and herpes simplex virus-2-coinfected African women. J Acquir Immune Defic Syndr 2003; 33:121–4.
56. Mole L, Ripich S, Margolis D, et al. The impact of active herpes simplex virus infection on human immunodeficiency virus load. J Infect Dis 1997;176:766–70.
57. Lingappa JR, Baeten JM, Wald A, et al. Daily aciclovir for HIV-1 disease progression in people dually infected with HIV-1 and herpes simplex virus type 2: a randomised placebo-controlled trial. Lancet 2010;375:824–33.
58. Chen KT, Segu M, Lumey LH, et al. Genital herpes simplex virus infection and perinatal transmission of human immunodeficiency virus. Obstet Gynecol 2005; 106:1341–8.
59. Lunney KM, Iliff P, Mutasa K, et al. Associations between breast milk viral load, mastitis, exclusive breast-feeding, and postnatal transmission of HIV. Clin Infect Dis 2010;50:762–9.
60. King SM. Evaluation and treatment of the human immunodeficiency virus-1-exposed infant. Pediatrics 2004;114:497–505.
61. McGuire W, Anthony MY. Donor human milk versus formula for preventing necrotising enterocolitis in preterm infants: systematic review. Arch Dis Child Fetal Neonatal Ed 2003;88:F11–4.
62. ACOG committee opinion number 304, November 2004. Prenatal and perinatal human immunodeficiency virus testing: expanded recommendations. Obstet Gynecol 2004;104(5 Pt 1):1119–24.
63. Bulterys M, Jamieson DJ, O'Sullivan MJ, et al. Rapid HIV-1 testing during labor: a multicenter study. JAMA 2004;292:219–23.
64. Hepatitis C. virus infection. American Academy of Pediatrics. Committee on Infectious Diseases. Pediatrics 1998;101(3 Pt 1):481–5.
65. Mofenson LM. Technical report: perinatal human immunodeficiency virus testing and prevention of transmission. Committee on Pediatric Aids. Pediatrics 2000; 106:E88.
66. Mofenson LM. U.S. Public Health Service Task Force recommendations for use of antiretroviral drugs in pregnant HIV-1-infected women for maternal health and interventions to reduce perinatal HIV-1 transmission in the United States. MMWR Recomm Rep 2002;51(RR-18):1–38 [quiz: CE31–4].
67. Van Rompay KK, Otsyula MG, Marthas ML, et al. Immediate zidovudine treatment protects simian immunodeficiency virus-infected newborn macaques against rapid onset of AIDS. Antimicrobial Agents Chemother 1995;39:125–31.
68. Tsai CC, Follis KE, Sabo A, et al. Prevention of SIV infection in macaques by (R)-9-(2-phosphonylmethoxypropyl)adenine. Science 1995;270:1197–9.
69. Bottiger D, Johansson NG, Samuelsson B, et al. Prevention of simian immunodeficiency virus, SIVsm, or HIV-2 infection in cynomolgus monkeys by pre- and postexposure administration of BEA-005. AIDS 1997;11:157–62.
70. Schneider E, Whitmore S, Glynn KM, et al. Revised surveillance case definitions for HIV infection among adults, adolescents, and children aged <18 months and for HIV infection and AIDS among children aged 18 months to <13 years—United States, 2008. MMWR Recomm Rep 2008;57(RR-10):1–12.

71. Recommended childhood immunization schedule—United States, 2002. MMWR Morb Mortal Wkly Rep 2002;51:31–3.
72. Measles immunization in HIV-infected children. American Academy of Pediatrics. Committee on Infectious Diseases and Committee on Pediatric AIDS. Pediatrics 1999;103(5 Pt 1):1057–60.

Antiretroviral Pharmacology: Special Issues Regarding Pregnant Women and Neonates

Mark Mirochnick, MD[a],*, Brookie M. Best, PharmD, MAS[b],
Diana F. Clarke, PharmD[c]

KEYWORDS

• Antiretrovirals • Pharmacology • Pregnant women • Neonates

Much progress has been made in recent years in treating human immunodeficiency virus (HIV) infection and preventing mother-to-child transmission (PMTCT) of HIV. In areas of the world where combination regimens of potent antiretroviral agents are available, the use of these regimens has resulted in dramatically increased survival of HIV-infected individuals and rates of transmission of HIV from infected pregnant women to their infants as low as 1%. In areas of the world where potent combination antiretroviral regimens are not available, the use of less intensive antiretroviral regimens has resulted in lesser but still significant reductions in the rate of mother-to-child transmission of HIV. Currently more than 25 antiretroviral agents in 5 classes have been approved by the US Food and Drug Administration (FDA) (**Table 1**), with new drugs and classes in development. This article reviews current knowledge of the pharmacology of these drugs during pregnancy and in the newborn period, highlighting those pharmacologic issues critical to the safe and effective use of antiretrovirals in these populations.

[a] Division of Neonatology, Department of Pediatrics, Boston University School of Medicine, 771 Albany Street – Dowling 4111, Boston, MA 02118, USA
[b] Department of Pediatrics – Rady Children's Hospital San Diego, Skaggs School of Pharmacy and Pharmaceutical Sciences, University of California, San Diego, 9500 Gilman Drive, MC 0719, La Jolla, CA 92093-0719, USA
[c] Section of Pediatric Infectious Diseases, Department of Pediatrics, Boston Medical Center, 670 Albany Street – Room 613, Boston, MA 02118, USA
* Corresponding author.
E-mail address: markm@bu.edu

Clin Perinatol 37 (2010) 907–927
doi:10.1016/j.clp.2010.08.006
0095-5108/10/$ – see front matter © 2010 Elsevier Inc. All rights reserved.

Table 1
FDA-approved antiretrovirals listed by class and approval date

Generic Name	Brand Name	Originator Name	Approval Date	FDA Pregnancy Category
Nucleoside/Nucleotide Reverse Transcriptase Inhibitors				
Zidovudine (ZDV), azidothymidine (AZT)	Retrovir	GlaxoSmithKline	19-Mar-87	C
Didanosine, dideoxyinosine (ddI)	Videx	Bristol-Myers Squibb	9-Oct-91	B
Zalcitabine, dideoxycytidine (ddC) (no longer marketed)	Hivid	Hoffmann-La Roche	19-Jun-92	—
Stavudine (d4T)	Zerit	Bristol-Myers Squibb	24-Jun-94	C
Lamivudine (3TC)	Epivir	GlaxoSmithKline	17-Nov-95	C
Abacavir sulfate (ABC)	Ziagen	GlaxoSmithKline	17-Dec-98	C
Enteric-coated didanosine (ddI EC)	Videx EC	Bristol-Myers Squibb	31-Oct-00	B
Tenofovir disoproxil fumarate (TDF)	Viread	Gilead Sciences	26-Oct-01	B
Emtricitabine (FTC)	Emtriva	Gilead Sciences	02-Jul-03	B
Nonnucleoside Reverse Transcriptase Inhibitors				
Nevirapine (NVP)	Viramune	Boehringer Ingelheim	21-Jun-96	B
Delavirdine mesylate (DLV) (no longer marketed)	Rescriptor	Pfizer	4-Apr-97	—
Efavirenz (EFV)	Sustiva	Bristol-Myers Squibb	17-Sep-98	D
Etravirine (ETR)	Intelence	Tibotec	18-Jan-08	B
Protease Inhibitors				
Saquinavir mesylate hard gel capsule (SQV)	Invirase	Hoffmann-La Roche	6-Dec-95	B
Ritonavir (RTV)	Norvir	Abbott Laboratories	1-Mar-96	B
Indinavir sulfate (IDV)	Crixivan	Merck	13-Mar-96	C
Nelfinavir mesylate (NFV)	Viracept	Agouron Pharmaceuticals	14-Mar-97	B
Saquinavir soft gel capsule (SQV) (no longer marketed)	Fortovase	Hoffmann-La Roche	7-Nov-97	—

Amprenavir (APV) (no longer marketed)	Agenerase	GlaxoSmithKline	15-Apr-99	–
Lopinavir and ritonavir (LPV/RTV)	Kaletra	Abbott Laboratories	15-Sep-00	C
Atazanavir sulfate (ATV)	Reyataz	Bristol-Myers Squibb	20-Jun-03	B
Fosamprenavir calcium (fAPV)	Lexiva	GlaxoSmithKline	20-Oct-03	C
Tipranavir (TPV)	Aptivus	Boehringer Ingelheim	22-Jun-05	C
Darunavir ethanolate (DRV)	Prezista	Tibotec	23-Jun-06	C
Fusion/Entry Inhibitors				
Enfuvirtide (ENF), T-20	Fuzeon	Hoffmann-La Roche & Trimeris	13-Mar-03	B
Maraviroc (MVC)	Selzentry	Pfizer	06-August-07	B
HIV Integrase Strand Transfer Inhibitors				
Raltegravir potassium (RAL)	Isentress	Merck	12-Oct-07	C
Combination Products				
Lamivudine and zidovudine	Combivir	GlaxoSmithKline	27-Sep-97	–
Abacavir, zidovudine, and lamivudine	Trizivir	GlaxoSmithKline	14-Nov-00	–
Abacavir and lamivudine	Epzicom	GlaxoSmithKline	02-Aug-04	–
Tenofovir disoproxil fumarate and emtricitabine	Truvada	Gilead Sciences	02-Aug-04	–
Efavirenz, emtricitabine, and tenofovir disoproxil fumarate	Atripla	Bristol-Myers Squibb and Gilead Sciences	12-July-06	–

FDA pregnancy categories are as follows: category A, adequate and well-controlled studies have failed to show a risk to the fetus in the first trimester of pregnancy (and there is no evidence of risk in later trimesters); category B, animal reproduction studies have failed to show a risk to the fetus and there are no adequate and well-controlled studies in pregnant women; category C, animal reproduction studies have shown an adverse effect on the fetus and there are no adequate and well-controlled studies in humans, but potential benefits may warrant use of the drug in pregnant women despite potential risks; category D, there is positive evidence of human fetal risk based on adverse reaction data from investigational or marketing experience or studies in humans, but potential benefits may warrant use of the drug in pregnant women despite potential risks; category X, studies in animals or humans have shown fetal abnormalities and/or there is positive evidence of human fetal risk based on adverse reaction data from investigational or marketing experience, and the risks involved in use of the drug in pregnant women clearly outweigh potential benefits.

PHARMACOKINETICS
Pregnancy Effects on Drug Disposition

Maternal physiologic changes associated with pregnancy may have a considerable effect on all 4 components of drug disposition: absorption, distribution, metabolism, and excretion. Nausea and vomiting, especially pronounced in early pregnancy, may decrease drug absorption. Intestinal motility decreases by 30% to 50%, increasing gastric emptying and intestinal transit times.[1] Acid secretion is reduced by 40%, increasing gastric pH, which may affect the ionization and absorption of weak acids and bases.[2] These physiologic changes would likely result in delayed drug absorption and reduced peak maternal blood concentrations.[3]

During an average pregnancy total body water increases by 8 L, plasma volume enlarges by 50%, and body fat stores increase, changing volume of distribution of both hydrophilic and lipophilic drugs.[4] In general, volume of distribution increases and peak drug concentrations decrease during pregnancy. Competitive inhibition from steroid hormones and a dilutional decrease in serum albumin result in decreased protein binding.[5] These changes may result in an increase in the free fraction of drug, which is the pharmacologically active moiety.

The effect of pregnancy on drug elimination is variable but may be significant. Progesterone may induce hepatic metabolic activity, increasing drug metabolism.[6] Conversely, drug metabolism may be reduced because of competition with estrogen and progesterone for metabolic binding sites.[7] Renal function increases during pregnancy, with 25% to 50% increases in renal plasma flow and glomerular filtration rate. Clearance of renally excreted drugs and drug metabolites increases during pregnancy.[8] Although the disposition of most drugs is measurably changed by the physiologic changes of pregnancy, multiple and contradictory effects may coexist.[2] The need for dosing adjustment is determined by the magnitude of these changes and the pharmacokinetic-pharmacodynamic relationship for each drug.

Nucleoside/tide Reverse Transcriptase Inhibitors in Pregnancy

When comparing pharmacokinetics during pregnancy and postpartum in the same women, abacavir, didanosine, emtricitabine, tenofovir, and zidovudine had decreased exposure during pregnancy.[9–13] Because concentrations of plasma nucleoside/tide reverse transcriptase inhibitors (NRTIs) do not directly correlate with the concentrations of intracellular phosphorylated metabolites or effects, the clinical significance of these differences in pregnancy is unknown.[14] No significant differences in lamivudine and stavudine concentrations have been found during pregnancy.[15,16] Standard adult doses of NRTIs are recommended for chronic dosing during pregnancy. Abacavir, emtricitabine, lamivudine, stavudine, tenofovir, and zidovudine all have roughly equivalent concentrations in cord blood and maternal plasma at delivery, whereas didanosine cord blood concentration averages 38% of maternal delivery concentration.[9–13,15,16] When starting an NRTI during labor, higher loading doses should be used for emtricitabine, tenofovir, and zidovudine to achieve rapid therapeutic concentrations.[17–19]

Nonnucleoside Reverse Transcriptase Inhibitors in Pregnancy

Nevirapine pharmacokinetic parameters are not significantly altered with chronic dosing during pregnancy.[20,21] When initial doses are administered during labor, volume, clearance, and half-life increase and area under the curve (AUC) and maximum concentrations decrease.[22] With single doses to the mother during labor, cord blood/maternal plasma ratio is approximately 80%.[23] Average cord blood concentration doubles with chronic maternal dosing during the last trimester of pregnancy.[24] No data are available describing delavirdine, efavirenz, or etravirine pharmacokinetics during pregnancy.

Protease Inhibitors in Pregnancy

All protease inhibitors (PIs) studied to date show decreased exposure during pregnancy, including atazanavir, fosamprenavir, indinavir, lopinavir, nelfinavir, ritonavir, and saquinavir.[25–30] Higher doses should be considered in later stages of pregnancy, particularly for women who have extensive experience of antiretrovirals or those with resistant strains of HIV. The ratio of PI cord blood concentration to maternal serum concentration at the time of delivery averages 0% to 30%.[26,30–33] No pharmacokinetic or safety data during pregnancy are available for the newer PIs darunavir and tipranavir.

Other Antiretroviral Drug Classes

Placental transfer of the viral entry inhibitor enfuvirtide is low, with mean cord blood to maternal plasma concentration ratios of 8%.[34] No pharmacokinetic or safety data during pregnancy are available for the viral entry inhibitor maraviroc or for the integrase inhibitor raltegravir.

Antiretroviral Transfer into Breast Milk

A simple, practical regimen to prevent mother-to-child HIV transmission via breast milk in resource-poor areas of the world where formula feeding is not safe and practical would be a major therapeutic advance. Although preliminary studies have reported that administration of nevirapine to nursing infants or treatment of the lactating mother with combination antiretroviral therapy both seem to provide protection against infection of the infant, the most effective regimen to prevent breast-milk transmission is not known.[35–37] Infant treatment studies have used a reduced-dose infant nevirapine regimen of 2 mg/kg once daily for the first 2 weeks of life followed by 4 mg/kg once daily for 24 weeks, which is well tolerated and maintains infant nevirapine concentrations more than 100 ng/mL, 10 times the nevirapine IC50 (half maximal inhibitory concentration) of wild-type HIV.[38] Zidovudine, lamivudine, nevirapine, and efavirenz can all be found in breast milk when administered to lactating women.[39–41] Nursing infants whose mothers receive zidovudine do not have detectable plasma zidovudine concentrations because of the small amount in breast milk and rapid elimination by the infant. In contrast, when lactating mothers receive lamivudine, nevirapine, or efavirenz, biologically significant plasma concentrations of these drugs can be found in their infants.[40,41] More studies are required to delineate the benefits and risks of infant nevirapine and maternal combination antiretroviral therapy for the prevention of transmission of HIV via breast milk.

Drug Disposition in the Neonate

The unique and developing physiology of newborns has a tremendous effect on drug distribution in the neonatal period. Gastric pH is between 6 and 8 at birth (essentially neutral), and falls within hours to 1.5 to 3 in most infants, although some infants may not produce much gastric acid for several weeks after birth.[42] Motility is irregular and unpredictable. Newborns have decreased synthesis and a smaller pool of bile salts, and decreased intestinal transport of bile acids. Lipase activity increases 5-fold in the first week of life and 20-fold during the first 9 months, whereas amylase is low even after birth.[43] In addition to irregular and changing gastrointestinal function, and differences between term and premature infants, neonates also have irregular feeding and diet routines. These physiologic and environmental factors may increase or decrease drug absorption compared with older children and adults.

High body-water content contributes to increased dose requirements in infants and children for some agents. In addition, body composition is different between term and preterm infants. In the neonate, total plasma protein concentration is decreased and binding to proteins may be less avid.[44] The resulting higher free fraction of drug necessitates a lower dose in the neonate.

In general, drug metabolism pathways are less active in newborns than in older children and adults, increase to peak activity in young children, and decline to adult levels in older children and adolescents.[44] The many different metabolic pathways all mature at different rates with a great deal of interindividual variation. Primary routes of metabolism may switch from one pathway to another during development. For example, cytochrome P450 (CYP) 3A7 expression peaks at 2 weeks postnatal age in neonate, and substrate metabolism switches primarily to CYP 3A4 in infants and older children/adults. Sulfation is a major drug biotransformation pathway in utero, whereas glucuronidation activity increases quickly after birth. Glomerular filtration is directly proportional to gestational age beyond 34 weeks, and develops rapidly after birth, reaching adult activity by 3 years of age. Tubular secretion increases 2-fold in the first week of life and 10-fold in the first year of life.[44] In addition to maturation variability, genetic and environmental variability influence organ function, making determination of age-appropriate doses difficult. Developmental changes interact in combination to create complex environments, limiting extrapolation from data in older populations.

NRTIs in Neonates

Both hepatic glucuronidation and renal function are depressed in infants immediately after birth; therefore, the clearance of NRTIs is prolonged in this period.[16,45–47] Elimination of didanosine, emtricitabine, lamivudine, stavudine, and zidovudine increase rapidly in the first month of life, requiring dose increases between 2 and 4 weeks of age.[12,15,46,47] NRTI clearance is further decreased in premature infants, and usually requires reduced doses in this infant group.[48] Pharmacokinetic data about abacavir and tenofovir in neonates are not available and no dosing recommendations can be made.

Nonnucleoside Reverse Transcriptase Inhibitors in Neonates

In areas of the world where combination antiretroviral regimens are not available, a regimen of a single maternal dose of nevirapine during labor and a single infant nevirapine dose at 2 to 3 days of life has been shown to result in infant nevirapine concentrations more than 100 ng/mL through the first week of life and to reduce mother-to-child HIV transmission by around 40%.[49,50] However, if the interval between maternal dosing and delivery is less than 2 hours, cord blood nevirapine concentrations are less than 100 ng/mL in many infants. These infants should receive an extra dose of nevirapine immediately after birth and then the standard infant dose at 48 to 72 hours.[22,51] Chronic maternal nevirapine dosing before delivery seems to accelerate nevirapine elimination in the infant after birth, presumably because of in utero autoinduction of nevirapine elimination.[24] If a pregnant woman receives prolonged nevirapine therapy before delivery, then an additional nevirapine dose should be given to the newborn at around day 5 of life to maintain infant nevirapine concentrations more than 100 ng/mL throughout the first week of life. Pharmacokinetic data for delavirdine, efavirenz, and etravirine in neonates are not currently available.

PIs in Neonates

Low and extremely variable nelfinavir plasma concentrations are seen in neonates.[47] Dosing with a weight-band dosing regimen that provided an average dose of nearly 60 mg/kg twice daily in newborns during the first 2 weeks of life showed adequate median AUC. However, interpatient variability was extreme, with AUC and trough concentrations less than the therapeutic drug monitoring targets in 44% of the infants.[52] No pharmacokinetic data are available describing other PIs, viral entry inhibitors, or integrase inhibitors in neonates.

SAFETY

The current approach to prevention of mother-to-child HIV transmission through the use of antiretrovirals to the mother during pregnancy and to the infant after birth can reduce the rate of mother-to-child HIV transmission to as low as 1%.[53,54] It is estimated that fewer than 200 HIV-infected infants are currently born each year in the United States.[55,56] Because most fetuses exposed to antiretrovirals during pregnancy are not infected with HIV, the safety of these agents for both fetus and mother is of paramount importance. However, the potentially life-threatening consequences of HIV infection to mother and fetus have compelled the use of many antiretroviral agents, generally as part of combination regimens, in pregnant women and their newborns in the absence of definitive safety data.

Maternal Toxicity

The physiologic changes of pregnancy may make the mother more susceptible to toxicities described in nonpregnant adults or may lead to toxicities unique to pregnancy, such as premature delivery. Abnormalities in carbohydrate metabolism are common side effects in nonpregnant adults receiving combination antiretroviral regimens, especially those including PIs, raising concerns about an increase in gestational carbohydrate intolerance in pregnant women receiving antiretrovirals.[57] However, several studies have shown no significant association between type of antiretroviral treatment and gestational diabetes, including a recent prospective study that performed detailed evaluations for glucose intolerance and insulin resistance in HIV-infected pregnant women receiving PI-containing and nonprotease-inhibitor-containing regimens.[58,59]

Pregnancy may also predispose to mitochondrial dysfunction associated with nucleoside exposure. Lactic acidosis and hepatic steatosis are rare and generally reversible nucleoside toxicities attributed to mitochondrial dysfunction from nucleoside analogue exposure.[60] Acute fatty liver and HELLP syndrome (hemolysis, elevated liver enzymes, and low platelets), 2 rare but life-threatening syndromes that occur during pregnancy, have been associated with abnormal mitochondrial fatty acid oxidation in mother and/ or fetus.[61] Pregnancy may possibly predispose to the mitochondrial dysfunction leading to all 3 syndromes: acute fatty liver of pregnancy, HELLP syndrome, and nucleoside-associated lactic acidosis/hepatic steatosis. Three fatal and several less severe cases of lactic acidosis and hepatic steatosis have been reported in pregnant or postpartum women whose antiretroviral regimen during pregnancy included stavudine and didanosine.[62,63] The combination of stavudine and didanosine should be avoided during pregnancy and used only if no other alternatives are available.[64]

Susceptibility to nevirapine toxicity may also be increased during pregnancy. Long-term therapy with nevirapine is associated with rare but significant toxicities in nonpregnant HIV-infected adults, including severe, life-threatening hypersensitivity skin reactions, including Stevens-Johnson syndrome, and severe, life-threatening, and in some cases, fatal hepatotoxicity, including fulminant and cholestatic hepatitis, hepatic necrosis, and hepatic failure.[65] Severe nevirapine-associated skin rash and hepatic toxicity are more common in women than men, and have been reported during pregnancy.[66–70] Risk of nevirapine-associated hepatic toxicity is related to CD4 cell count, with risk increased nearly 10-fold in women with CD4 cell counts more than 250 cells/mm^3 compared with those less than 250 cells/mm^3.[71] Although there have been several reports of deaths as a result of hepatic failure in HIV-infected pregnant women receiving nevirapine, other studies suggest that although pregnancy is associated with an increased risk of hepatic toxicity in HIV-infected women, nevirapine use does not increase that risk.[69,70,72,73] Current US recommendations are that initiation of nevirapine therapy should be avoided if at all possible in pregnant women, especially those with CD4 cell counts more than 250 cells/mm^3, but that if nevirapine is used during pregnancy, close clinical and laboratory monitoring for hepatic toxicity is necessary.[74]

The relationship between antiretroviral use and preterm delivery is a subject of much controversy. Several reports from Europe have shown an increased rate of preterm delivery in HIV-infected women receiving antiretrovirals, especially combination antiretroviral regimens.[75–77] In contrast, several US studies have shown no association between antiretroviral use and preterm delivery or other adverse pregnancy outcomes.[78,79] A meta-analysis of 14 European and US studies that examined the association between antiretroviral therapy during pregnancy and premature delivery found no increased risk of premature delivery associated with antiretroviral use compared with no use, but a small increase (odds ratio 1.35, 95% confidence interval 1.08–1.70) in women who received combination therapy including PIs compared with combination therapy without PIs.[80] Although no clear explanation is available for the inconsistency among these studies, the potential for an increased risk of premature birth in HIV-infected pregnant women receiving combination antiretroviral therapy during pregnancy should be recognized and included in clinical discussions of the risks and benefits of antiretroviral therapy.[81]

Teratogenicity and Fetal/Newborn Toxicity

The effect on the fetus of drugs used by the mother during pregnancy may be difficult to assess. Preclinical drug evaluations include in vitro and animal in vivo studies for carcinogenicity, mutagenicity, and reproductive and teratogenic effects. Direct extrapolation of the results of these preclinical studies to humans is of uncertain value. Of approximately 1200 known animal teratogens, only about 30 have been shown to be teratogenic in humans.[82] However, in at least one case, that of isotretinoin, animal studies showing severe teratogenicity prevented widespread use of this agent in pregnant women and averted a likely epidemic of birth defects.[83] A summary of preclinical data relevant to perinatal antiretroviral use can be found in the US Guidelines for the Use of Antiretrovirals in Pregnancy.[64]

Human perinatal phase I, II, and III antiretroviral studies are too small and of too limited duration to definitively assess for adverse fetal effects, especially those effects that are uncommon or first appear outside infancy. The largest amount of data are available for zidovudine, which has been consistently associated with transient neonatal anemia but otherwise seems to be without harmful effects after in utero and postnatal exposure.[84,85] Lamivudine also causes bone marrow suppression, and anemia may be worse in neonates exposed to the combination of zidovudine and lamivudine.[86] Monitoring of clinical experience is ongoing in epidemiologic cohort studies and in the Antiretroviral Pregnancy Registry, a postmarketing surveillance registry sponsored by the pharmaceutical industry to collect information about major teratogenic effects with prenatal exposure to more than 25 antiretroviral agents (http://www.apregistry.com/). No overall increased risk of birth defects has been seen with antiretroviral use in the most recent report of the Registry, which includes data from more than 10,000 predominantly US live births, and in separate surveillance of HIV-infected pregnancies in the United Kingdom and Ireland.[87,88] Although these cohorts include large numbers of exposures and provide useful information, their subjects have exposure to a large variety of drug combinations, making it difficult to establish safety assessments for individual agents. These monitoring studies are also limited by ethnic, social, and clinical differences in the populations studied, possible bias associated with voluntary reporting, the lack of randomized comparator groups, inadequate information about confounding variables, and uncertain accuracy of outcomes.[89]

Preclinical animal studies of antiretrovirals are especially concerning for efavirenz, delavirdine, and tenofovir. Administration of efavirenz to 20 pregnant cynomolgus monkeys resulted in 3 with severe malformations, including anencephaly, anophthalmia, microphthalmia, and cleft palate.[90] Several cases of myelomeningocele and 1 case of anophthalmia have been reported in infants born to women receiving efavirenz early in pregnancy.[91-93] The use of efavirenz should be avoided during pregnancy, especially during the first trimester.[64] Administration of delavirdine to pregnant rats at doses that produced systemic exposures equal to or lower than typical human exposures caused ventricular septal defects and increased infant mortality.[94] No human data describing delavirdine pharmacokinetics during pregnancy are available, but this drug is no longer commercially available. In primate studies, tenofovir exposure is associated with osteomalacia and renal toxicity with prolonged high-dose exposure in adults and fetal growth retardation and reduction in bone porosity after chronic prenatal exposure.[95-97] Renal toxicity has been described in HIV-infected adults taking tenofovir, and decreased bone mineral density has been reported in some, but not all, studies of adult and pediatric patients using tenofovir.[98-103] The clinical significance of these findings is uncertain. Although tenofovir is recommended as a first-line NRTI in nonpregnant adults, its use during pregnancy is recommended only in special cases such as zidovudine intolerance or resistance.[64,104]

Nucleoside reverse transcriptase inhibitors are known to inhibit mitochondrial function.[105] Their long-term use may result in toxicity associated with depletion of mitochondrial DNA, although these toxicities generally resolve with cessation of use.[106] Investigators in France reported that 8 of 1754 uninfected infants with in utero and postnatal nucleoside reverse transcriptase exposure had persistent mitochondrial dysfunction proved by biopsy.[107] All 8 infants were exposed to zidovudine, 4 as zidovudine monotherapy and 4 in combination with lamivudine. Five, of whom 2 died, presented with delayed onset of neurologic symptoms, whereas 3 were symptom free but had laboratory abnormalities.[107] This report stimulated a worldwide search for other uninfected infants with perinatal antiretroviral exposure and evidence of mitochondrial toxicity. The only other definitive case that has been discovered is a US infant who was exposed to antiretrovirals including zidovudine and lamivudine for the last 4 weeks of pregnancy; this infant had severe neurologic symptoms present at birth, and a muscle biopsy confirmed mitochondrial dysfunction.[108] Otherwise no cases consistent with mitochondrial dysfunction could be found among the uninfected antiretroviral exposed children in several research cohorts, including 3 US cohorts totaling 19,486 children, an African cohort of 1798 children, a Thai cohort of 330 children, and a European cohort of 1008 children.[109-113] Although the difficulty in finding cases fitting the description of mitochondrial dysfunction in these other cohorts from around the world is encouraging, the limitations in diagnosing mitochondrial dysfunction without prospective neurologic and laboratory evaluations prevents a definitive conclusion about the relationship between perinatal nucleoside exposure and persistent mitochondrial toxicity from being drawn.[114]

With current diagnostic testing algorithms, some HIV-infected infants are identified shortly after birth. Although these infants often have high plasma HIV viral loads, the lack of neonatal pharmacokinetic and safety data and appropriate formulations makes treatment difficult in the immediate newborn period. The only nonnucleoside reverse transcriptase inhibitor (NNRTI) with sufficient safety data for use in the term newborn is nevirapine, but its use is often undesirable because of the possibility of preexisting NNRTI resistance. Nelfinavir is the only PI with pharmacokinetic data in the newborn period, but a reliable dosing regimen has not yet been developed.[52] Even fewer data support the use of antiretrovirals in HIV-infected infants born prematurely. Zidovudine is the only antiretroviral with adequate safety and dosing information for use in a premature infant and is the only antiretroviral commercially available in an intravenous formulation.[48] Nevirapine elimination has been shown to be prolonged in preterm infants receiving single doses for prevention of mother-to-child transmission but no data are available describing its pharmacokinetics with chronic use in premature infants.[115] The dangers in using antiretrovirals in premature infants in the absence of adequate pharmacokinetic and safety data are highlighted by the recent reports of 4 HIV-infected premature infants who were treated with lopinavir/ritonavir and developed life-threatening cardiomyopathy and heart block.[116,117]

PHARMACOLOGIC CONSIDERATIONS AND CLINICAL CARE

Several clinical management issues are important in caring for pregnant women with HIV and their infants. Care of the HIV-infected pregnant woman and her infant requires coordination among caregivers with multiple areas of expertise, including high-risk obstetrics, adult HIV care, clinical pharmacology, and pediatric HIV care. Current recommendations for care of HIV infected pregnant women and their infants can be found at www.aidsinfo.nih.gov. Education of the mother on what to expect during pregnancy, about the use of antiretrovirals for prevention of mother-to-child transmission, treatment during labor and delivery, infant testing and prophylaxis with antiretrovirals, and postpartum and infant follow-up is extremely important.

Caring for HIV-infected Pregnant Women

In areas of the world where antiretrovirals are readily available, all pregnant women should receive antiretrovirals during pregnancy regardless of CD4 count or viral load.[64] Women who require antiretrovirals for their own health should begin therapy as soon as possible. For women who do not meet antiretroviral treatment criteria and are initiating therapy for prevention of mother-to-child transmission, initiation of therapy may be delayed until after 10 to 12 weeks' gestation when the risk of teratogenicity is lower and management of antiretroviral-related side effects less problematic. The antiretroviral regimen currently recommended for use during pregnancy is the combination of lamivudine, zidovudine, and lopinavir/ritonavir.[64] For women who become pregnant while receiving other antiretrovirals for their own health, decisions about whether to continue with or change regimens need to be made based on safety issues, concerns for teratogenicity, viral suppression, CD4 count, pharmacokinetics, and availability of dosing information during pregnancy. Because of the risk of teratogenicity, efavirenz is not routinely prescribed to women who may become pregnant and its use during the first trimester should be avoided. Monitoring for potential complications of antiretrovirals during pregnancy include routine hematologic tests and chemistries including liver function tests and glucose screening.

Adherence to antiretroviral therapy is necessary for HIV viral suppression and to prevent the development of viral resistance.[118] Inadequate control of viral replication during pregnancy can result in a higher risk of transmission to the infant and the potential development of viral resistance in the mother, which may affect future treatment options. For PI-based regimens, adherence rates of 90% are required to maintain adequate viral suppression.[119,120] Many barriers to adherence exist, including issues surrounding disclosure to sexual partners and secrecy within the household. A recent large cohort study of HIV-1-infected women and their infants assessed adherence rates in 445 pregnant women.[121] Only 75% of pregnant women in this study reported perfect adherence (defined as no missed doses 4 days before their study visit) during their pregnancy. Postpartum rates of perfect adherence declined to 64% to 66% at their 6-, 24-, and 48-week postpartum visits. Factors found to be associated with perfect adherence included the initiation of antiretrovirals during pregnancy, not having an AIDS-defining condition, perfect adherence with prenatal vitamins, no marijuana use, and feeling happy most of the time.[121] The importance of adherence during pregnancy should be stressed at all clinic visits.

Common side effects of the PIs and zidovudine include nausea and vomiting. Many women experience nausea and vomiting in early pregnancy, which is exacerbated with the initiation of antiretrovirals. Control of the symptoms of nausea and vomiting promotes adherence and avoids drug malabsorption. The management of nausea and vomiting in early pregnancy depends on the severity of symptoms. For some patients lifestyle modifications and nonpharmacologic treatments adequately manage symptoms. Patients should be instructed to ingest only small amounts of fluids or foods at a time at frequent intervals, to avoid rich, fatty, spicy foods, and to avoid an empty stomach.[122,123] Ginger has been shown to be an effective remedy for the treatment of mild symptoms of nausea and vomiting.[122,123] Acupressure and acupuncture may be helpful in some women. Phenothiazines such as prochlorperazine and promethazine are effective antiemetics but sedation is a common side effect that limits their use on a regular basis. Metoclopromide at a dose of 5 to 10 mg every 6 to 8 hours is recommended for women who need antiemetic medication on a regular basis. Ondansetron at a dose of 4 to 8 mg every 6 to 8 hours is another effective alternative antiemetic that can be used in patients unresponsive to other therapies.[122,123] For women unable to tolerate antiretroviral medications because of hyperemesis, all drugs should be stopped at the same time and reinstituted at the same time.[64] Diarrhea is another common side effect often seen when initiating PI-based antiretroviral therapy. Women should be instructed to drink adequate amounts of fluids to avoid dehydration and eat binding foods such as bananas, rice, toast, and apple sauce to help control diarrheal symptoms. For diarrheal symptoms not adequately controlled with dietary modifications, loperamide is often prescribed as needed for management.

Many drug interactions are associated with antiretroviral agents, especially the PIs and NNRTIs, and drug interaction resources should be consulted before prescribing additional medications. A useful Web site for drug interactions is http://www.hiv-druginteractions.org/. Patients should be instructed not to take any over-the-counter medications or herbal preparations without consulting their caregiver. Because so many herbal preparations are taken by pregnant women, providers should ask whether any of these products have been taken by the patient to ensure that there are no significant interactions. A Web site about natural products that can be used to search for potential drug interactions is http://www.naturalstandard.com/.

HIV-infected pregnant women are more likely to have inadequate nutrition and to gain less weight during pregnancy when compared with noninfected pregnant women.[124] Both macronutrient and micronutrient deficiencies are more common, especially iron deficiency, which can lead to anemia. Anemia may be exacerbated by antiretroviral agents such as zidovudine and lamivudine, which are bone marrow suppressants.[64,124] Infants born to mothers who are receiving zidovudine and lamivudine during pregnancy are more likely to become anemic while receiving zidovudine for PMTCT. During pregnancy it is important to ensure that the woman eats a nutritious diet and takes prenatal vitamins. For women who become iron deficient, treatment with iron supplements may be necessary but problematic. Nausea and constipation are common side effects with iron preparations.

Women with extensive experience of treatment are more likely to have HIV drug-resistant mutations requiring newer antiretrovirals that have limited safety and dosing information available in pregnancy. Regimens for patients with treatment experience generally have a higher pill burden with more frequent dosing, and pill fatigue may pose a significant barrier to adherence.[125,126]

During Delivery

Intravenous zidovudine is standard for PMTCT and women should be instructed that if they are transported to another hospital for delivery they inform the medical providers about their HIV-positive status so that they and their infants receive appropriate therapy. Women on PI-based regimens experiencing postpartum hemorrhage as a result of uterine atony should not be administered oral or parenteral methergine or other ergot alkaloids. The PIs are potent CYP3A4 enzyme inhibitors and interfere with the metabolism of the ergot compounds, potentially resulting in an exaggerated vasoconstrictor response. Alternative agents such as prostaglandin $F_{2\alpha}$, misoprostol, or oxytocin are recommended.[64]

Infant

Six weeks of zidovudine chemoprophylaxis regimen is recommended for all neonates exposed to HIV to reduce perinatal HIV transmission.[64] Zidovudine should be initiated as soon as possible, preferably within 6 to 12 hours of delivery. Zidovudine is dosed orally at 2 mg/kg every 6 hours for 6 weeks in infants of 35 weeks' gestation or greater. Reduced doses are recommended for premature infants and an intravenous preparation is available for infants unable to tolerate oral medications.[48] The importance of adherence in the infant should be stressed. Twice-daily dosing (4 mg/kg every 12 hours) instead of 4-times-daily dosing may be considered when adherence is a concern. Neonatal zidovudine prophylaxis is limited to 4 weeks in the United Kingdom. [127,128] Limiting zidovudine prophylaxis to 4 weeks may be considered if there are concerns about adherence or toxicity.

In situations with an increased risk of transmission, such as inadequate viral suppression during pregnancy, poor adherence, maternal HIV infection occurred during pregnancy, diagnosis at delivery or just before delivery, or inadequate prenatal care, additional drugs may be added to zidovudine in the infant prophylaxis regimen. A pediatric HIV specialist should be consulted to determine the potential risks and benefits to the infant. Safety and dosing information for antiretrovirals in the neonate are available for zidovudine, lamivudine, nelfinavir, and nevirapine.

After delivery and before discharge from the hospital, the mother or caregiver should be able to demonstrate how to draw up the medication in an oral syringe and administer the medication to the infant, and should be given a follow-up appointment for the infant for HIV testing, monitoring of safety of zidovudine, and dosage adjustments based on weight. If other caregivers are involved, it is important for them to be able to administer the medications to the infant. Any insurance issues that affect coverage for infant medications should be resolved before discharge from the hospital. A calendar that includes when all the zidovudine doses should be administered to the infant is a helpful adherence tool. Dose calculations should be rounded up to the nearest one-tenth of a milliliter for ease of administration. Flexibility in the timing of administration and what to do if a dose is missed should be explained to the mother or caregiver. Providing the parent with oral syringes and bottle adapters and marking the oral syringes to indicate the dose size further ensure the proper doses are administered to the infant. Clear instructions with contact information about who to call with questions about medications should be provided before discharge.

Transient hematologic toxicity with anemia and/or neutropenia is the most common toxicity seen in infants receiving zidovudine for PMTCT. The combination of zidovudine plus lamivudine may be associated with increased hematologic toxicity compared with that observed with zidovudine alone.[129–131] Laboratory monitoring for anemia, neutropenia, or liver abnormalities should be obtained at the regularly scheduled clinic visits. Infants with low birth hemoglobin and hematocrit may require more frequent monitoring, because these infants are at the greatest risk of developing symptomatic anemia. If symptomatic anemia occurs, treatment with erythropoietin or transfusion should be considered. For infants who have received at least 4 weeks of zidovudine, consideration to shorten the duration of prophylaxis to 4 weeks instead of completing the usual 6-week course may be given.

Infants with NRTI exposure should be followed for the development of mitochondrial toxicity, which may be more common with exposure to multiple versus single NRTIs.[129] For infants who develop severe clinical symptoms of unknown cause, particularly neurologic symptoms, serum lactate levels should be obtained to rule out hyperlactemia and mitochondrial toxicity. It is unclear if long-term risks are associated with in utero and/or neonatal antiretroviral exposure. Because of theoretic concerns for potential carcinogenicity from antiretrovirals, especially NRTIs, follow-up of children with antiretroviral exposure should continue into adulthood.

SUMMARY

Although significant advances have been made in our understanding of the perinatal pharmacology of antiretrovirals, there remain many critical unanswered questions. Additional studies describing the pharmacokinetics of antiretrovirals in pregnant women and their newborns and evaluating their safety and efficacy in preventing mother-to-child transmission of HIV and in treating HIV disease in infected mothers and infants are urgently needed.

REFERENCES

1. Morgan DJ. Drug disposition in mother and foetus. Clin Exp Pharmacol Physiol 1997;24(11):869–73.
2. Loebstein R, Lalkin A, Koren G. Pharmacokinetic changes during pregnancy and their clinical relevance. Clin Pharmacokinet 1997;33(5):328–43.
3. Wright LL, Catz CS. Drug distribution during fetal life. In: Polin RA, Fox WW, editors. Fetal and neonatal physiology. Philadelphia: WB Saunders; 1998. p. 169.
4. Krauer B, Krauer F, Hytten FE. Drug disposition and pharmacokinetics in the maternal-placental-fetal unit. Pharmacol Ther 1980;10(2):301–28.
5. Krauer B, Dayer P, Anner R. Changes in serum albumin and alpha 1-acid glycoprotein concentrations during pregnancy: an analysis of fetal-maternal pairs. Br J Obstet Gynaecol 1984;91(9):875–81.

6. Davis M, Simmons CJ, Dordoni B, et al. Induction of hepatic enzymes during normal human pregnancy. J Obstet Gynaecol Br Commonw 1973;80(8): 690–4.
7. Juchau MR, Mirkin DL, Zachariah PK. Interactions of various 19-nor steroids with human placental microsomal cytochrome P-450 (P-450hpm). Chem Biol Interact 1976;15(4):337–47.
8. Zaske DE, Cipolle RJ, Strate RG, et al. Rapid gentamicin elimination in obstetric patients. Obstet Gynecol 1980;56(5):559–64.
9. Watts DH, Brown ZA, Tartaglione T, et al. Pharmacokinetic disposition of zidovudine during pregnancy. J Infect Dis 1991;163(2):226–32.
10. Best BM, Mirochnick M, Capparelli EV, et al. Impact of pregnancy on abacavir pharmacokinetics. AIDS 2006;20(4):553–60.
11. Burchett SK, Best B, Mirochnick M, et al, for the PACTG P1026s Team. Tenofovir pharmacokinetics during pregnancy, at delivery and postpartum [abstract 738b]. 14th Conference on Retroviruses and Opportunistic Infections. Los Angeles (CA), February 25–28, 2007.
12. Wang Y, Livingston E, Patil S, et al. Pharmacokinetics of didanosine in antepartum and postpartum human immunodeficiency virus-infected pregnant women and their neonates: an AIDS clinical trials group study. J Infect Dis 1999; 180(5):1536–41.
13. Best BM, Stek A, Hu C, et al, for the PACTG/IMPAACT P1026s Team. High-dose lopinavir and standard-dose emtricitabine pharmacokinetics during pregnancy and postpartum [abstract #629]. The 15th Conference on Retroviruses and Opportunistic Infections Boston, February, 2008. Available at: http://www.retroconference.org/2008/PDFs/629.pdf. Accessed November 14, 2008.
14. Sale M, Sheiner LB, Volberding P, et al. Zidovudine response relationships in early human immunodeficiency virus infection. Clin Pharmacol Ther 1993; 54(5):556–66.
15. Moodley J, Moodley D, Pillay K, et al. Pharmacokinetics and antiretroviral activity of lamivudine alone or when coadministered with zidovudine in human immunodeficiency virus type 1-infected pregnant women and their offspring. J Infect Dis 1998;178(5):1327–33.
16. Wade NA, Unadkat JD, Huang S, et al. Pharmacokinetics and safety of stavudine in HIV-infected pregnant women and their infants: pediatric AIDS Clinical Trials Group protocol 332. J Infect Dis 2004;190(12):2167–74.
17. Hirt D, Urien S, Rey E, et al. Population pharmacokinetics of emtricitabine in HIV-infected pregnant women and their neonates: TEmAA ANRS 12109 [abstract 626]. 15th Conference on Retroviruses and Opportunistic Infections. Boston (MA), February 3–6, 2008.
18. O'Sullivan MJ, Boyer PJ, Scott GB, et al. The pharmacokinetics and safety of zidovudine in the third trimester of pregnancy for women infected with human immunodeficiency virus and their infants: phase I acquired immunodeficiency syndrome clinical trials group study (protocol 082). Zidovudine Collaborative Working Group. Am J Obstet Gynecol 1993;168(5):1510–6.
19. Rodman J, Shapiro D, Jean-Philippe P, et al. Pharmacokinetics (PK) and safety of tenofovir disoproxil fumarate (TDF) in HIV-1-infected pregnant women and their infants. In: 13th Conference on Retroviruses and Opportunistic Infections. Denver (CO), February 6, 2007.
20. Taylor GP, Lyall EG, Back D, et al. Pharmacological implications of lengthened in-utero exposure to nevirapine. Lancet 2000;355(9221):2134–5.

21. Capparelli EV, Aweeka F, Hitti J, et al. Chronic administration of nevirapine during pregnancy: impact of pregnancy on pharmacokinetics. HIV Med 2008; 9(4):214–20.
22. Mirochnick M, Clarke DF, Dorenbaum A. Nevirapine: pharmacokinetic considerations in children and pregnant women. Clin Pharmacokinet 2000;39(4): 281–93.
23. Musoke P, Guay LA, Bagenda D, et al. A phase I/II study of the safety and pharmacokinetics of nevirapine in HIV-1-infected pregnant Ugandan women and their neonates (HIVNET 006). AIDS 1999;13(4):479–86.
24. Mirochnick M, Siminski S, Fenton T, et al. Nevirapine pharmacokinetics in pregnant women and in their infants after in utero exposure. Pediatr Infect Dis J 2001; 20(8):803–5.
25. Acosta EP, Zorrilla C, Van Dyke R, et al. Pharmacokinetics of saquinavir-SGC in HIV-infected pregnant women. HIV Clin Trials 2001;2(6):460–5.
26. Capparelli EV, Stek A, Best B, et al. Boosted fosamprenavir pharmacokinetics in pregnancy. In: 17th Conference on Retroviruses and Opportunistic Infections. San Francisco (CA), February 19, 2010.
27. Kosel BW, Beckerman KP, Hayashi S, et al. Pharmacokinetics of nelfinavir and indinavir in HIV-1-infected pregnant women. AIDS 2003;17(8):1195–9.
28. Mirochnick M, Stek A, Capparelli E, et al, and PACTG 1026s Protocol Team, Atazanavir pharmacokinetics with and without tenofovir during pregnancy. The 16th Conference on Retroviruses and Opportunistic Infections, Montreal (Canada), February 2, 2009.
29. Read JS, Best BM, Stek AM, et al. Pharmacokinetics of new 625 mg nelfinavir formulation during pregnancy and postpartum. HIV Med 2008;9(10):875–82.
30. Stek AM, Mirochnick M, Capparelli E, et al. Reduced lopinavir exposure during pregnancy. AIDS 2006;20(15):1931–9.
31. Acosta EP, Bardeguez A, Zorrilla CD, et al. Pharmacokinetics of saquinavir plus low-dose ritonavir in human immunodeficiency virus-infected pregnant women. Antimicrob Agents Chemother 2004;48(2):430–6.
32. Ripamonti D, Cattaneo D, Maggiolo F, et al. Atazanavir plus low-dose ritonavir in pregnancy: pharmacokinetics and placental transfer. AIDS 2007;21(18): 2409–15.
33. Scott GB, Rodman JH, Scott WA, et al, Pharmacokinetic and virologic response to ritonavir (RTV) in combination with zidovudine (ZDV) and lamivudine (3TC) in HIV-1-infected pregnant women and their infants [abstract 794-W]. 9th Conference on Retroviruses and Opportunistic Infections. Seattle (WA), February 24–28, 2002. Available at: http://www.retroconference.org/2002/Abstract/13702.htm. Accessed November 26, 2008.
34. Haberl A, Linde R, Reitter A, et al. Use of enfuvirtide in HIV+ pregnant women. 15th Conference on Retroviruses and Opportunistic Infections [abstract 627b]. Boston (MA), February 3–6, 2008.
35. Bedri A, Gudetta B, Isehak A, et al. Extended-dose nevirapine to 6 weeks of age for infants to prevent HIV transmission via breastfeeding in Ethiopia, India, and Uganda: an analysis of three randomised controlled trials. Lancet 2008; 372(9635):300–13.
36. Giuliano M, Guidotti G, Andreotti M, et al. Triple antiretroviral prophylaxis administered during pregnancy and after delivery significantly reduces breast milk viral load: a study within the Drug Resource Enhancement Against AIDS and Malnutrition Program. J Acquir Immune Defic Syndr 2007;44(3):286–91.

37. Kumwenda NI, Hoover DR, Mofenson LM, et al. Extended antiretroviral prophylaxis to reduce breast-milk HIV-1 transmission. N Engl J Med 2008;359(2): 119–29.

38. Shetty AK, Coovadia HM, Mirochnick MM, et al. Safety and trough concentrations of nevirapine prophylaxis given daily, twice weekly, or weekly in breast-feeding infants from birth to 6 months. J Acquir Immune Defic Syndr 2003; 34(5):482–90.

39. Shapiro RL, Holland DT, Capparelli E, et al. Antiretroviral concentrations in breast-feeding infants of women in Botswana receiving antiretroviral treatment. J Infect Dis 2005;192(5):720–7.

40. Mirochnick M, Thomas T, Capparelli E, et al. Antiretroviral concentrations in breast-feeding infants of mothers receiving highly active antiretroviral therapy. Antimicrob Agents Chemother 2009;53(3):1170–6.

41. Schneider S, Peltier A, Gras A, et al. Efavirenz in human breast milk, mothers', and newborns' plasma. J Acquir Immune Defic Syndr 2008;48(4):450–4.

42. Marciano T, Wershil BK. The ontogeny and developmental physiology of gastric acid secretion. Curr Gastroenterol Rep 2007;9(6):479–81.

43. Grand RJ, Sutphen JL, Montgomery RK. The immature intestine: implications for nutrition of the neonate. Ciba Found Symp 1979;70:293–311.

44. Anderson GD, Lynn AM. Optimizing pediatric dosing: a developmental pharmacologic approach. Pharmacotherapy 2009;29(6):680–90.

45. Blum MR, Ndiweni D, Chittick G, et al. Steady-state pharmacokinetic evaluation of emtricitabine in neonates exposed to HIV in utero [abstract 568]. 13th Conference on Retroviruses and Opportunistic Infections. Denver (CO), February 5–9, 2006.

46. Moodley D, Pillay K, Naidoo K, et al. Pharmacokinetics of zidovudine and lamivudine in neonates following coadministration of oral doses every 12 hours. J Clin Pharmacol 2001;41(7):732–41.

47. Rongkavilit C, Thaithumyanon P, Chuenyam T, et al. Pharmacokinetics of stavudine and didanosine coadministered with nelfinavir in human immunodeficiency virus-exposed neonates. Antimicrob Agents Chemother 2001;45(12):3585–90.

48. Capparelli EV, Mirochnick M, Dankner WM, et al. Pharmacokinetics and tolerance of zidovudine in preterm infants. J Pediatr 2003;142(1):47–52.

49. Mirochnick M, Fenton T, Gagnier P, et al. Pharmacokinetics of nevirapine in human immunodeficiency virus type 1-infected pregnant women and their neonates. Pediatric AIDS Clinical Trials Group Protocol 250 Team. J Infect Dis 1998;178(2):368–74.

50. Guay LA, Musoke P, Fleming T, et al. Intrapartum and neonatal single-dose nevirapine compared with zidovudine for prevention of mother-to-child transmission of HIV-1 in Kampala, Uganda: HIVNET 012 randomised trial. Lancet 1999;354(9181):795–802.

51. Mirochnick M, Dorenbaum A, Blanchard S, et al. Predose infant nevirapine concentration with the two-dose intrapartum neonatal nevirapine regimen: association with timing of maternal intrapartum nevirapine dose. J Acquir Immune Defic Syndr 2003;33(2):153–6.

52. Mirochnick M, Nielsen-Saines K, Pilotto JH, et al, and NICHD/HPTN 040/PACTG 1043 Protocol Team. Nelfinavir pharmacokinetics with an increased dose during the first two weeks of life. The 15th Conference on Retroviruses and Opportunistic Infections, Boston (MA), February 4, 2008.

53. Townsend CL, Cortina-Borja M, Peckham CS, et al. Low rates of mother-to-child transmission of HIV following effective pregnancy interventions in the United Kingdom and Ireland, 2000-2006. AIDS 2008;22(8):973–81.

54. Boer K, Nellen JF, Patel D, et al. The AmRo study: pregnancy outcome in HIV-1-infected women under effective highly active antiretroviral therapy and a policy of vaginal delivery. BJOG 2007;114(2):148–55.

55. Centers for Disease Control Prevention (CDC), Mofenson LM, Taylor AW, et al. Achievements in public health. Reduction in perinatal transmission of HIV infection–United States, 1985–2005. MMWR Morb Mortal Wkly Rep 2006;55(21):592–7.

56. McKenna MT, Hu X. Recent trends in the incidence and morbidity that are associated with perinatal human immunodeficiency virus infection in the United States. Am J Obstet Gynecol 2007;197(Suppl 3):S10–6.

57. Dube MP, Sattler FR. Metabolic complications of antiretroviral therapies. AIDS Clin Care 1998;10(6):41–4.

58. Watts DH, Balasubramanian R, Maupin RT Jr, et al. Maternal toxicity and pregnancy complications in human immunodeficiency virus-infected women receiving antiretroviral therapy: PACTG 316. Am J Obstet Gynecol 2004; 190(2):506–16.

59. Hitti J, Andersen J, McComsey G, et al. Protease inhibitor-based antiretroviral therapy and glucose tolerance in pregnancy: AIDS Clinical Trials Group A5084. Am J Obstet Gynecol 2007;196(4). 331 e1–331 e7.

60. Powderly WG. Long-term exposure to lifelong therapies. J Acquir Immune Defic Syndr 2002;29(Suppl 1):S28–40.

61. Ibdah JA, Bennett MJ, Rinaldo P, et al. A fetal fatty-acid oxidation disorder as a cause of liver disease in pregnant women. N Engl J Med 1999;340(22):1723–31.

62. Food and Drug Administration. Important drug warning: retyped text of a letter from Bristol-Myers Squibb. January 5, 2001. Available at: http://www.fda.gov/medwatch/safety/2001/zerit&videx_letter.htm. Accessed October 15, 2002.

63. Sarner L, Fakoya A. Acute onset lactic acidosis and pancreatitis in the third trimester of pregnancy in HIV-1 positive women taking antiretroviral medication. Sex Transm Infect 2002;78(1):58–9.

64. Panel on Treatment of HIV-Infected Pregnant Women and Prevention of Perinatal Transmission. Recommendations for use of antiretroviral drugs in pregnant HIV-1-infected women for maternal health and interventions to reduce perinatal HIV transmission in the United States. May 24, 2010:1–117. Available at: http://aidsinfo.nih.gov/ContentFiles/PerinatalGL.pdf. Accessed May 24, 2010.

65. Patel SM, Johnson S, Belknap SM, et al. Serious adverse cutaneous and hepatic toxicities associated with nevirapine use by non-HIV-infected individuals. J Acquir Immune Defic Syndr 2004;35(2):120–5.

66. Mazhude C, Jones S, Murad S, et al. Female sex but not ethnicity is a strong predictor of non-nucleoside reverse transcriptase inhibitor-induced rash. AIDS 2002;16(11):1566–8.

67. Bersoff-Matcha SJ, Miller WC, Aberg JA, et al. Sex differences in nevirapine rash. Clin Infect Dis 2001;32(1):124–9.

68. Knudtson E, Para M, Boswell H, et al. Drug rash with eosinophilia and systemic symptoms syndrome and renal toxicity with a nevirapine-containing regimen in a pregnant patient with human immunodeficiency virus. Obstet Gynecol 2003; 101(5 Pt 2):1094–7.

69. Hitti J, Frenkel LM, Stek AM, et al. Maternal toxicity with continuous nevirapine in pregnancy: results from PACTG 1022. J Acquir Immune Defic Syndr 2004;36(3): 772–6.

70. Lyons F, Hopkins S, Kelleher B, et al. Maternal hepatotoxicity with nevirapine as part of combination antiretroviral therapy in pregnancy. HIV Med 2006;7(4): 255–60.

71. Baylor MS, Johann-Liang R. Hepatotoxicity associated with nevirapine use. J Acquir Immune Defic Syndr 2004;35(5):538–9.

72. Ouyang DW, Shapiro DE, Lu M, et al. Increased risk of hepatotoxicity in HIV-infected pregnant women receiving antiretroviral therapy independent of nevirapine exposure. AIDS 2009;23(18):2425–30.

73. Ouyang DW, Brogly SB, Lu M, et al. Lack of increased hepatotoxicity in HIV-infected pregnant women receiving nevirapine compared with other antiretrovirals. AIDS 2010;24(1):109–14.

74. Public Health Service Task Force. Recommendations for use of antiretroviral drugs in pregnant HIV-infected women for maternal health and interventions to reduce perinatal HIV transmission in the United States. July 8, 2008:1–98. Available at: http://aidsinfo.nih.gov/contentfiles/PerinatalGL. Accessed November 11, 2008.

75. Grosch-Woerner I, Puch K, Maier RF, et al. Increased rate of prematurity associated with antenatal antiretroviral therapy in a German/Austrian cohort of HIV-1-infected women. HIV Med 2008;9(1):6–13.

76. Thorne C, Patel D, Newell ML. Increased risk of adverse pregnancy outcomes in HIV-infected women treated with highly active antiretroviral therapy in Europe. AIDS 2004;18(17):2337–9.

77. Townsend CL, Cortina-Borja M, Peckham CS, et al. Antiretroviral therapy and premature delivery in diagnosed HIV-infected women in the United Kingdom and Ireland. AIDS 2007;21(8):1019–26.

78. Tuomala RE, Shapiro DE, Mofenson LM, et al. Antiretroviral therapy during pregnancy and the risk of an adverse outcome. N Engl J Med 2002;346(24): 1863–70.

79. Tuomala RE, Watts DH, Li D, et al. Improved obstetric outcomes and few maternal toxicities are associated with antiretroviral therapy, including highly active antiretroviral therapy during pregnancy. J Acquir Immune Defic Syndr 2005;38(4):449–73.

80. Kourtis AP, Schmid CH, Jamieson DJ, et al. Use of antiretroviral therapy in pregnant HIV-infected women and the risk of premature delivery: a meta-analysis. AIDS 2007;21(5):607–15.

81. Watts H. Management of human immunodeficiency virus infection in pregnancy. N Engl J Med 2002;346:1879–91.

82. Mills JL. Protecting the embryo from X-rated drugs. N Engl J Med 1995;333(2): 124–5.

83. Lammer EJ, Chen DT, Hoar RM, et al. Retinoic acid embryopathy. N Engl J Med 1985;313(14):837–41.

84. Culnane M, Fowler M, Lee SS, et al. Lack of long-term effects of in utero exposure to zidovudine among uninfected children born to HIV-infected women. Pediatric AIDS Clinical Trials Group Protocol 219/076 Teams. JAMA 1999; 281(2):151–7.

85. Chotpitayasunondh T, Vanprapar N, Simonds RJ, et al. Safety of late in utero exposure to zidovudine in infants born to human immunodeficiency virus-infected mothers: Bangkok. Bangkok Collaborative Perinatal HIV Transmission Study Group. Pediatrics 2001;107(1):E5.

86. Chaisilwattana P, Chokephaibulkit K, Chalermchockcharoenkit A, et al. Short-course therapy with zidovudine plus lamivudine for prevention of mother-to-child transmission of human immunodeficiency virus type 1 in Thailand. Clin Infect Dis 2002;35(11):1405–13.

87. Antiretroviral Pregnancy Registry Steering Committee. Antiretroviral Pregnancy Registry international interim report for 1 Jan 1989-31 July 2009. Wilmington

(NC): Registry Coordinating Center; 2009. Available at: http://www.APRegistry. com. Accessed May 5, 2010.

88. Townsend CL, Tookey PA, Cortina-Borja M, et al. Antiretroviral therapy and congenital abnormalities in infants born to HIV-1-infected women in the United Kingdom and Ireland, 1990 to 2003. J Acquir Immune Defic Syndr 2006; 42(1):91–4.

89. Fleming TR. Evaluating the safety of interventions for prevention of perinatal transmission of HIV. Ann N Y Acad Sci 2000;918:201–11.

90. Sustiva [package insert]. Wilmington, DE: Dupont Pharmaceuticals Company; 2000.

91. Fundaro C, Genovese O, Rendeli C, et al. Myelomeningocele in a child with intrauterine exposure to efavirenz. AIDS 2002;16(2):299–300.

92. De Santis M, Carducci B, De Santis L, et al. Periconceptional exposure to efavirenz and neural tube defects. Arch Intern Med 2002;162(3):355.

93. Saitoh A, Hull AD, Franklin P, et al. Myelomeningocele in an infant with intrauterine exposure to efavirenz. J Perinatol 2005;25(8):555–6.

94. Rescriptor [package insert]. La Jolla, CA: Agouron Pharmaceuticals; 2001.

95. Antoniou T, Park-Wyllie LY, Tseng AL. Tenofovir: a nucleotide analog for the management of human immunodeficiency virus infection. Pharmacotherapy 2003;23(1):29–43.

96. Tarantal AF, Marthas ML, Shaw JP, et al. Administration of 9-[2-(R)-(phosphonomethoxy)propyl]adenine (PMPA) to gravid and infant rhesus macaques (Macaca mulatta): safety and efficacy studies. J Acquir Immune Defic Syndr Hum Retrovirol 1999;20(4):323–33.

97. Tarantal AF, Castillo A, Ekert JE, et al. Fetal and maternal outcome after administration of tenofovir to gravid rhesus monkeys (Macaca mulatta). J Acquir Immune Defic Syndr 2002;29(3):207–20.

98. Lanzafame M, Lattuada E, Rapagna F, et al. Tenofovir-associated kidney diseases and interactions between tenofovir and other antiretrovirals. Clin Infect Dis 2006;42(11):1656–7 author reply 1658.

99. Antoniou T, Raboud J, Chirhin S, et al. Incidence of and risk factors for tenofovir-induced nephrotoxicity: a retrospective cohort study. HIV Med 2005;6(4): 284–90.

100. Izzedine H, Hulot JS, Villard E, et al. Association between ABCC2 gene haplotypes and tenofovir-induced proximal tubulopathy. J Infect Dis 2006;194(11): 1481–91.

101. Gafni RI, Hazra R, Reynolds JC, et al. Tenofovir disoproxil fumarate and an optimized background regimen of antiretroviral agents as salvage therapy: impact on bone mineral density in HIV-infected children. Pediatrics 2006;118(3): e711–8.

102. Purdy JB, Gafni RI, Reynolds JC, et al. Decreased bone mineral density with off-label use of tenofovir in children and adolescents infected with human immunodeficiency virus. J Pediatr 2008;152(4):582–4.

103. Giacomet V, Mora S, Martelli L, et al. A 12-month treatment with tenofovir does not impair bone mineral accrual in HIV-infected children. J Acquir Immune Defic Syndr 2005;40(4):448–50.

104. Panel on Antiretroviral Guidelines for Adults and Adolescents. Guidelines for the use of antiretroviral agents in HIV-1-infected adults and adolescents. Department of Health and Human Services. December 1, 2009; 1–161. Available at: http://www.aidsinfo.nih.gov/ContentFiles/AdultandAdolescentGL.pdf. Accessed May 5, 2010.

105. Martin JL, Brown CE, Matthews-Davis N, et al. Effects of antiviral nucleoside analogs on human DNA polymerases and mitochondrial DNA synthesis. Antimicrob Agents Chemother 1994;38(12):2743–9.

106. Brinkman K, ter Hofstede HJ, Burger DM, et al. Adverse effects of reverse transcriptase inhibitors: mitochondrial toxicity as common pathway. AIDS 1998; 12(14):1735–44.

107. Blanche S, Tardieu M, Rustin P, et al. Persistent mitochondrial dysfunction and perinatal exposure to antiretroviral nucleoside analogues. Lancet 1999; 354(9184):1084–9.

108. Cooper ER, DiMauro S, Sullivan M, et al. Biopsy-confirmed mitochondrial dysfunction in an HIV-exposed infant whose mother received combination antiretrovirals during the last 4 weeks of pregnancy [abstract TUPEB4394 2004]. Presented at the 15th International AIDS Conference. Bangkok (Thailand), July 11–16, 2004.

109. Bulterys M, Nesheim S, Abrams EJ, et al. Lack of evidence of mitochondrial dysfunction in the offspring of HIV-infected women. Retrospective review of perinatal exposure to antiretroviral drugs in the Perinatal AIDS Collaborative Transmission Study. Ann N Y Acad Sci 2000;918:212–21.

110. Lindegren ML, Rhodes P, Gordon L, et al. Drug safety during pregnancy and in infants. Lack of mortality related to mitochondrial dysfunction among perinatally HIV-exposed children in pediatric HIV surveillance. Ann N Y Acad Sci 2000;918: 222–35.

111. Dominguez K, Bertolli J, Fowler M, et al. Lack of definitive severe mitochondrial signs and symptoms among deceased HIV-uninfected and HIV-indeterminate children < or = 5 years of age, Pediatric Spectrum of HIV Disease project (PSD), USA. Ann N Y Acad Sci 2000;918:236–46.

112. Lange J, Stellato R, Brinkman K, et al. Review of neurological adverse events in relation to mitochondrial dysfunction in the prevention of mother to child transmission of HIV: PETRA Study. Presented at the Second Conference on Global Strategies for the Prevention of HIV Transmission from Mothers to Infants [abstract]. Montreal (Canada), September 1–6, 1999.

113. European Collaborative Study. Exposure to antiretroviral therapy in utero or early life: the health of uninfected children born to HIV-infected women. J Acquir Immune Defic Syndr 2003;32(4):380–7.

114. Blanche S, Tardieu M, Benhammou V, et al. Mitochondrial dysfunction following perinatal exposure to nucleoside analogues. AIDS 2006;20(13):1685–90.

115. Mugabo P, Cotton M, Smith J, et al. Nevirapine pharmacokinetics in premature infants. Can J Clin Pharmacol 2008;15:e420–781.

116. McArthur MA, Kalu SU, Foulks AR, et al. Twin preterm neonates with cardiac toxicity related to lopinavir/ritonavir therapy. Pediatr Infect Dis J 2009;28(12):1127–9.

117. Lopriore E, Rozendaal L, Gelinck LB, et al. Twins with cardiomyopathy and complete heart block born to an HIV-infected mother treated with HAART. AIDS 2007;21(18):2564–5.

118. Haubrich RH, Little SJ, Currier JS, et al. The value of patient-reported adherence to antiretroviral therapy in predicting virologic and immunologic response. California Collaborative Treatment Group. AIDS 1999;13(9):1099–107.

119. Maggiolo F, Ravasio L, Ripamonti D, et al. Similar adherence rates favor different virologic outcomes for patients treated with nonnucleoside analogues or protease inhibitors. Clin Infect Dis 2005;40(1):158–63.

120. Bangsberg DR. Less than 95% adherence to nonnucleoside reverse-transcriptase inhibitor therapy can lead to viral suppression. Clin Infect Dis 2006;43(7):939–41.

121. Bardeguez AD, Lindsey JC, Shannon M, et al. Adherence to antiretrovirals among US women during and after pregnancy. J Acquir Immune Defic Syndr 2008;48(4):408–17.

122. King TL, Murphy PA. Evidence-based approaches to managing nausea and vomiting in early pregnancy. J Midwifery Womens Health 2009;54(6):430–44.

123. Badell ML, Ramin SM, Smith JA. Treatment options for nausea and vomiting during pregnancy. Pharmacotherapy 2006;26(9):1273–87.

124. Kunstel K. AIDS/HIV in pregnancy. In: Lammi-Keefe CJ, Couch SC, Philipson EH, editors. Handbook of nutrition and pregnancy. Totowa (NJ): Humana Press; 2008. p. 161–76.

125. Ostrop NJ, Hallett KA, Gill MJ. Long-term patient adherence to antiretroviral therapy. Ann Pharmacother 2000;34(6):703–9.

126. Hazra R, Siberry GK, Mofenson LM. Growing up with HIV: children, adolescents, and young adults with perinatally acquired HIV infection. Annu Rev Med 2010; 61:169–85.

127. de Ruiter A, Mercey D, Anderson J, et al. British HIV Association and Children's HIV Association guidelines for the management of HIV infection in pregnant women 2008. HIV Med 2008;9(7):452–502.

128. Ferguson W, Good M, Walksh A, et al. Four weeks of neonatal antiretroviral therapy (ART) is sufficient to optimally prevent mother to child transmission (PMTCT) of HIV [abstract H-459]. 48th Annual ICAAC/IDSA 46th Annual Meeting. Washington, DC, October 25–28, 2008. p. 400.

129. Mandelbrot L, Landreau-Mascaro A, Rekacewicz C, et al. Lamivudine-zidovudine combination for prevention of maternal-infant transmission of HIV-1. JAMA 2001;285(16):2083–93.

130. Lambert JS, Nogueira SA, Abreu T, et al. A pilot study to evaluate the safety and feasibility of the administration of AZT/3TC fixed dose combination to HIV infected pregnant women and their infants in Rio de Janeiro, Brazil. Sex Transm Infect 2003;79(6):448–52.

131. Mirochnick M, Stek A, Acevedo M, et al. Safety and pharmacokinetics of nelfinavir coadministered with zidovudine and lamivudine in infants during the first 6 weeks of life. J Acquir Immune Defic Syndr 2005;39(2):189–94.

Index

Note: Page numbers of article titles are in **boldface** type.

A

Abacavir
  FDA category of, 908
  for infected infants, 876–877
  in breastfeeding, 814–815
  pharmacokinetics of, 910
  prophylactic, 768, 814–815
Adaptive immunity, HIV transmission and, 725
AIDS Clinical Trials Group study, 831
ALVAC vaccines, 792, 813, 816
Amprenavir, FDA category of, 908
Anemia, in antiretroviral therapy, 891, 899, 919
Antibodies
  HIV, in breast milk, 808
  HIV transmission and, 726
Antibody-based assays, 753–754
Antiretroviral drugs, 758, **765–776**
  adherence to, 917
  disposition of, in neonates, 911–913
  drug interactions of, 917
  FDA-approved, 907–909
  for exposed infants, 868
  for infants, 769–770, 918–919
  for infected infants, 875–878
  for labor and delivery, 918
  for premature infants, 898–899
  in breast milk, 835, 911
  in breastfeeding, 810–816
  in pregnancy, 916–918
  in resource-limited settings, 771–772
  intrapartum, 769
  mechanisms of action of, 766
  monitoring of, 770–771, 877–878
  pharmacokinetics of, 918
  pharmacology of, **907–927**
  resistance to, 743–744, **825–842,** 878, 918
    in drug-naive women, 828
    in industrialized countries, 830–834, 836–837
    in infants, 828–830
    in resource-limited countries, 831, 835, 838
    principles of, 825–826

Clin Perinatol 37 (2010) 929–938
doi:10.1016/S0095-5108(10)00121-1
0095-5108/10/$ – see front matter © 2010 Elsevier Inc. All rights reserved.

perinatology.theclinics.com

United States Postal Service
Statement of Ownership, Management, and Circulation
(All Periodicals Publications Except Requestor Publications)

1. Publication Title	2. Publication Number	3. Filing Date
Clinics in Perinatology	0 0 1 - 7 4 4	9/15/10

4. Issue Frequency	5. Number of Issues Published Annually	6. Annual Subscription Price
Mar, Jun, Sep, Dec	4	$239.00

7. Complete Mailing Address of Known Office of Publication (Not printer) (Street, city, county, state, and ZIP+4®)

Elsevier Inc.
360 Park Avenue South
New York, NY 10010-1710

Contact Person
Stephen Bushing
Telephone (Include area code)
215-239-3688

8. Complete Mailing Address of Headquarters or General Business Office of Publisher (Not printer)

Elsevier Inc., 360 Park Avenue South, New York, NY 10010-1710

9. Full Names and Complete Mailing Addresses of Publisher, Editor, and Managing Editor (Do not leave blank)

Publisher (Name and complete mailing address)

Kim Murphy, Elsevier, Inc., 1600 John F. Kennedy Blvd. Suite 1800, Philadelphia, PA 19103-2899

Editor (Name and complete mailing address)

Carla Holloway, Elsevier, Inc., 1600 John F. Kennedy Blvd. Suite 1800, Philadelphia, PA 19103-2899

Managing Editor (Name and complete mailing address)

Catherine Bewick, Elsevier, Inc., 1600 John F. Kennedy Blvd. Suite 1800, Philadelphia, PA 19103-2899

10. Owner (Do not leave blank. If the publication is owned by a corporation, give the name and address of the corporation immediately followed by the names and addresses of all stockholders owning or holding 1 percent or more of the total amount of stock. If not owned by a corporation, give the names and addresses of the individual owners. If owned by a partnership or other unincorporated firm, give its name and address as well as those of each individual owner. If the publication is published by a nonprofit organization, give its name and address.)

Full Name	Complete Mailing Address
Wholly owned subsidiary of	4520 East-West Highway
Reed/Elsevier, US holdings	Bethesda, MD 20814

11. Known Bondholders, Mortgagees, and Other Security Holders Owning or Holding 1 Percent or More of Total Amount of Bonds, Mortgages, or Other Securities. If none, check box ☐ None

Full Name	Complete Mailing Address
N/A	

12. Tax Status (For completion by nonprofit organizations authorized to mail at nonprofit rates) (Check one)
The purpose, function, and nonprofit status of this organization and the exempt status for federal income tax purposes:
☐ Has Not Changed During Preceding 12 Months
☐ Has Changed During Preceding 12 Months (Publisher must submit explanation of change with this statement)

PS Form 3526, September 2007 (Page 1 of 3 (Instructions Page 3)) PSN 7530-01-000-9931 PRIVACY NOTICE: See our Privacy policy in www.usps.com

---

13. Publication Title	14. Issue Date for Circulation Data Below
Clinics in Perinatology	September 2010

15. Extent and Nature of Circulation		Average No. Copies Each Issue During Preceding 12 Months	No. Copies of Single Issue Published Nearest to Filing Date
a. Total Number of Copies (Net press run)		3156	2982
b. Paid Circulation (By Mail and Outside the Mail)	(1) Mailed Outside-County Paid Subscriptions Stated on PS Form 3541. (Include paid distribution above nominal rate, advertiser's proof copies, and exchange copies)	1710	1600
	(2) Mailed In-County Paid Subscriptions Stated on PS Form 3541 (Include paid distribution above nominal rate, advertiser's proof copies, and exchange copies)		
	(3) Paid Distribution Outside the Mails Including Sales Through Dealers and Carriers, Street Vendors, Counter Sales, and Other Paid Distribution Outside USPS®	745	756
	(4) Paid Distribution by Other Classes Mailed Through the USPS (e.g. First-Class Mail®)		
c. Total Paid Distribution (Sum of 15b (1), (2), (3), and (4))	▶	2455	2356
d. Free or Nominal Rate Distribution (By Mail and Outside the Mail)	(1) Free or Nominal Rate Outside-County Copies Included on PS Form 3541	85	61
	(2) Free or Nominal Rate In-County Copies Included on PS Form 3541		
	(3) Free or Nominal Rate Copies Mailed at Other Classes Through the USPS (e.g. First-Class Mail)		
	(4) Free or Nominal Rate Distribution Outside the Mail (Carriers or other means)		
e. Total Free or Nominal Rate Distribution (Sum of 15d (1), (2), (3) and (4))	▶	85	61
f. Total Distribution (Sum of 15c and 15e)	▶	2540	2417
g. Copies not Distributed (See Instructions to publishers #4 (page #3))		616	565
h. Total (Sum of 15f and g)	▶	3156	2982
i. Percent Paid (15c divided by 15f times 100)		96.65%	97.48%

16. Publication of Statement of Ownership

If the publication is a general publication, publication of this statement is required. Will be printed in the December 2010 issue of this publication. ☐ Publication not required

17. Signature and Title of Editor, Publisher, Business Manager, or Owner

Stephen R. Bushing

Stephen R. Bushing – Fulfillment/Inventory Specialist

Date: September 15, 2010

I certify that all information furnished on this form is true and complete. I understand that anyone who furnishes false or misleading information on this form or who omits material or information requested on the form may be subject to criminal sanctions (including fines and imprisonment) and/or civil sanctions (including civil penalties).

PS Form 3526, September 2007 (Page 2 of 3)

Moving?

Make sure your subscription moves with you!

To notify us of your new address, find your **Clinics Account Number** (located on your mailing label above your name), and contact customer service at:

Email: journalscustomerservice-usa@elsevier.com

800-654-2452 (subscribers in the U.S. & Canada)
314-447-8871 (subscribers outside of the U.S. & Canada)

Fax number: 314-447-8029

Elsevier Health Sciences Division
Subscription Customer Service
3251 Riverport Lane
Maryland Heights, MO 63043

*To ensure uninterrupted delivery of your subscription, please notify us at least 4 weeks in advance of move.

Printed in the United States
By Bookmasters

Printed in the United States
By Bookmasters